Praise for Doctor Yourself: Natural Healing that Works

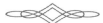

"One of the best. An enormous amount of information on the use orthomolecular medicine—in treating almost all disease. Saul coats his medical advice with wit and humor—important information that is also fun to read about. If every American had a copy of this book, it could change the world as we know it."
—*TOWNSEND LETTER FOR DOCTORS AND PATIENTS*

"Up to date, well put, easy to follow, and if followed, will help readers enhance their degree of health and decrease the possibility of developing serious disease."
—ABRAM HOFFER, M.D., PHD.

"What a superb book *Doctor Yourself* is. I applaud the work, especially its forthright manner of presentation. It should be of enormous value to a vast number of people."
—HUGH D. RIORDAN, M.D.

"Fabulous and brilliant. Andrew Saul is educating us to educate ourselves."
—MARGOT KIDDER

"Really good advice and loads of it. Thank you for all that you're doing to educate the public about the most important aspects of how to stay healthy, and avoid medical consequences of the traditional healthcare system."
—DR. JOSEPH MERCOLA

"Provocative and exciting. *Doctor Yourself: Natural Healing that Works* is nutritional medicine in action, and as such deserves a prominent place in the library of anyone serious about self health care."
—*VITALITY* MAGAZINE

"Expertly written. *Doctor Yourself* is filled from cover to cover with gems of information that aren't usually discussed in most other nutrition books."
—MIDWEST BOOK REVIEW

Doctor Yourself

Second Edition

Natural Healing That Works

Andrew W. Saul, Ph.D.

Foreword by Abram Hoffer, M.D.

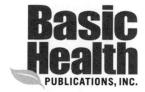

Basic Health
PUBLICATIONS, INC.

DISCLAIMER: The information in this book is not in any way offered as prescription, diagnosis, nor treatment for any disease, illness, infirmity, or physical condition. Any form of self-treatment or alternative health program necessarily must involve an individual's acceptance of some risk, and no one should assume otherwise. Persons needing medical care should obtain it from a physician. Consult your doctor before making any health decision.

Neither the author nor the publisher has authorized the use of their names or the use of any material contained within in connection with the sale, promotion, or advertising of any product or apparatus. Such use is strictly prohibited.

The opinions offered in this book are those of the author, who is not a physician, and are not necessarily the views of the publisher.

Basic Health Publications, Inc.
885 Claycraft Road
Columbus, OH 43230
800-334-9969 • www.basichealthpub.com

Library of Congress Cataloging-in-Publication Data

Saul, Andrew W.
    Doctor yourself : natural healing that works / Andrew W. Saul ;
foreword by Abram Hoffer. — 2nd ed.
        p. cm.
    Includes bibliographical references and index.
    ISBN 978-1-59120-310-0
    1. Orthomolecular therapy—Popular works. 2. Naturopathy—Popular works.
I. Title.
    RM235.5.S38   2012
    615.5'35—dc23

                                                           2012026758

Editor: Carol Rosenberg
Typesetter: Gary A. Rosenberg
Cover design: Mike Stromberg

Printed in the United States of America

10   9   8   7

Contents

PART ONE   Natural Healing Protocols

PART TWO   Natural Healing Tools and Techniques

For Michael, Gabriel, and Raphael

Foreword

by Abram Hoffer, M.D.

In 1952 when we first began to study the therapeutic properties of vitamin B_3 for the treatment of schizophrenia, my colleagues and I did not think that we were blazing new trails. We merely used much larger amounts of this vitamin than were required to keep anyone free from pellagra. At that time, it was forbidden for medical doctors to have any professional interaction with alternative medicine professions such as homeopathy, chiropractic, and naturopathy. Even sharing an office with them could lead to the financial death of losing one's license to practice. So we happily carried on with our work, gathering more and more data showing how powerful niacin and niacinamide were in helping to treat the schizophrenias, among the worst of all human diseases.

We were rudely awakened when we began to publish our findings in the psychiatric literature. To my surprise, I discovered that our conclusions were not accepted with grace and interest. They were rejected with boredom, or hostility and anger. At the time I was both a professor of psychiatry and director of psychiatric research. But because of the vitamin research I was doing, I was in an awkward situation. I could not be politically loyal to the medical school and to the profession of psychiatry if I continued to advocate megadoses of niacin. I chose to give my loyalty to my patients.

Gradually, a few brave physicians, mostly American psychiatrists previously trained as analysts, began to use the treatment we had described and slowly we began to make some headway. The medical associations fought us tooth and nail every step of the way, but interest in our work continued to grow. We were far from the first to point out the importance of good food, but we were the first to show that very large "megadoses" of some vitamins were therapeutic when usual vitamin doses were not. (Actually, the first controlled experiment that showed the importance of good food was published in the Bible, in the first chapter of the Book of Daniel. It was an open study.)

Today, orthomolecular medicine is beginning to flourish. "Orthomolecular" means using a therapeutic substance that is natural to the human body, such as a vitamin or mineral. There has been a major paradigm shift away from the "old school," which maintained that a few easy dietary rules as promoted by governments and medical associations would ensure everyone's good health. Every year, more and more authors join the orthomolecular field, publishing good books that set the record straight about vitamins and put power into the hands of patients.

Doctor Yourself is one of these. In it, the reader will find information on a large number of conditions, ranging from attention deficit disorder in children to Alzheimer's, arthritis, women's health issues, alcoholism, cancer, diabetes, the problems with vaccination, and many more. As Dr. Saul shows, all of these conditions are treatable through natural means. In fact, they are best treated that way.

It is high time somebody said this, because natural means have been almost totally ignored. The body is composed of innumerable molecules developed over billions of years by the toughest test of all: survival. We are finely tuned organisms, with a dizzying number of different compounds and reactions. To think that one can insert a strange molecule that has never before been there, and hope to correct some malfunction, is the height of folly. The only molecules that are therapeutic are orthomolecular ones—those that are normally present and with which the body is familiar. I can't think of a single toxic molecule that has ever truly cured anything. The only compounds that have been used successfully in chronic ailments are the nutrients, vitamins, minerals, amino acid, essential fatty acids, and hormones. And when one tries to replace natural hormones by compounds that are slightly different in order to have patent protection, the results are dismal.

By writing this foreword, I mean to give Dr. Saul, and the other writers in this field, the recognition and honor due to them for preparing for the eventual takeover of all health care by safe, effective nutritional medicine. *Doctor Yourself* represents a new type of comprehensive medical reference book. With this book, Dr. Saul is making a major contribution toward consolidating what is known in the huge and growing field of natural, orthomolecular medicine. Some day it will be considered malpractice for any healer anywhere to ignore the vast importance of nutrition and the optimum use of nutrients in preventing and healing disease, as is detailed in this book. I urge all readers to promote *Doctor Yourself* to their physicians. Some of them will be grateful.

Acknowledgments

I would like to thank a whole lot of teachers who had so much to do with what and how I write, and who I am today. I had an extraordinarily good series of public school teachers, followed by some really outstanding college, graduate, and doctoral professors. Australian National University Professor Wilfrid Douglas Laidlaw Crow, way back in 1973, succeeded in teaching me undergrad organic chemistry through an inspired combination of his brilliance, humor, kindness, and patience. Masters faculty Drs. Walter Brautigan, Betsy Balzano, Hugh Ratigan, and John Mosher taught me to teach. Frances Newburg, Donald Lee, and Martha Palmer, three of the most excellent grade school teachers that ever lived, are responsible for first setting me on the course to be an author, speaker, and science editor. I would also like to thank the memory of Richard Hicks, the man who, against all aeronautical odds, taught me to pilot an aircraft. He was not onboard at the time, but his words were in my mind when I had to land a plane with a flat tire—and did it. A special appreciation is owed to Norman Goldfind, my publisher, for doing for me what no one else had the moxie to do: encourage, print, and distribute my work in over twenty books.

Many decades have passed since my parents taught me so much about life so early in mine. My mother, bless her heart, the very afternoon she learned she was unexpectedly pregnant with me, was so delighted that she ran all the way home from the doctor's office, nearly a mile. An expert teacher, she taught a four-year-old me to read using the comic pages. My father showed me how to do hundreds of things by letting me watch him do them thousands of times. He bought me my first microscope when I was twelve, but also gave me my favorite gift of all time when I was eight: a complete set of genuine Army surplus field equipment.

I would like to thank Steven Carter and Dr. Jonathan Prousky for kind permission to use material that was first published in the *Journal of Orthomolecular Medicine*. I also thank Richard Bennett, Jack Challem, Rev. James R. Hughes, Drs. Robert G. Smith, Thomas E. Levy, Steve Hickey, Hilary Roberts, William B. Grant, Erik Paterson, Damien Downing, Atsuo Yanagisawa, Gert E. Schuitemaker, Jagan N. Vaman, and all other colleagues who have encouraged and contributed to this book. My appreciation is extended to the editorial board and writers of the Orthomolecular Medicine News Service, some of whose articles have been incorporated here. Robert K. McClain, Robert Sarver, Bob C. Kennedy, Dr. Ahmed Nuriye, and Mike Stewart have kept me updated and computer literate. A cosmic thank-you to the memories of Drs. Hugh Riordan and Abram Hoffer, my colleagues and mentors. And I wish to very much thank my far better half, Colleen, my number-one fan.

Introduction to the Second Edition

Over the past almost ten years, I have compiled quite a "request list" from readers worldwide. *Doctor Yourself* has gone through eleven printings and has been published in several foreign languages, including Chinese. So, in this new updated and expanded edition, I will yield to your wonderful persistence and try to tackle just what alternatives may be worth trying for a number of ailments not discussed in the previous edition. As the list is fairly long, some of my suggestions will necessarily be brief.

Commonsense caution: I am not a physician, and these are opinions and options to consider. There is rarely a short answer to any illness, and no one should think that what follows is anything close to being the whole story. But if an idea presented here is new to you, and especially if it is new to your doctor, it is time to look into the matter further. (This really *is* a singularly annoying book, isn't it?)

We simply must be curious and follow up on our curiosity, if we are to plot the best course for our family's health. Renowned scientist and Nobel Prize–winner Linus Pauling famously said, "The way to have a good idea is to have a lot of ideas." And when physician and biochemist Dr. Abram Hoffer was a first-year student, his very first medical school lecture began with the professor saying: "Half of what we teach you is wrong . . . and we do not know which half."

Does this worry you? It well might. But do you know what worries me? The United States is spending close to $3 trillion each year on disease care that so very often does not work . . . and is almost always paying for some other therapy than nutrition. Half a century ago, Dr. Roger J. Williams said, "When in doubt, use nutrition first." Today we give a nod to the preventive value of good eating and a healthy lifestyle. But when there is illness, we still tend to use drugs first. In the doctor's office, the prescriptions written are almost always for drugs, not vitamins.

This needs to change today, and you can make it happen.

Once I won a Scrabble game with my adult daughter . . . by one point. She said it was hardly a win at all, but of course I made a lot of the fact that I still was the winner.

You may remember from history class that America's seventeenth president, Andrew Johnson, avoided impeachment by just one senate vote. More recently, Al Gore lost the presidency by the smallest of margins. A small margin, but plenty big enough to keep him from redecorating the White House. Many a world series has been decided by just one game of seven, and perhaps more importantly, many a Supreme Court decision has been decided by one vote, five to four.

You might have already guessed where I am going with all this: one person really matters.

Legend has it that back in the 1930s, humorist Will Rogers was on the board of directors of an airline. At a board meeting he was attending, corporate big shots were discussing the possibility of issuing parachutes to passengers for use in case of emergency. They also mentioned that if parachutes *were* available, most passengers would not be able to put them on in time, and those that did might not have time or room to get to an exit. They concluded by saying that of the dozen or so passengers on a flight, probably only one would be saved. Rogers leaned back in his chair, put his boots up on the conference table, tipped his hat down over his eyes, and said: "But wouldn't *he* be just tickled."

Naysayers are fond of pointing out that natural healing methods do not always work on everybody. But they don't have to: they only have to work on you, or one of your family, to make the biggest possible difference.

Modern drug-and-cut medicine is at least the third leading cause of death in the USA. Some estimates place medicine as the number-one cause of death.

Null G, Dean C, Feldman M, Rasio D. 2005. Death by medicine. *J Orthomolecular Med* 20(1):21–34 http://orthomolecular.org/library/jom/2005/pdf/2005-v20n01-p021.pdf.

Linus Pauling estimated that disease and mortality could be reduced by at least 25 percent if people took large daily quantities of essential vitamins. Let's say he was way off, and the improvement was only 5 percent. If upwards of two million Americans die each year, a five percent improvement will save 100,000 people. That is a lot of funerals that will not occur.

When I die, I would very much like to know that I saved a life or two. One hundred thousand lives would please me better. Linus Pauling was right, though. With time, the real savings in life will be in the millions.

There are two kinds of people who buy Cadillacs: those that can afford them, and those that cannot. There are two kinds of sick people: those that do not want to change their lifestyle, and those that do but don't know where to start. Prospecting for gold and seeking better health are similar in three ways:

1. You need the motivation to get rich.

2. You need information on where to dig.

3. You need to do the digging.

So dig. Be a health nut, and show the world. You really do make a difference, and don't you forget it.

As you go forth, consider this book for your knapsack. At the very least, the pages may come in handy if there is no toilet paper. On the other hand, consider this: using megadoses of vitamin C, board-certified chest physician Frederick Klenner, M.D., cured acute hepatitis in two days and viral pneumonia in three.

I love this job.

—Andrew W. Saul
June 2012

Warning:
Do Not Read This Page

In fact, do not read this book. Put it back right now, because you are only going to get into trouble for reading it. Your family, your doctor, your professor, your druggist, your newscaster, your TV set, and your undertaker will all oppose what you'll learn inside here: how to get healthy, naturally, and affordably.

As a teacher for some years, I found that most folks never read the instructions on a test (or on anything else, for that matter). You could label a part of any exam INSTRUCTIONS and then you could put all the answers right there, safe in the knowledge that no one would see a single one.

Well, now you've done it. You are still holding my book even after all this. Glad to have you aboard, but don't say I didn't warn you.

And about those answers: please read "How to Use This Book" for a jump-start on getting yourself well.

Gripes and Grievances

*"If you could kick the person in the pants responsible for most of your trouble,
you wouldn't sit for a month."*
—THEODORE ROOSEVELT

Today, it is called "customer service." But when I was a boy, every department store had a full-blown Complaint Department. Nice, straightforward, honest labeling appeals to me. If the premise of this book bugs you, read on to have your doubts weighed in:

"You are just promoting products you make money on."

Nope. I do not sell any health products or vitamins, or supplements. I have absolutely no financial connection with the health products industry. I deliberately avoid vitamin company/health product affiliations, because it would reduce my credibility to zero. By not selling what I might recommend, I may be losing out on some ready cash, but I am gaining hundreds of thousands of readers who appreciate information without the hype.

"You write with an awful lot of 'attitude.' "

You bet I do. Over many years, I have told students and would-be writers that they should have more attitude, not less. This book is provocative for a reason: "The function of a civil resister is to provoke response," said Mahatma Gandhi. "We will continue to provoke until they respond. They are not in control. We are." My worst critics are my biggest asset: they stimulate me to write more books. You can thank them for this second edition.

"Not much on herbs in this book."

As Maynard G. Krebs of *Dobie Gillis* fame said, "True." Although I am a biologist, I am not a medical herbologist. The first rule of writing is, "Write about what you know well." I continue my attempt to keep to that policy in this new edition. I do include some useful and possibly unique material on comfrey, calendula, and hypericum.

"The author is not a physician."

And I'm not, believe me. Physicians often write strikingly weak health books. I have looked through many doctor-authored books on depression, infectious diseases, arthritis, heart disease, fertility, ADHD, lupus, allergies, and countless other topics without finding any serious consideration of natural healing or therapeutic nutrition. These doctors, and therefore the public, are largely unaware of the proven value of natural healing in treating serious disease. *Doctor Yourself* contains enough scientific references that a reader will either say, "Wow, this is it!" or,

"They are all liars . . . liars by the hundreds." I think the public is tired of medication, and ready for education. If delivered with style, we will read.

To misquote one Dr. Leonard McCoy: "Damn it, Jim, I'm a teacher, not a doctor!" I do not prescribe; I describe. People need alternative health information. Here's some good stuff. What you do with it is up to you.

"There are health books like this on the market already."

And good ones, too. My bibliography lists dozens and dozens. So go ahead: put this book down and go read them.

One reason you may not jump to do that is because even the best natural health books share a common fault. Most are fine references, but make for dry reading. Not *Doctor Yourself.* You are going to like this one. Though I hardly understand why, my writing has been described as "outrageous," among other epithets. You may coin a few of your own before you're through.

Health self-help books should be fun to read. Most of the best scientific natural therapeutics information has not reached the people who need it most because it's too hard to understand. People need health research presented for them the way a sports announcer describes a ball game. That's what I try to do. At the same time, a health book needs to be full of practical how-to techniques, backed by specific medical references, and to be based on considerable experience. You'll get plenty of that here. As a college lecturer, I liked to rock the scientific boat, trotting out study after study showing proven natural alternatives to pharmaceutical medicine.

"Hey, where's my illness?"

If you searched the Contents and Index and did not find the topic you're looking for, you might suppose that perhaps this book is not for you. There are thousands of illnesses. You know I cannot cover them all. Plus, your arms are not strong enough to carry home the library big enough to present all knowledge of all healing of all ailments.

However, I am trying to do my part to build your book-lugging biceps. I have written another book, *Fire Your Doctor: How to Be Independently Healthy.* Topics not covered in this book are discussed in that one, with similar attitude as *Doctor Yourself.* By way of disclaimer, I am also the editor of Basic Health Publications' *The Vitamin Cure* book series. Individual volumes are devoted to expanding on specific disease topics, including (in alphabetical order): alcoholism, allergies, children's health problems, chronic fatigue, depression, diabetes, eye diseases, heart disease, infant's health issues, migraines, and women's health problems. More are in the works as well.

While it has been my experience that most people like an "organized-by-illness" format, a fundamental natural-healing premise is "treat the person, not the disease." This means that there is a lot of topic overlap in *Doctor Yourself,* and that information applicable to one illness may be extended to another. More generally, diet and lifestyle changes benefit a broad spectrum of chronic illnesses. If you live, breathe, and know anyone who ever gets sick, this book is for you.

"There's too much emphasis in this book on vitamin C."

No there isn't. Dr. Abram Hoffer taught me that vitamin C was Linus Pauling's favorite vitamin. Dr. Pauling had two more Nobels than I do, so that's good enough for me.

"Vitamins are a promising area in health care, but more research is needed before they can be used therapeutically."

Nonsense. Already by 1953, there were literally thousands of studies compiled in one textbook alone, *The Vitamins in Medicine,* by Bicknell and Prescott. Physicians using vitamin therapy (often dismissed as "quacks") developed successful protocols for curing pneumonia, fibromyalgia, arthritis, cardiovascular disease, chronic fatigue, encephalitis, and even polio. The work is already done; but the word has yet to get out. Want to believe this but can't?

It is not a matter of belief. Vitamin therapy is a matter of observed fact. There is no longer any doubt that a century of vitamin research has demonstrated this to any medical physician who reads her or his own journals. They don't, of course. After you listen to enough detail men from the pharmaceutical companies, and read dietitians' drivel in the newspapers or nutrition texts, you'll see why. I know; I've taught thousands of students. Most immediately see the value of supplements as primary therapy. Try and see for yourself. Results are what matter, and vitamins get them. Pharmaphilic (drug lovin') doctors and food-groups dietitians will see the light eventually, but can you afford to wait?

Again and again relentless science meets megavitamin therapy, and again and again the evidence is overwhelmingly in favor of using vitamin and mineral therapeutics now. Still more proof is to be found every day, usually on the Internet. There simply just isn't any longer any serious argument: the world is round, headache is not due to an aspirin deficiency, and vitamins in sufficiently high quantity cure disease.

I offer my readers what I've learned, tried and verified in preventing and also treating real illnesses with safe, inexpensive, and effective drugless techniques. I have been very satisfied with the science behind, and the results gained, with natural healing.

My own kids made it all the way into college and never, not once ever, had a single dose of any antibiotic. One television interviewer told me that this was the best lead-in she had ever had for a guest.

And the best part of it is that it's true.

How to Use This Book

1. You can look up an illness in the Contents or Index, or;

2. You can read the book straight through because I am such a witty and fascinating writer, or;

3. You can read it straight through for a holistic picture of a natural lifestyle, and then make your own overall healthy lifestyle changes.

Nobody is interested in vitamins. For that matter, nobody is all that whooped up about health. What people want to know is how to cure disease. This goes for preoccupied doctors as much as for desperate patients. In more than thirty-five years of lecturing on natural health care, I have almost never had anyone come up to me afterward and say, "Tell me more about the biochemistry of vitamin therapy." Rather, the ubiquitous follow-up question is, "What vitamins should I use for (such and such an illness)?"

This book is not about vitamins; it is about diseases treatable with vitamins. It is also about any number of other ways you can, as I say, "fire your doctor." Should you ever want to put someone to sleep, just start lecturing on nutrition with the ever-boring "vitamins A through E and foods that contain them" approach. I guarantee that heads will be nodding long before you finish with the B complex.

I hope this book, and the bibliography at the close of it, proves useful to patients who are struggling upstream to convince their pharmaphilic (drug-lovin') physicians to at least give vitamin therapy the time of day. There is nothing quite like pulling out a whole pile of medical references to shorten physicians' "supplements might hurt you so just eat a good diet" speeches. Even the most ostrichlike orthodox practitioner cannot long resist the call of the peer-reviewed journal reference.

For a real blast of information, trot out Abram Hoffer's *Orthomolecular Medicine for Everyone* and Linus Pauling's *How to Live Longer and Feel Better* next time somebody tries to tell you that more research is needed before vitamins can be used to treat illness.

Still, there remains the real possibility that your doctor will recoil when presented with all these references. This reaction, true to human nature, is nevertheless unscientific. It is embarrassing to doctors when patients know more about their case than they do. Yet there is no other rational choice. If therapy exists, and is reasonably well-tested and safe, it is inexcusable not to try it. Doctors know this, but are so uneducated on nutrition that they are usually not in a position to supervise such therapy. Hence the embarrassment. Let us therefore provide the continuing education they so sorely need.

Obviously, you need to do some reading first, but you do not have to read it all. Do you read the dictionary cover to cover? (You don't have to, because, as comic Steven Wright says, "The zebra did it.") Just look up the diseases that are closest to home.

Most people pick up health books because they want immediate information about a disease, either their own or that of a loved one. So *Doctor Yourself* presents many protocols (instructions) for the natural treatment of illnesses. The balance of the book consists of personal experiences and case stories. I like writing these the best.

The Doctor Yourself Laws of Natural Therapeutics

People often want to know where I'm coming from. After all, some will say, "If this "natural healing" stuff was so good, my doctor would have already told me about it." My college students frequently wondered why the content of my lectures was so "different" from their other health classes. And certainly all readers of this book deserve to know, up front, just which garden path I am going to lead them down. Fair enough. Here are my "Laws of Natural Therapeutics":

LAW: Generally, the price of a food is inversely proportional to its nutritional value. That is, the best foods in the supermarket are often the cheapest; the worst foods usually cost the most. Brown rice, dry beans, vegetables from your garden, sprouts from your own countertop jars, fruits from your own trees and bushes . . . all are superior to prepared convenience foods that cost a fortune.

LAW: Most illness is due to malnutrition. This not only includes the chronic diseases, but also viral and bacterial acute illnesses, which are greatly aggravated by inadequate nutrition.

LAW: Adding drugs to a sick body to cure it is like adding poison to a polluted lake to clean it. Killing microorganisms, or masking the cause of symptoms, is no more than a temporary answer.

LAW: Restoring health must be done nutritionally, not pharmacologically. All cells in all persons are made exclusively from what we drink and eat. Not one cell is made out of drugs.

LAW: Neither the chemical spraying of a sick plant nor the chemical dosing of a sick child can substitute for really good nutrition.

LAW: Nutrient therapy increases individual resistance to disease. Drug therapy generally lowers resistance to disease. Healthy plants, healthy animals, and healthy people do not get sick. Doctors do not admit to this, because healthy people make poor customers. What if word got out?

LAW: With vitamin therapy, speed of recovery is proportional to the dosage given. As there is a certain, large amount of fuel needed to launch an aircraft, there is a certain, large amount of nutrients needed to cure a sick body.

11

LAW: The quantity of a nutritional supplement that cures an illness indicates the patient's degree of deficiency. It is therefore not a megadose of the vitamin, but rather a megadeficiency of the nutrient that we are dealing with.

LAW: Nutritional therapy is inexpensive, effective, and, most important, safe. There is not even one death per year from vitamins.

LAW: Vitamin supplementation is not the problem. It is under-nutrition that is the problem. Vitamins are the solution.

LAW: Vitamin C can replace antibiotics, antihistamines, antipyretics, antitoxins, and antiviral drugs at saturation (bowel tolerance) levels. "Saturation" means vastly higher doses than you ever imagined, and "bowel tolerance" means exactly what you think it means.

LAW: The reason one nutrient can cure so many different illnesses is because a deficiency of one nutrient can cause many different illnesses.

LAW: A vitamin can act as a drug, but a drug can never act as a vitamin.

LAW: With vitamin therapy, at any given quantity, frequently divided doses are more effective. This is especially true with the water-soluble B and C vitamins.

LAW: What you need to do to doctor yourself is less than you might think but more than you might want. There are no free rides in life.

LAW: Health recovered is proportional to effort expended. You do not have to live an inflexibly perfect life to have a much healthier body . . . but it sure helps to try.

LAW: Most confusion over what constitutes proper health care arises from partisans. Bias against vitamin supplements proceeds from people who stand to lose when cheap, natural health care succeeds. Hospitals, physicians, nurses, dietitians, politicians, pharmaceutical companies, and others have a vested interest in disease.

LAW: Many conflicting reports about vitamin therapy come from natural health partisans. These include vitamin distributors, individual supplement companies, brands, and even practitioners trying to corner as much of the market as they can for themselves. Ignore them. I have no financial connection whatsoever to the health products industry or to any part of it.

LAW: Health knowledge worth having does not go out of date in ten years or even one hundred years. "New" does not automatically mean more accurate or more valuable. "Old" research and clinical studies are often superior references. What works is never out of date. Fasting, near-vegetarian diet, use of nutritional supplements, and other nonpharmaceutical methods have stood the test of time, as have Einstein's theories and the Bill of Rights.

Fire Your Doctor!

"The art of medicine consists in amusing the patient while nature cures the disease."
—VOLTAIRE

If you want something done right, you have to do it yourself. This especially applies to your health care.

I fired my first doctor when I was fifteen. I was away at school and experiencing some anxiety symptoms. Without hesitation and without explanation, the school physician gave me a little white envelope containing half a dozen little green capsules. Before leaving the infirmary, I took two of them, as directed. By the time I got to the campus dining hall, I was higher than a kite. I still remember walking over to the table by the window where my roommate and best friend, Dean, always sat. As I approached, he looked at me quizzically. Me, I just smiled. And I mean *all* I did was smile. Everything was absolutely, positively fine; there are no worries when you are as heavily doped up as I was. Of course I could do nothing *but* smile in that state. I did not care if I ate and I do not remember if I did; I had no interest in schoolwork, conversation, or anything else, either. Those little green capsules turned out to contain a very powerful tranquilizer.

It was odd, really, for the year was 1970, and seemingly every student I knew (except Dean and me) was perpetually in search of any way at all to purchase the kind of high I had just received, legally, entirely paid for by health insurance, and dispensed from the wise hands of the good ol' school doc.

I never took a second dose of that tranquilizer. Maybe this is because I was a straight-laced good boy. Maybe. More likely, though, the real reason was because I wanted a healthy life. This was a major realization, a truly big step: I realized that the doctor's treatment was seriously amiss. I never went back to the infirmary.

Firing a doctor need not assume the conventional image of a pink slip and a bootprint on the keester. Rather, to fire your doctor means to not need him, to outgrow her, to decide that the doctor's information is incomplete or wrong, and to determine his skill to be insufficient to bet your life on.

To fire your doctor is to hire yourself as your chief physician.

You probably think you are not up to the job. After all, who are you? You didn't go to medical school. That's true, of course. Neither did I. But consider what the limitations of "medicine" are. Drugs and surgical treatments have always been the focus of medical school. Any physician will confirm that, even today, the rest of the curriculum runs far, far behind. Ask your doctor how many courses in clinical nutrition she has completed. Ask you doctor how many hours of homeopathic medicine, herbal medicine, and orthomolecular medicine he has logged. You are likely to find that those "medicines" aren't even counted worthy of time in the medical school syllabus.

Big mistake. Homeopathy has been successfully practiced by physicians the world over for 200 years. Homeopaths were giving tiny, nontoxic amounts of natural substances to effect a cure while "regular" doctors were drugging people to a premature death with stiff quantities of arsenic and mercury. Herbal medicine goes back for centuries, when practitioners (mostly women) used plants to heal instead of taking blood by the quart from the arms of anybody unfortunate enough to come within the reach of a surgeon's lancet. If anything, drug-and-cut "medicine" is an alternative to the natural health disciplines—and not a very good alternative at that.

And orthomolecular (megavitamin) medicine? There are tens of thousands of references to support it. I have more than 4,000 at my doctoryourself.com website alone. Can all of those successful vitamin-study authors, all those researchers and physicians, be dumber than the reporter you have heard intone that "vitamins may be dangerous and just give you expensive urine"?

Of course not. And far-thinking doctors are beginning to come around to what they were initially taught, and then taught to forget: *vis medicatrix naturae:* the healing power of nature. They have been led back to this timeless principle by their patients, the majority of which see a natural-health practitioner at least once in a given year. The market favors success, and savvy doctors can see the handwriting on the wall.

Now they are trying to learn "natural health," which they want to call "complementary medicine" to keep it in their shop. Monopolistic concerns aside, we should focus on this point: your doctor probably doesn't know any more about natural healing than you do . . . and is likely to know a good deal less. It is a fair race when all parties start at the same time and place. You can learn whatever your doctor learns, just as fast and just as well. You even have several advantages:

First, you have the Home Team Advantage. Your body is better known to you than Yankee Stadium was to Babe Ruth. You live inside you every minute of every day. You can better monitor and adjust your needs than can anyone else.

Second, you only have to learn what you and your family specifically need to know. You have to study up on your own particular health problems, but you do not have to spend time learning about everyone else's. This makes you a specialist in the same time it will make your new study-buddy doctor a poor generalist.

Third, you have the personal, altruistic advantage: you are doing this for your family. Unlike the doctor, you are working for love and life, not money.

Together, these make one tough starting lineup. This is a very powerful, healthy combination, and it will serve you well.

Hire Your Doctor

Now that you have fired your doctor and taken charge of your own health care, it is the perfect time to hire him back. After all, just like a roofer or a plumber, he can be useful for certain things. But, as with those professions, whenever you consult him, remember that your doctor works for you and not the other way around. It is your body. You run the show; your doctor is a subcontractor.

In order for this to work, you need to be on an equal footing with your physician. This is where a lot of people balk and are more than willing to sit down, shut up, and behave. To be on a level playing field with your doctor, first you need to read. Knowledge is power. Read like mad about your condition and the alternatives available for it. Search the library and search the Internet, and do not rest until you have the references to back yourself up.

Next, you need to have a workable physician. If your doctor is not providing you with the care you want, there are two possibilities. One: you have a miscommunication, meaning you have not made it sufficiently clear to your doctor what you do in fact want. Two: you have a disagreement, meaning you have made it clear all right, and the physician is not cooperating with you.

Both of these problems are common, though it is far easier to clear up a miscommunication than a disagreement. I am not saying that you should jettison every doctor that does not knuckle under, but you simply must have a baseline agreement, or any attempts to share information will be futile.

Even polite, personable doctors can still be very paternalistic, sweetly telling you to leave the complicated stuff to them. Hogwash. I would not accept that phrase from a mechanic, plumber, or politician. Neither should you, and in this case your life depends on it. Pleasant office or bedside manner is no substitute for thoroughness.

Do not accept vagueness, either. Nail down a deal, and get your doctor to clearly and unequivocally state his or her acceptance of your wishes. There is no excuse for not trying alternatives with a physician as your copilot. Herbs and vitamins are not perfect, but they are a million times safer than drugs.

With these goals in mind, I offer the following checklist to help you modify and improve the doctor you choose:

Ten Ways to Make Your Doctor into a Naturopath

1. *Pick a workable doctor.* How do you know if a doctor is workable? Interview them. I screen any physician I'm thinking of consulting with. Since there may actually be a charge for this "initial consultation," I carry this out by asking the office manager, nurse or assistant to please relay these three questions to the doctor: 1) "I take vitamin supplements. How do you feel about that?" 2) "I feel that my doctor should work with me, but that I am in charge of my health. Is this compatible with your philosophy of care?" 3) "I choose to decline immunizations. Are you willing to accept this viewpoint?" If the doctor agrees to all three position statements, you are in business. If not, keep looking. Be prepared to spend some time on this process. It pays off.

2. *Not all doctors that promote themselves as "holistic," "alternative," or "complementary" will be as advertised.* Lip service to a natural philosophy is not the same as actually prescribing a fast for obesity or treating pneumonia with vitamin C. Hiring a doctor requires an in-depth evaluation that only personal experience can provide. Word of mouth is a way to capitalize on others' experience with this doctor. Ask around.

3. *Make it easy for your doctor.* Stay healthy. Eat right. Do not smoke. Avoid alcohol and illegal drugs. Keep fit. Show that you take care of yourself.

4. *Do your homework.* Prepare your case before you go in for an office visit. Look up your ailment in the *Merck Manual* to learn what the conventional medical approach to such an illness is. Then read up on the alternatives. You might start with the sizable bibliography at the end of this book. There is no substitute for being well informed.

15

5. *If you need a diagnosis, get one*. Be responsible. Use technology. Listen to what your doctor has to say, but do not *do* it until you complete step 4, above.

6. *Use the "suggestive selling" technique*. Suggest a natural alternative to any medical treatment you may be offered. Or, instead of one or the other, suggest both. Know what you want and see that you get it.

7. *Look at your situation from the doctor's perspective*. If you were legally bound and professionally constrained to the extent that most physicians are, how would you react to a know-it-all upstart patient who marched into your office and began to dictate terms? To not create a defensive physician, avoid backing your doctor into any corners. Instead, bring along materials written by other physicians who treat naturally. If such-and-such a doctor already does it successfully, it takes the pressure off your doctor in trying it with you. Ask for a "therapeutic trial."

8. *Try the good cop, bad cop approach*. Offer to sign a paper stating that you will not sue the doctor if the natural treatment you request is unsuccessful. At the same time, subtly point out that a patient could sue if the doctor refused a patient's natural treatment request.

9. *Compromise*. Half a pie is better than none. Your doctor does not have to meet you 100% on every issue. It is generally sufficient to hear any of the following phrases, which indicate an open-minded physician:

"Vitamins aren't likely to do you any harm."

"I've heard of more and more people doing this."

"I attended a seminar on this recently."

"Let's try it."

"Let me know how this works out for you."

"I told my other patients about this."

10. *Provide positive feedback*. Doctors love to be told that "their" therapy is successful. Whenever appropriate, tell your doctor that you are feeling great. You are likely to be rewarded with, "Whatever you are doing, keep doing it." That is the sweet sound of self-reliant success.

Your Money or Your Health?

As should already be clear, making pharmaceuticals available to everyone won't solve our disease problem any more than making guns available to everyone will solve our crime problem. More vaccinations will do little for the cardiovascular diseases that are responsible for one half of all deaths in the United States. At least half of all illnesses are avoidable, being entirely due to unhealthy lifestyles and eating habits. Only lip service has been paid to preventive medicine, even though America's chronic-or-crisis style of medicine is the very trillion-dollar-per-year boondoggle that got us into this mess in the first place.

I feel very strongly that there is an alternative, a nutritional "road less traveled" that we should have taken long before this. That road is the one of personal responsibility for health, complete dietary overhaul, and, when needed, aggressive high-dose vitamin therapy in place of drugs. The closest professional description of this approach is naturopathy, the organized science of natural healing. There is still time to reverse our steps and take this other path. I perceive a keen need for a direct appeal to individual doctors, students, and patients to improve their health by changing their own lives.

It will not be easy, however. I have personally known more than one physician who was run out of New York State by his peers for practicing naturopathy. This is not a new phenomenon. Since the nineteenth century, the AMA and its clones have declared war on their competitors, eager for a monopoly of the lucrative health field. Has it worked? You decide. One of my most repetitive readers' questions remains "Can you tell me where I can find a natural healing physician near where I live?"

America's expensive and ineffective health care system is fundamentally unworkable. Even the most creative of financial makeovers will not save it. Merely by avoiding megavitamin therapies and downplaying vegetarian diet, it is doomed. Merely by assigning our health responsibility out to someone else rather than to ourselves, it is doomed again. The only way to have health care for all individuals is for all individuals to take responsibility for their own health. People need specific instruction on how exactly to do this, and they have not been getting it.

Most of what we do to our bodies we do ourselves, daily, by the lifestyle choices we make. There is no outside enemy to fight. We do not need "further study" on mineral and vitamin therapy. The work has already been done, the results are in print, and the public is cheerfully ignorant. How did we miss it?

One possible explanation is the cozy relationship between mainstream medicine and the media. There is more than a hint of collusion. Major wire services are continually fed articles reflecting the positions of the largest, most vocal, and best funded health lobbies and professional trade groups. What is politically correct, popular, and easily reduced to a sound byte is what gets publicity. What gets publicity tends to get funded, and what is funded gets done. Medical witch hunts for a test-tube, magic-bullet cure for cancer or AIDS fit this description. Since pharmaceutical industry investment in such projects is very high, there is funding. Media cooperation is equally high, for a heroic, new celebrity-style medical crusade easily sells papers and commercial air time. On top of that, the American Medical Association has the biggest-spending professional lobby in the country. Politicians know a bandwagon when they see it, and the result is more laws favoring orthodox medicine . . . and still more funding.

Considering the paucity of interest (and funding), it is quite remarkable how much good nutrition research has been done, and how almost all of it points to three embarrassingly simple conclusions:

1. The average American's diet is truly terrible, being superabundant in chemicals, calories, and animal protein and very deficient in fiber and diverse major vitamins and minerals.

2. Higher U.S. Recommended Dietary Allowances, plus nutritional supplements, are clearly needed, and even modest increases in vitamin and mineral intake regularly result in both disease prevention and clinical cure.

3. Most citizens, and their doctors, are vaguely aware of item 1, unaware of item 2, and not concerned enough to act on either.

I continue to be amazed at the number of people who actually do not know that huge doses of vitamin C can safely be used as an antibiotic, antiviral, and antihistamine. Most surprising is

17

the nutritional misinformation level among doctors, who ought to read their own journals but apparently don't. Busy physicians tend to rely on the sales force from pharmaceutical houses the way TV viewers rely on news anchorpersons: just give us the summary. Patent drug companies make money from patented drugs, not generic vitamins. There is much more money to be made with prednisone than with pyridoxine (vitamin B_6). Doctors' prescriptions generate patent drug sales without the doctor having to pay a cent. Whether nutrition disinterest results from a lack of financial interest, a lack of political clout, or a lack of inclination, the end product is the same: patients are the losers.

My purpose is to help correct this problem by placing both the facts and the motivation directly into your hands. From that point, it is up to you to live healthfully using all available tools to do so. Thorough knowledge of megavitamin nutrition mixed with our own keen need for personal health improvement is such a combustible mixture that a single, well-placed spark will start a good fire. To help provide that initial spark, I have written this book, which blends personal conviction, motivation, and all-too-seldom-seen scientific literature into a guide for students and patients. This project has evolved over thirty-five years as a medical writer and naturopathic educator.

In the Sixties, one slogan was "What if they gave a war, and nobody came?" Enough individual actions could add up to peace. Well, what if each person eats right, exercises, eradicates bad habits, and starts taking vitamins? Might our new slogan be: "What if they gave everybody health insurance, and nobody needed it?" The result would be nothing less than total national health, gained one person at a time.

Oddly enough, it may be that we've had trouble seeing the trees because of the forest. Health care is such an enormous issue that we tend to bite off more than we can chew. Getting a nation to be healthy is one tall order. To think we can ever gain national health by refinancing the same old disease model is ludicrous.

As difficult as it truly is to change our own personal habits, it remains the only sure method to gain back our health, and to positively influence another person to do the same. This book is really about education and motivation in just one person's health behavior, and that is yours.

In the end, education may be reduced to an option, and motivation may be reduced to an offer: there is a way out, and you are free to try it. Many of the lifeboats on the *Titanic* were launched when less than half full. There was a way for hundreds more to be saved, but only for those who 1) knew early that the ship was sinking, and 2) climbed into a boat. Too many of those lost never knew their options until it was too late.

Today, Americans have real health options but are largely unaware of the safety, the scientific validity, and the real curative power of simple nutrients. I have written this book to help people make the discovery, on their own, that there is a way off the sinking ship of conventional drug-and-surgery disease care. That small lifeboat, no matter how flimsy it looks, is a better bet than staying on any big, solid, doomed ship.

18

Part One

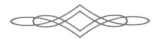

Natural Healing Protocols

*"The world cares very little about what a person knows;
it is what the person is able to do that counts."*

—BOOKER T. WASHINGTON

The solution to a problem is not always found at the level of the problem. Chasing symptoms can be a dead-end street unless your goal is to personally enrich the stockholders of pharmaceutical companies.

If you suffer from acid reflux or a hiatus hernia, you might want to give these ideas a try.

1. **Make your midday meal your largest**, and do not eat at all after 5 P.M. It is amazing how many indigestion symptoms go away when you do so.

2. **Chew your food very thoroughly**. This sounds too simple to work, so a lot of folks ignore it and miss the benefits. Don't be one of them.

3. **Eat easily digestible food**. This includes fruits, rice, steamed vegetables, sprouted seeds and grains, well-cooked beans, aged cheeses, yogurt, cottage cheese, and *especially* vegetable juices. Avoid fried food. Stop eating meat. (And if you can't manage that completely, at least avoid the worst offenders: cold cuts, ham, pastrami, and pepperoni.)

INDIGESTION, OR SIMPLY INDIGESTIBLE?

A young man with indigestion mentioned to me that he really liked hot dogs. He stopped eating them. His indigestion went away. No, this is not a Henny Youngman routine. It is true just as written. There may be a solid reason. In landfills, "Whole hot dogs have been found, some of them in strata suggesting an age upwards of several decades" (*Smithsonian*, July 1992, p. 5).

There is a lesson in there somewhere.

4. **Try multiple digestive enzyme tablets**, particularly if you did not follow the advice in step 2, above.

5. Better yet, **eat lots of figs, pineapples, kiwis, mangoes, and papayas**. These fruits are simply loaded with natural digestive enzymes that do half the work for you. *These fruits must be fresh, not canned.* That's because the digestive enzymes are destroyed by cooking temperatures. Dried fruits processed at low temperatures may be okay. A simple way is to try and see.

6. You might also want to **up your consumption of good-quality yogurt**, which contains beneficial digestive bacteria. Make sure you buy a brand that lists live cultures on the label. An old trick from India is to dilute the yogurt in an equal amount of water. This makes it even easier to digest and reduces nose stuffiness.

7. **Raise your head at night**. Sleep on a thicker pillow, or stack up two thin ones. Some people prefer a foam rubber, wedge-shaped bolster pillow.

8. **Chiropractic adjustments** may help. Try three visits and see.

9. **Try the homeopathic remedy (and Schuessler cell salt) Natrum Phos 6X**.

10. **Reduce stress**. Yeah, right! Easier said than done. But the truth is, meditation, relaxation, massage, music, reading, or just some plain old time alone can really make a difference.

11. If your symptoms are really troublesome, **see your physician**. While you are waiting for the appointment, you could go on a vegetable-juice-only diet for three to seven days. Many an appointment has been cancelled by a juice fast.

12. That includes even some serious cases. I have met people who had acid reflux for so long that there was scarring of the esophagus. I acquainted them with the **four-glasses-of-cabbage-juice-a-day** hospital-tested protocol of Garnett Cheney, M.D. While originally used primarily on stomach and lower gastrointestinal conditions, cabbage juice proved effective above the tummy as well. Dr. Cheney found that the entire gastrointestinal tract, from throat to colon, benefits from fresh raw cabbage juice, taken regularly and in quantity. His articles are far from new, but what has changed about cabbage?

FOOD POISONING

"Greetings from Mexico. Just wanted to write and report my latest success with vitamin C. I've been reading Pauling's *How to Live Longer and Feel Better*, which I happened to have bought just a few days before you recently recommended it. It was in a used book store for 25 pesos. Talk about serendipity!

"I have lived here in Mexico for over ten years and I have learned that when I have food poisoning I'd better head for the antibiotic powder that I've always had to use. This time, though, I decided to grab my vitamin C instead. So I took 2,000 to 4,000 milligrams every few hours and it really worked. Here I am at the end of only one day, and I seem to be pulling out of the ordeal quite nicely.

"The first time I got this I lost about 15 pounds in three or four days. Montezuma does not mess around. *¡Mil gracias! ¡Salud y saludos!*"

Recommended Reading

Cheney G. Antipeptic ulcer dietary factor. *American Dietetics Association* 26 (1950): 9.

Cheney G. The nature of the antipeptic ulcer dietary factor. *Stanford Medical Bulletin* 8 (1950): 144.

Cheney G. Prevention of histamine-induced peptic ulcers by diet. *Stanford Medical Bulletin* 6 (1948): 334.

Cheney G. Rapid healing of peptic ulcers in patients receiving fresh cabbage juice. *California Medicine* 70 (1949): 10.

Cheney G. Vitamin U therapy of peptic ulcer. *California Medicine* 77, no. 4 (1952).

"No illness which can be treated by diet should be treated by any other means."

—MOSES MAIMONIDES, TWELFTH-CENTURY PHYSICIAN

Nutritional supplements have been used, with considerable success, to help overcome learning disabilities in children. In a well-designed clinical trial, megadoses of vitamins were seen to be safe and remarkably effective, even offering improvement in Down's syndrome children.

Dr. Ruth F. Harrell and associates published their important findings in *Proceedings of the National Academy of Sciences*—in 1981! Although *Medical Tribune* picked the story up, your doctor is likely as unaware of this research as I was until one of my chiropractic students showed it to me in 1993.

What worked then works now.

The Harrell study was successful because her team gave learning-disabled kids much larger doses of vitamins than other researchers: more than 100 times the *adult* (not child's) RDA for riboflavin; 37 times the RDA for niacin (given as niacinamide); 40 times the RDA for vitamin E; and 150 times the RDA for thiamin. These are the quantities that evidently get results, and get them safely. Safety and effectiveness are the rule, not the exception, with therapeutic nutrition. I urge you to read the full paper: Harrell RF, Capp RH, Davis DR, Peerless J, and Ravitz LR. "Can nutritional supplements help mentally retarded children? An exploratory study." *Proc Natl Acad Sci USA* 78 (1981): 574–8.

Dr. Harrell, who had been publishing on vitamin effects on learning for over thirty years, was not inventing the idea of megavitamin therapy in one paper. Psychiatrist Abram Hoffer pioneered megavitamin research and treatment back in the early 1950s. Half a century later, his work still has been largely ignored by the medical profession. Dr. Hoffer has treated a whole lot of ADHD kids with vitamins.

It works.

I know a ten-year-old boy who was having considerable school and behavior problems. Interestingly enough, the child was already on physician-prescribed doses of niacin, but the total daily dose was only 150 mg. Not a bad beginning, since the RDA for kids is less than 20 mg per day. But it wasn't enough to be effective, and the boy was slated for the Ritalin-for-lunch bunch. Dr. Hoffer suggested giving him 500 mg niacinamide three times a day (1,500 mg total). That's a lot, but niacinamide is a comfortable, flush-free form of vitamin B_3. So Mom tried it. It helped greatly.

Then, she upped the dose to 3,000 mg per day. What a difference! The boy slept better, and his nightmares went away. He had fewer emotional meltdowns during the day and was less argumentative, less hyper, and less aggressive. He was warmer and more loving with his parents and more tolerant of changes in his routine. Basically, he reverted to the normal, happy-kid behavior that you just cannot buy in a Ritalin bottle.

People often ask, "If this treatment is so good, how come my doctor doesn't know about it? How come it is not on the news?" The answer may have more to do with medical politics than with medical science. Dr. Hoffer writes this about attention deficit hyperactivity disorder: "The DSM system [the standard of the American Psychiatric Association] has little or no relevance to diagnosis. It has no relevance to treatment, either, because no matter which terms are used to classify these children, they are all recommended for treatment with drug therapy" combined, sometimes, with other non-megavitamin approaches. "If the entire diagnostic scheme were scrapped today, it would make almost no difference to the way these children were treated, or to the outcome of treatment. Nor would their patients feel any better or worse." Statements like these do not exactly endear one to the medical community.

> *"Freedom of the press is guaranteed only to those who own one."*
> —ABBOTT JOSEPH LIEBLING
>
> When psychiatric journals refused to publish Abram Hoffer's controlled studies showing that niacin cured many forms of mental illness, Dr. Hoffer started his own *Journal of Orthomolecular Medicine.* You may access over forty years' worth of the *Journal's* archive free of charge at http://orthomolecular.org/library/jom/.

As if such statements are not enough, Dr. Hoffer has devoted an entire book (*Dr. Hoffer's ABC of Natural Nutrition for Children,* Quarry Press, 1999) to setting out genuine nutritional alternatives to drug therapy for ADHD children. He provides vitamin dosage details, food tables, and more than 150 references. In addition, 120 case histories are included, along with a "bad foods" list, numerous research summaries, precise recommendations for optimum diet, comparisons of drugs and vitamins, a discussion of allergies and food additives, behavioral self-tests, and, most important, a wealth of professional experience.

Criticisms and even lawsuits over the hazards of tranquilizers, Ritalin, and behavior-modifying pharmaceuticals are on the rise, but neither court nor controversy can cure your child. "Battered parents" (Hoffer's term) need to know what to do, and *now*. Saying no to drugs also requires saying "yes" to something else. That something else is nutrition, properly employed.

For example: Supplemental magnesium and vitamin B_6 given to 52 hyperexcitable children produced the following results: "In all patients, symptoms of hyperexcitability (physical aggressivity, instability, scholar attention, hypertony, spasm, myoclony) were reduced after 1 to 6 months treatment" (Mousain-Bosc, et al. 2004).

And that's just using two nutrients.

For those who say there is insufficient scientific evidence to support high-dose nutritional therapy for children's behavior disorders, I say they haven't been looking hard enough. Hoffer and his colleagues conducted the first double-blind controlled vitamin trials in psychiatric history in 1952. He was among the first to employ vitamin C as an antioxidant, to use the B vitamins against heart disease, and to employ niacin to treat behavioral disorders.

In light of this, organized medicine's "try everything but megavitamins" philosophy remains a puzzler, but it isn't the bottom line. This, however, is: the simple way to determine whether vitamins will help your child is to try them.

"I read a book about the evils of drinking, so I gave up reading."

—HENNY YOUNGMAN

She was a very nice lady, the wife of a surgeon, and an incurable alcoholic. Betty, age fifty-six, had been in and out of every rehab facility you can name. The famous ones, the expensive ones: all the king's horses and all the king's men couldn't seem to stop her from drinking again.

But it's no joke, not at all. One in three American adults does not drink any alcoholic beverages. One third drinks very moderately and responsibly. And one third of all American adults drinks too much. Ten percent of our population can be classified as very heavy drinkers, putting down half of all alcohol consumed in the nation.

So Betty is not alone. But it seemed strange at first as she sat there in front of me, gracious and poised, telling me of her misery. Most of my experience with alcoholics came from volunteering at an urban soup kitchen. There the winos fit the stereotype much better: disheveled men slurping from bottles of blackberry brandy in filthy paper bags. Truth is, you will not recognize most alcoholics. Most manage, somehow, to cope. This is easiest if they have money and free time, which means that many have gray hair. Believe it or not, "70 percent of elderly hospitalizations in 1991 were for alcohol-related problems." (*Newsletter of the New York State Office of Alcoholism and Substance Abuse Services,* Sept–Oct 1992)

"Is there anything you can do for me?" Betty asked.

Yeah, right, I thought to myself. Nobody had had any lasting luck getting this lady off the sauce. And you think you're gonna do it, fella? Pull the other leg.

Then the little cartoon angel whispered in my other ear. Roger J. Williams!

"There is a proven nutritional treatment for alcoholism," I said. "Roger Williams, a chemistry professor at the University of Texas and former president of the American Chemical Society, has written extensively on the subject. His work dates as far back as the 1950s, but is still as practical as if written yesterday."

"What does he recommend?" Betty asked.

"Megadoses of vitamins and an amino acid called L-glutamine. You might want to write this down. Thousands of milligrams of vitamin C a day, in divided doses; all the B vitamins, especially thiamin, in a B-complex supplement, five times a day; and about three grams of L-glutamine. This, plus a general good diet, with an avoidance of sugar, is essentially it. Can you do it?"

Betty smiled. "The real question is, *will* I do it, isn't it?"

"Yes," I said. "You've tried everything else."

Some weeks later I got an encouraging phone call from Betty. "Things are going great," she said. "Haven't had a drink since the day I saw you."

"Terrific!" But will she keep it going? I wondered. "Remember that the supplements won't do any good in the bottle. You've got to stay with this permanently, you know."

Months passed. A Christmas card from Betty: she was still clean and sober, she wrote. Next year, another Christmas card told of her continued success. "I'm going back to school," she wrote. Nice! "I've been able to have a drink or two now and again," Betty added, and the bottom fell right out of my happy mood. "But I stop when I choose, and do not want any more than that. I'm still taking all the vitamins. Thank you again!"

Once more, my understanding of alcoholism was overturned. Professional dogma tells us that "once an alcoholic, always an alcoholic." I've taught alcohol and substance abuse classes at the college level as part of a certified alcohol counselor training program. I know the drill, and Betty's experience did not fit well. She should not drink at all! Never!

Yet here she was, able to have a drink just like a normal person. She could choose to have a drink, and then stop. No compulsion, no addiction. Betty wasn't just coping better; she wasn't just recovering. Betty was cured.

Dr. Williams is responsible for the key nutritional concept, ignored by the medical and dietetic professions, that different people need differing amounts of nutrients. One size never fits all; anyone who has ever bought underwear will tell you this. Even people the same size and age will require differing amounts of nutrients, due to lifestyle and genetic factors. An alcoholic, for example, needs vastly more of certain vitamins than a non-drinker. There is a reason for this.

Beverage alcohol is ethanol, C_2H_5OH. It is a simple carbohydrate, much like sugar, supplying lots of energy and no other nutrients. Thiamin (vitamin B_1) is needed for carbohydrate metabolism. Extra carbos, including extra alcohol, require extra thiamin. Because alcohol is filling, it displaces more nourishing foods in the diet, causing malnutrition and specifically causing thiamin deficiency.

So the heavy drinker is much less likely to get even the usual dietary amount of thiamin, at a time when she needs much more. Add to this the fact that alcohol destroys the liver and brain gradually, but profoundly. This damage increases the need for nutrients to repair the body at a time when the drinker is eating fewer and fewer good foods. Still worse, alcohol causes poor absorption and utilization of what few B vitamins are coming in. Alcohol can literally destroy folic acid.

A deficiency of thiamin, just thiamin, produces the following symptoms, according to the respected textbook *Nutrition and Diet Therapy:*

Gastrointestinal: anorexia, indigestion, severe constipation, gastric atony, and insufficient stomach-acid secretion. All of these result mostly from a lack of energy to the GI tract cells: no thiamin, no energy, no function.

Cardiovascular: dilation of peripheral blood vessels (edema), weakened heart muscle, and heart failure.

Neurological: diminished reflex response, reduced alertness, fatigue, apathy. Continued deficiency produces damage or degeneration to myelin sheaths (fatty nerve-cell insulation material).

If you see an obvious tie-in to multiple sclerosis, you are right. A lack of thiamin causes increased nerve irritation, pain, prickly sensations, deadening sensations, and, if unchecked, paralysis. Thiamin-deficiency nerve damage can result in the DTs and hallucinations.

All this, mind you, from a deficiency of just one vitamin.

The U.S. thiamin RDA of a milligram or two is not remotely enough. A very strong case can be made for 25 to 65 mg per day even for nonalcoholics. The heavy drinker's poor diet plus ensuing alcohol damage plus increased thiamin need proportional to carbohydrate intake points to an optimum B_1 intake of several hundred mg per day.

One study of about 2,000 households for a full year showed that more than 65 percent of adults got less than the RDA of thiamin. This means that half to two-thirds of Americans probably are thiamin-deficient even if they do not drink at all. Thiamin is found in almost all natural foods, but in tiny amounts. Precious few sober Americans, let alone alcoholics, eat large quantities of the whole grains and legumes (peas, beans, and lentils) that are modest food sources of thiamin.

Therefore, vitamin B_1 supplements are essential. To get maximum results, additional nutrients must also be provided in abundance through supplementation.

Which ones, specifically?

1. Vitamin C in great quantity (on the order of 10,000 to 20,000 mg per day and more). High doses of vitamin C chemically neutralize the toxic byproducts of alcohol metabolism. Vitamin C also increases the liver's ability to reverse the fatty buildup so common in alcoholics.

2. B complex, consisting of 50 mg of each of the major B vitamins, six times daily. The B-complex vitamins work best in concert with each other.

3. L-glutamine, 2,000 to 3,000 mg per day. This amino acid helps decrease physiological cravings for alcohol.

4. Lecithin, 2 to 4 tablespoons daily. This provides inositol and choline, which are related to the B complex. Lecithin also helps mobilize fats out of the liver.

5. Chromium, at least 200 to perhaps 400 mcg chromium polynicotinate daily. Chromium greatly improves carbohydrate metabolism and helps control blood sugar levels. Many, if not most, alcoholics are hypoglycemic.

6. A good high-potency multivitamin, multimineral supplement as well, containing magnesium (400 mg) and the antioxidants carotene and vitamin E (d-alpha-tocopherol).

27

Another reader says:

"I am the wife of an alcoholic who came out of a thirty-day detox two months ago; has not been back to work for weeks; and was showing no promise of doing so, relapsing every three to four days—up until this past week. On the brink of divorce, I sent out to the universe a serious intention . . . a prayer . . . an absolute letting go to find an answer. So recently, he has been taking the vitamins you mention, in the dosages suggested, plus eating whole-grain foods, vegetables, fruits, *no* sugar, and plenty of water. He had indicated no alcohol cravings for the past four to five days, but decided to get 'a shot and a beer' this afternoon. Normally this would have led to a relapse, ending up in three to five shots and five to six beers and a lot of headache and heartache for me (and him too). Guess what?! He took the one shot, one beer, said it tasted disgusting, didn't give him the pleasurable physical response, and threw away the second shot and beer!! That's huge, almost unbelievable! It's the early evening here. He's drinking water and sipping tea (has a headache and is generally remorseful), but he's not drunk, and he controlled the drinking and stopped the cycle. On behalf of my husband, in memory of my father (another alcoholic), and the millions of very wonderful human beings who think this 'disease' is incurable and they just have to 'manage' their symptoms, I am militant about getting the word out about this program."

Dr. Ruth Harrell elegantly confirmed Dr. Williams's theory when she gave huge doses of vitamins, especially B complex, to severely mentally handicapped children. She obtained extraordinary improvement in learning and IQ in a matter of months, including spectacular advances in Down's syndrome children. This work was done in 1981 and published in the *Proceedings of the National Academy of Sciences.*

Why, then, does the medical establishment keep Dr. Williams's knowledge filed away, out of sight? The answer is classic: follow the money.

In America, there is a vested interest in disease. There is no profit in prevention. You make a whole lot more money treating alcoholism than you do not having alcoholism. It is the very "social cost" of this, and other diseases, that makes them profitable. It is a tough concept, but think about it: There is a shortage of special-education teachers! America's courts and prisons are backlogged and overcrowded! Nursing homes have waiting lists! There are waiting lists for organ transplants! Medical costs are through the roof! What can we conclude? Simple: business is good! In a PBS news program entitled *Affluenza,* the point is made that every time a person is diagnosed with cancer, the nation's gross domestic product goes up.

So what are we to do, at least those of us who want results? The first rule of fishing is to put your hook in the water, for that is where the fish are. Try Roger Williams's protocol, and see what I saw with Betty.

When someone becomes unconscious from ethanol, they may have had just enough to pass out, or they may have had just enough to die. One cannot afford to take a chance and see if they sleep it off, or never wake. To stop such emergencies from occurring, we also cannot afford to ignore vitamin therapy.

Another reader says:

"One day, not so long ago, I went searching online for a miracle to help me stop drinking. I have been a closet drinker for twenty-five years and spent much of every day thinking about picking up a bottle of wine on the way home and getting "relaxed." I hid bottles in my studio, my closet, and in the basement. When I felt ashamed of how much I drank, I refilled the bottles to make it look as if I had only had a glass instead of an entire bottle. If I had a day off, I would start drinking at eleven in the morning. By the time my husband came home from work, I would already be on my second bottle of the day. I very rarely remembered conversations I had had with others from the night before.

"People just thought I was a bit of a wine snob and even my children purchased nice wine for me for my birthday. Honestly, I could have cared less about how it tasted.

"Every morning I hated myself as I nursed my hangover and promised to only have one or two glasses that day, but once I started, there was no stopping and my cravings became impossible to ignore by six in the evening.

"Then I saw your article on vitamin therapy, bought the book, and decided to try it, thinking, Oh well, at least it won't cost much or hurt me if it doesn't work. But it worked! Oh my God, it worked! It has now been a whole month with no drinking and no cravings. I am absolutely faithful about taking the vitamins and supplements. I am even starting to let go of the thought that I might fail again, because it is different this time. I am not feeling at a loss for the alcohol. I am not feeling deprived, and I am not mourning the fact that I will never have a drink again. I am hopeful for the first time in years. Thank you for making something that seemed insurmountable something achievable."

For Further Reading

Hoffer A. and Saul A. W. *The Vitamin Cure for Alcoholism.* Laguna Beach, CA: Basic Health Publications, 2009.

28

"I don't know if the world is full of smart men bluffing or imbeciles who mean it."

—ATTRIBUTED TO MORRIE BRICKMAN

Food allergies now affect about one in thirteen children in the U.S. That is almost six million kids (Gupta et al. 2011; Tanner 2011).

As Jack Benny famously said, with hand-to-cheek, in scenery-chewing shock: "Well!"

Many an allergy will disappear while you wait if you use the safest, cheapest, and most effective antihistamine-antitoxin in existence: vitamin C. I know, you don't believe me. How could a simple vitamin replace a medical specialty? Yet it's true. You could start a drive-in allergy clinic with only one prescription: "Take C. Forty dollars, please. Do you want fries with that?"

Wisdom is inherent in simplicity and safety. Hippocrates, the father of so-called medicine, said, "Of several remedies, the physician should choose the least sensational." That is genius, and it is practical advice good for modern man. Vitamin C therapy is safe, simple, and effective.

So you question this naive approach? Naturally, since we've all been taught that anything safe and simple cannot possibly be medically effective. So I give you the case of my friend Tim.

Tim brought in his wife and family to talk about scarlet fever. They'd had a touch of it in their family—and a touch is enough of that. We discussed vitamin C's role as an antipyretic (fever-reducer) and value as an antibiotic. They were keen to focus on this. In passing, Tim also mentioned some unspecified allergy problems. I briefly mentioned that vitamin C had great usefulness there as well.

A reader says:

"I am a twenty-six-year-old male skeptical of all things in life. I came across your site because I was under a spell of lethargy I couldn't resolve for the life of me. I followed your chronic fatigue guide and within a few weeks I was no longer yawning or tired. I've had blood in my stool for years due to hemorrhoids and even that cleared up. But I especially wanted to mention I've had shellfish allergies since childhood. Last time I tried lobster, my face exploded into some disfigured swollen state of affairs, which as you can imagine, wasn't very pleasant and has traumatized me now in adulthood. I read your words on allergies and your take on them. I upped my vitamin C dosage and convinced my significant other to allow me to sample shrimp, much to her dismay.

"Nothing. Not even the slightest reaction. My heart was racing, my palms were clammy. I attribute this to nerves from the experiences I've had with shellfish. Then came crab.

"Nothing.

"My allergies are now for naught. I can actually enjoy seafood, something I've yearned to do for years. My significant other still is a bit skeptical and keeps a case supply of Benadryl and the ER on speed dial whenever we sample seafood, but I'm confident that my allergies have subsided as I haven't had the slightest reaction. Since my realizations of how important vitamin therapy is, I always take my vitamins even though sometimes I'm ridiculed at work ("why are you taking so many pills?", etc.). It really is the only thing that has ever worked for me. Shame on the medical community to overlook this; just goes to show the amount of influence big Pharma has."

Tim called me a few weeks later. "Good resolution with the fever," he said. "We gave all the kids grams of vitamin C and only one of them had scarlet fever symptoms. That was Jeffrey, and he got over it much faster than the doctor expected him to."

"That's really good, Tim," I said.

"There's more to tell," he responded. "I was stung by a bee last week."

"And?"

"And I'm allergic to bee stings."

Ulp. He hadn't previously told me that.

"I have medicine and an inhaler," Tim continued. "The whole kit and kaboodle. When I was stung, I took 25,000 mg of vitamin C in the first hour. By the end of the day, I'd taken 100,000 mg. No symptoms at all. Not even any swelling. You had to look hard to find where the sting was."

"But you used your medicine, right?"

"No!" Tim said. "That's the amazing thing. Normally I would have had to, or I would probably die. But this time, all I did was the C. Talk about an antitoxin-antihistamine! That stuff really works."

I was unnerved at the high stakes Tim had played for, but impressed with his findings.

Allergy, like most disease names, tells you little about cause and nothing about cure. Robert F. Cathcart, M.D., looks at allergy (and many other conditions as well) simply in terms of how much vitamin C it takes to cure it. He has much experience as a clinician and has published numerous papers on the topic.

And he is correct.

A twenty-year-old woman once saw me about her allergies to horses and hay. Since she loved to ride, and her parents kept several horses in their barn, this was a big problem. The young lady was not readily going to change her eating habits, but was willing to take a lot of vitamin C. It was effective, as she tells it:

"Whenever I was taking 20,000 mg of vitamin C a day, I had no allergies at all. The only time I got them back was when I drank beer. So I either avoided beer, or if I drank, I took an extra 10,000 mg of C. I never had problems with horses or hay again."

I once had a client who was allergic to everything, literally. She'd tested out positive as allergic to seventy-two different substances. I'd never heard of that severe a condition before, and neither had her allergist. He said that she could take a "megadose" of perhaps 1,000 mg a day. It was not doing anything. I suggested she take vitamin C to bowel tolerance, and hold the C level just below the amount that caused loose stools. This turned out to be nearly 40,000 mg a day. She took all the C she could hold. That was the end of her seventy-two allergies.

And I've seen more of the same with children and teenagers, friends and neighbors, all ages and stages. Take enough C to be symptom free, whatever the amount might be . . . but stay a few thousand milligrams under the amount that causes diarrhea. That's about your only concern, because the safety of vitamin C therapy is unassailable. Dr. Frederick Robert Klenner writes, "Vitamin C is the safest substance available to the physician."

If these people can get rid of their allergies, perhaps your child can too. The leading allergies in children are to peanuts, milk, and shellfish. These can be very serious indeed. Let me make it clear that I am not suggesting that you trifle with your kids' health. What I do suggest is that, in addition to best-choice medication, you also give your child a Dr. Klenner amount of vitamin C daily. How much is that? The child's age in grams. That is 3,000 mg/day for a three-year-old; 8,000 mg/day for an eight-year-old. Some kids need less, and many need more.

Divide the dose for best absorption. (For more details on this approach, please see the chapter Vitamin C Megadose Therapy.) With your doctor's cooperation and maintained vitamin C supplementation, you may be able to wean your child off the medication.

I've got another story for you. Back in the 1970s, Dr. Benjamin Feingold, an allergist, noticed that some children seemed to be noticeably sensitive to artificial colors and other food additives. He worked primarily with hyperactive kids, had their parents clean up their diets and go chemical-free, and the hyperactive behavior stopped. From this came a classic book, *Why Your Child Is Hyperactive.*

Feingold was an M.D., credentialed in every way and then some. Feingold's diet was so effective that Feingold Associations—grassroots groups of parents—sprung up across the nation. Basically all they did was keep painted foods out of their children's stomachs.

The food industry's response was predictable. Study after study has been bankrolled to show that food additives—and sugar, for that matter—have no negative effect on children's behavior. Yeah, right! Been to a kid's birthday party lately? Ever taught school during the week following Halloween? Ever tried to nap a toddler full of M&M's? Most important, did you ever read Feingold's book? This man knows what he is talking about and got good results. As long as we let kids eat chemically dyed foods and drinks, we might just as well give them a can of Sherwin-Williams housepaint and a spoon.

FOOD ADDITIVES: WHAT? STILL?

Congress passed the U.S. Pure Food and Drugs Act in 1906. A physician, Harvey W. Wiley, M.D., was the first chief of the U.S. Bureau of Chemistry, the direct forerunner of the Food and Drug Administration (FDA). He oversaw extensive, detailed research on food additives to see if they were harmful to health. In his now rare and long out-of-print book, *A History of a Crime Against the Food Law* (1929), he describes his policy: "If there was any doubt that a food additive was harmful in any way, it could not be put in food at all." How things have changed.

Modern food science is the best money can buy, and it has been bought off. Read almost any processed food label, and prepare to be either bored or baffled. Bored, because the list of industrial ingredients is so very, very long. Baffled, because we can rarely pronounce (let alone understand) them all.

The ideal of really pure foods is not new. In the 1950s, the U.S. Congress pondered and actually passed the Delaney Amendment. Based on the work of Dr. Wiley, it argued that there is no such thing as a safe dose of a harmful substance. Lobbies were paid and even your federal tax dollars were all too often spent to be sure that safety standard was never adopted. That legislation has been buried by newer, permissive, food-manufacturer-friendly regulations.

A substance that may cause illness has no business being allowed, ever, in the food supply. Not even a little bit. If you question this, ask yourself: How many drops of rat urine would you accept in your next glass of lemonade? Twelve? Five? Two? Even half a drop of rat urine? Yet no case whatsoever can be made that a few drops of rat urine will kill you. Sanitation an issue, you say? Okay, we'll boil the rat urine first.

Now how many drops would you accept in your next glass of lemonade?

Ridiculous analogy? Maybe not. Consider that the public eats food paint (artificial colors) and consumes daily a variety of microbe poisons (preservatives). These substances will, in quantity, sicken or kill. Small amounts are used in foods. If foods were fresh, none would be needed. It is accepted as a given that your food will almost never be fresh. Look at any supermarket: the produce section is only a fraction of the store's floor space.

The worst that can be said about the Feingold approach is that it doesn't work for all children. Somewhere around half of all kids will improve on his program. Maybe it is no more than a placebo effect. But it is still worth a try because there is no harm to it. Doctors give chemotherapy with a success rate of under 30 percent, and chemo has serious side effects. What is the down side of not feeding kids food paint? How can it possibly hurt to try avoidance of unneeded chemicals?

What really rankles me is that allergists have made a subculture out of avoiding various molds, pollens, hairs, foods—all substances to which we have had millions of years of evolutionary exposure. Allergists will be quick to tell you that your child is allergic—but not, of course, to an industrial synthetic chemical dye. For it would somehow seem to them that only substances found in nature can produce an authentic allergy. Factory foods and artificial colors bearing molecular names a yard long cannot *possibly* cause hyperactivity.

And remember, everyone: giving sugar to a hyper child is perfectly okay! Logic like that does not even pass the straight-faced test.

Imagine what would actually happen if everyone were healthy. If each person ate right and took vitamins. If doctors and hospitals and pharmaceuticals, all of which prosper from sickness, were not needed. In America, there is a vested interest in disease. There is no profit in prevention.

The United States Recommended Dietary Allowances (or Reference Intakes, or whatever other claptrap they offer you) are forms of nutritional communism. According to them, the government-set levels are ample for all, and that's the end of it. A socialist state might say that you only need a subsistence income, say a few thousand dollars above the federal poverty level. Would your needs be met with ten thousand dollars a year? Would you be best off that way? Or would you like the right to try to get more? Does the government have either the knowledge, or the right, to decide either your financial needs or your nutritional needs?

When it comes to RDAs, one size fits nobody. Let's temporarily assume that orthodox dietitians are correct when they tell us that vitamin supplements can cure nothing but vitamin deficiency diseases. If this is true, then any symptom cured by supplements indicates a deficiency. If zinc speeds recovery from the common cold (and many studies confirm this), then people with colds are zinc-deficient. If lots of vitamin C shortens the intensity and duration of the common cold (and dozens of scientific studies prove this), then people with colds are vitamin C deficient as well. The RDAs and pitiful American intakes are therefore below the deficiency levels.

LAW: The quantity of a nutritional supplement that cures an illness indicates the patient's degree of deficiency. It is therefore not a megadose of the vitamin, but rather a megadeficiency of the nutrient, that we are dealing with.

Allergies evidently constitute one such megadeficiency.

ALLERGIES AND WATER DEFICIENCY

Your body is mostly water. Vegetable juice is mostly water. Food is mostly water. Even wood from your local lumberyard is 25 percent water.

Drink a lot of water and you will feel better immediately. Try it and see. Headaches vanish; stuffiness clears up pronto; your "plumbing" will work like a dream (less constipation; risk of kidney stones drops to near zero); water will even help you lose a bit of weight (especially in combination with vegetable juicing).

Do not take this as an excuse or an endorsement to spend money on water products, with the possible exception of an inexpensive device to clean up your drinking water if you live in an area where tap water is a bit dicey.

President Ronald Reagan's personal physician, Ralph Bookman, M.D., long urged his patients with asthma or allergies to drink lots of water to relieve their symptoms. In an interview, Dr. Bookman said, "Unquestionably, the single most important element in the treatment of asthma and other bronchial allergy symptoms is hydration." He added that without adequate fluids, bronchial mucous secretions are very difficult to bring up. "Liquids are medications," said Dr. Bookman. "Liquids make mucus liquid. I demand that my patients drink 10 full glasses of liquid every day. You must make a fetish of it."[1]

He is right. Sipping from a cute little bottled-water container, while at least a small step in the right direction, is not the same as drinking water by the glassful. Unless there is a clear medical requirement that you limit your fluids, then don't. Open the hatch and gulp it down! It is remarkably difficult to overhydrate yourself, but it is amazingly easy to get dehydrated. Though everyone knows that hot weather activity causes water loss, you need as much or more to replace water lost in cold weather activity. It is not just exercising (I'm for that, too) that causes water loss. Talking uses water: classroom teachers need an extra liter or two a day just for that. Airline travel dehydrates you, and there you just sit. In many ways, the old-time hydropathists were right: Water can be good for what ails you. Certainly the value is great, the safety high, and the price right.

Reference

1. Bookman, R. "101 Hints, Tips and Bits of Wisdom from the President's Allergist: Timely Help for People with Allergies and Asthma." Rodale's Allergy Relief 3:7 (July 1988), 1–8. Posted at: healthandenergy.com/ 101_allergy_tips. htm. See also: Bookman, R. *The Dimensions of Clinical Allergy,* Springfield, IL: Charles C. Thomas, 1985.

You must use vitamins correctly to get the job done. Large amounts work; small amounts don't. The dose depends on the patient. Dr. Klenner said, "If you want results, use adequate ascorbic acid. Don't send a boy to do a man's job." If I were to die tomorrow, I'd want you to remember that I told you this today: "Take enough C to be symptom-free, whatever that amount might be." (It even rhymes, making your job easier.)

I raised my kids all the way into college without either of them ever having a single dose of an antibiotic. Why? Because we used vitamins instead, that's why. And this especially meant lots of vitamin C. Vitamin C very effectively treated their influenzas and mononucleosis; it promptly stopped their coughs and bronchitis; it lowered their fevers and cured their sore throats. I repeat: they never once had an antibiotic. Because of the C, they never once needed an antibiotic.

FLU, VIRUSES, AND VITAMIN C MEGADOSES
By Robert G. Smith, Ph.D.

Like most Americans, throughout most of my life I have occasionally been down with a virus. But for a long time, a simple cold for me started as a headache, sore throat and congestion in my nasal passages, and typically progressed to prolonged infection in my lungs, and a terrible cough. The whole experience took up to two weeks for recovery from the virus, and several more weeks for my lungs to recover.

In his book *Vitamin C and the Common Cold*[1], Linus Pauling explained that vitamin C, taken at the proper dose, can prevent a virus from taking hold in the body. This pioneering book, written back in 1970, was ignored by many doctors but was well-received by the public. One chemistry professor told me that he had heard of Pauling's book and the vitamin C therapy but didn't think taking a big dose of an acid, even a mild one like ascorbic acid, would be good for the body. As for me, I imagined Pauling was probably correct about the details he had researched, because he was a renowned scientist and knew much more than most about biochemistry. Perhaps, I thought, he had simply gotten some of the medical details wrong or had missed some of the important studies about the effects of vitamins. But I started taking 1,000 mg of vitamin C every day and kept this up for several decades.

Two years ago, I decided to look further for myself. I looked online and found a recent book by Hickey and Roberts[2] that summarized 60 years of vitamin C research and revisited the issue of Dr. Pauling's rejection by the medical establishment. Pauling and a few brave physicians had continued research into the use of vitamin C to prevent illness and had gained a lot of new knowledge and intuition about its use. The book explained that all of the studies showing little effect of vitamin C had serious flaws. It also carefully debunked the myths about hazards of vitamin C use. I also read Pauling's newer book on vitamin therapy, *How to Live Longer and Feel Better*[3], and was amazed at his clear explanation of individual differences in the need for essential nutrients. Pauling had been right all along, and now there was a lot of new knowledge about how to use vitamin C for best benefit. Next, I found a book by Thomas Levy on the use of vitamin C to cure infectious disease.[4] All of these books contained numerous references to the scientific literature.

So I started taking 2,000–3,000 milligrams of vitamin C *every few hours*, and more when I went to bed at night. This caused no discomfort and only occasionally produced a minor laxative effect from vitamin C that was unabsorbed. Then, if I ever got an infection, I followed Dr. Robert Cathcart's instructions about going to "bowel tolerance" of vitamin C.[5] Usually when I get a cold or the flu there is an initial period of several hours when I feel tired, with a slight headache, sometimes with a slight sore throat or sniffle. As the books described, I could stop the symptoms of the oncoming infection within an hour or two by taking a higher dose of vitamin C at shorter intervals (3,000–5,000 milligrams *every 20 minutes*). Did it work? Well, that first year I didn't get any colds or flu, though in previous years I usually had 2–3 colds.

Continuing to read about vitamin C and its effects, I read the new Hickey and Saul[6] book. The authors presented a very clear rationale for ingesting vitamin C at a high level to bowel tolerance. Normally, the body does not take up vitamin C from the gut very efficiently at high doses. However, when the body is stressed with bacteria, viruses, or toxins, the need for vitamin C goes up tremendously, and the gut absorbs proportionately more.

Now, after two years of taking high doses of vitamin C whenever I feel symptoms of a cold or flu, I haven't had any colds or flu. I have found, exactly as Hickey and Saul report, that it is possible to feel the symptoms wax and wane in one's body in inverse proportion to the dose that one takes throughout the day. This is a helpful scientific observation that anyone can verify whenever one treats a cold or influenza with vitamin C. Although in previous years I typically got a secondary bacterial infection in my lungs, requiring antibiotics and another two weeks for recovery beyond the duration of the cold, now with my vitamin C therapy I simply don't get a cough at all, much less a prolonged bacterial infection. From this experience, it is obvious to me that vitamin C helps to strengthen the immune response.

It is also now obvious to me that all the years I had been taking 1,000 mg/day and continued to get two or three colds, the amount was simply not enough. I ride my bicycle in to work throughout the year, even when it is freezing cold in the winter, and this puts a severe stress on my lungs. The books I've read explain that any severe stress, for example, a low-grade bacterial infection, or an injury, increases the body's need for an anti-oxidant, and lowers the level of vitamin C in the blood. *Although 1,000 milligrams of vitamin C per day does some good, it simply is not enough to suffice for the body's needs when an infection comes on.*

Most animal species make in the neighborhood of 5,000–10,000 mg/day of vitamin C in their own bodies; this is the norm for all mammals except primates, some fruit eating bats, and guinea pigs. And it is known that during times of stress or illness, the majority of animal species dramatically increase their need and production of vitamin C. We humans can respond to this increased need by taking mega-doses of vitamin C when we start to feel a virus taking hold. When we do so, our bodies will be able to fight it off more readily.

Every year there are a few reports ostensibly showing some problem with mega-doses of vitamin C. But after close scrutiny none have held true, and the Hickey and Saul book explains why very clearly. Every individual 2,000–3,000 milligram dose I take allows my body, according to Hickey's dynamic flow model, to eliminate any excess after the vitamin performs its function. No heartburn, sometimes a little gas, very little laxative effect, and this is reduced by lower doses. For me, this is a small price to pay for not having several prolonged three- to four-week periods per year during which I'm essentially out of operation with congestion and a terrible cough. If everyone could read the Pauling, Levy and Hickey and Saul books, I imagine we'd have a lot less illness in our country. Does this mean that we could stop the current flu epidemic with vitamin C? I suspect that if clinics around the country could make the facts known about vitamin C and give some simple instructions about its use, then yes, this could be accomplished. That is, if we take large enough doses.

(Robert G. Smith is Research Associate Professor, University of Pennsylvania Department of Neuroscience. He is a member of the Institute for Neurological Sciences and the author of several dozen scientific papers and reviews.)

References

1. Pauling L. *Vitamin C and the Common Cold.* W.H. Freeman and Company, San Francisco, 1970. Also: *Vitamin C, the Common Cold, and the Flu.* W.H.Freeman, San Francisco, 1976.

2. Hickey S and Roberts H. *Ascorbate: The science of vitamin C.* 2004. Morrisville, NC: Lulu. An author interview is posted at www.doctoryourself.com/hickey.html

3. Pauling L. *How to Live Longer and Feel Better.* Corvallis, OR: Oregon State University Press, 2006. Originally published 1986. Reviewed in *J Orthomolecular Med* and posted at www.doctoryourself.com/livelonger.html

4. *Curing the Incurable: Vitamin C, Infectious Diseases, and Toxins,* by Thomas E. Levy (paperback, 2002). Reviewed in *J Orthomolecular Med* and posted at www.doctoryourself.com/levy.html

5. Robert F. Cathcart, MD: *Why a sick body need so much vitamin C:* www.doctoryourself.com/cathcart_thirdface.html

Robert F. Cathcart, MD: *How to determine a therapeutic dose of vitamin C:* www.doctoryourself.com/titration.html

6. Hickey S, Saul AW. *Vitamin C: The Real Story.* Laguna Beach, CA: Basic Health Publications, 2008. Reviewed at www.townsendletter.com/June2009/bc_vitc0609.htm

Reprinted by permission.

Vitamin C is but one of many vitamins, vitamins are but one part of nutrition, and nutrition is but one aspect of health. But look at what just one vitamin can do. *At saturation (bowel tolerance) levels, vitamin C replaces antibiotics, antihistamines, antipyretics, antitoxics, and antiviral drugs.* This is one of the most inflammatory statements in medicine.

An English friend of mine told me that he'd hardly even heard of allergies until he came to the United States. "Allergies were quite rare in Britain," he said. "In America it seems everyone has them, children especially." He's right. If you asked Grandma, she might say the whole allergy subculture, now a big business, is ridiculous. I agree with Grandma. I think there is only one genuine allergy, and that involves the fatal result of transfusing the wrong type of blood into a person. Anything else is simple by comparison, and deserving of nutritional therapy.

What we now label "allergies" could just as easily be called "undernutrition" and I think should be. The majority of Americans eat lousy diets; nine out of ten of us do not meet even the already low RDA levels for fruit and vegetable vitamins. Insufficient vitamin C results in exaggerated sensitivity to even average levels of irritants, toxins, chemicals, pollution, and microorganisms. Deficiencies of vitamins A, B complex, and E frequently manifest as skin problems or hypersensitivity to foods, stress, or germs. Millions of vitamin-deficient but overstuffed people are literally waiting to be allergic to something. Food that fills and fattens but doesn't fortify the body is like trying to build a wall with bricks but no mortar: it will hold up only until you lean upon it.

If your son got sweaty palms or hives every time he telephoned a girl to ask her for a date, would you conclude that he's allergic to women and send him to a monastery? Of course not. You'd find out why he got so nervous and strengthen him, encourage him, and most of all allow him to get over it. So why not do the same for your body?

An allergy is a symptom, and symptoms tell us that our body is not quite right. Naturopaths tell us that if our body is not quite right, we should take a good look at the way we take care of it. Check your diet first, not for the presence of allergens but for an absence of nutrients. You can start with a saturation test with vitamin C, as mentioned above.

Other questions to ask yourself: Are you avoiding chemical preservatives and other unnecessary food additives? Avoiding drugs, nonprescription and otherwise? Are you getting enough rest? Do you need a cleansing fast? These questions should replace battery after battery of allergy tests.

36

SUGAR IS NOT YOUR FRIEND

Pediatrician Lendon H. Smith, M.D., nationally famous as "The Children's Doctor," repeatedly said that sugar causes profound mood disorders. He specifically advised parents to give their children a "sugarless diet without processed foods."[1] It is not easy. The Center for Science in the Public Interest has reported that children between the ages of six and eleven drink nearly a pint of soda pop a day. Twenty percent of toddlers drink soda pop, nearly a cup daily.[2] And, of the seven best-selling soft drinks, six have caffeine in them. In sensitive persons, caffeine can cause psychotic behavior.[3]

Food colorings and benzoate preservatives increase childhood hyperactivity, according to research published in the *Archives of Disease in Childhood*, June 2004.[4] The study, involving 277 preschool children, also demonstrated that withdrawing these chemical additives decreased hyperactivity. When additives were reintroduced, there was once again an increase in hyperactivity. "Additives do have an effect on overactive behavior independent of baseline allergic and behavioral status," said lead author Dr. J. O. Warner. So many parents, and any of us who have taught school the day after Halloween, can verify this.

Health professionals are increasingly aware that the normal functioning of the brain and nervous system is nutrient-dependent and additive-sensitive. Ian Brighthope, M.D., says, "What is going on in the mind can be influenced by the nutrients and chemicals going into it. You can't get anywhere with a patient with psychiatric symptomatology if their brain is hungry, starved, or poisoned."[5]

References

1. Smith L. *Foods for Healthy Kids.* Berkley, 1991.

2. Jacobson M. F. Liquid Candy: How soft drinks are harming Americans' health. www.cspinet.org/sodapop/liquid_ candy. htm. Accessed Sept 18, 2008.

3. Whalen R. Welcome to the dance: caffeine allergy, a masked cerebral allergy and progressive toxic dementia. Trafford Publishing, 2005. Reviewed in *J Orthomolecular Med,* 2005. Vol 20, No 3, p 215–217 and at www.doctoryourself.com/ caffeine_allergy.html

4. Bateman B., Warner J. O., Hutchinson E., et al. The effects of a double blind, placebo controlled, artificial food colourings and benzoate preservative challenge on hyperactivity in a general population sample of preschool children. *Arch Dis Child.* 89(6): 506–11.

5. Interview in the documentary film *Food Matters.* Permacology Productions, 2008. www.foodmatters.tv

For Further Reading

Feingold B. F. *Why Your Child Is Hyperactive.* New York: Random House, 1985. List of Dr. Feingold's publications: www.doctoryourself.com/biblio_feingold.html

www.feingold.org/pg-research.html and www.feingold.org/pg-news.html. Free email newsletter available.

Hoffer A. *Healing Children's Attention & Behavior Disorders: Complementary Nutritional and Psychological Treatments.* Toronto: CCNM Press, 2004. List of Hoffer's publications: www.doctoryourself.com/biblio_hoffer.html See also: www.doctoryourself.com/review_hoffer_B3.html

In my opinion, the way to be healthy is deceptively simple:

1. Stop eating meat, sugar, and artificially colored junk food, or at least reduce intake of these substances as much as possible.

2. Instead, eat whole grains, fruits, nuts, beans, sprouts, lightly cooked or raw vegetables, and regularly take vitamin food supplements (especially vitamin C).

3. Clean out body wastes by occasional juice fasts and an everyday natural diet that is high in fiber and free of artificially colored or preserved foods.

This is more than folk medicine. It is a real remedy for all folks.

But don't just take my word for it. A whole host of reputable doctors have championed the virtues of C. Here are some of the best: *How to Live Longer and Feel Better,* by Linus Pauling; *Vitamin C, Infectious Diseases, and Toxins: Curing the Incurable,* by Thomas E. Levy, M.D., J.D.; *Clinical Guide to the Use of Vitamin C,* edited by Lendon Smith, M.D.; *The Vitamin C Connection,* by Emanuel Cheraskin, M.D.; *A Physician's Handbook on Orthomolecular Medicine,* edited by Roger Williams; and *Orthomolecular Psychiatry,* edited by David Hawkins, M.D., and Linus Pauling. Do not be dismayed by these highfalutin titles. "Orthomolecular" is simply another term for nutritional medicine.

Can you make your allergies disappear forever? There's only one way: try and see. If you are on medication, you can and should do so responsibly by having your doctor provide you with a gradually tapering reduction dosage schedule for your meds. It may just change your life. And think what you'll save on facial tissues.

Recommended Reading

Downing D. *The Vitamin Cure for Allergies.* Laguna Beach, CA: Basic Health Publications, 2010.

"If everyone were to start on a good nutritional program supplemented with optimum doses of vitamins and minerals before age fifty and were to remain on it the incidence of Alzheimer's disease would drop precipitously."

—ABRAM HOFFER, M.D.

Fact: More than half the nursing-home beds in the United States are occupied by Alzheimer's patients. Fact: Alzheimer's disease is the number-six killer of Americans, causing over 100,000 deaths each year. I believe that many of these deaths are unnecessary; aggressive use of therapeutic nutrition could substantially reduce the incidence and severity of Alzheimer's disease. Let's take a look on a nutrient-by-nutrient basis.

Vitamin B_{12}

B_{12} deficiency may be mistaken for, or perhaps cause, Alzheimer's disease. (Dommisse, John [1991] Subtle vitamin B-12 deficiency and psychiatry: a largely unnoticed but devastating relationship? *Med Hypotheses.* 34:131–140. See also: Dommisse, John [1990] Organic mania induced by phenytoin. *Can J Psychiatry.* 35:5, June.)

Note how closely these symptoms of B_{12} deficiency mirror those of Alzheimer's: ataxia, fatigue, slowness of thought, apathy, emaciation, degeneration of the spinal cord, dizziness, moodiness, confusion, agitation, delusions, hallucinations, and psychosis. B_{12} deficiency is easy to come by in the elderly: poor diet; poor intestinal absorption (due to less intrinsic factor being secreted by the aging stomach, and possibly due to calcium deficiency); digestive tract surgery; pharmaceutical interference, notably from Dilantin (phenytoin); and stress all decrease B_{12}. It is necessary to measure the cerebrospinal fluid, not the blood, to get accurate B_{12} readings.

Even marginal B_{12} deficiency over an extended time produces an increased risk of Alzheimer's disease; nearly three-quarters of the elderly deficient in B_{12} also have Alzheimer's disease. (Garrison Jr., Robert H. and Somer, Elizabeth. [1990]. *The Nutrition Desk Reference.* New Canaan, CT: Keats, p. 211.)

Over the years, many popular diet plans have proven to be B_{12} deficient, including the Pritikin, Scarsdale, and Beverly Hills diets. (Fisher and Lachance [1985] Nutrition evaluation of published weight reducing diets. *J Amer Dietetic Assn,* 85(4) 450–54.)

The elderly are often "dieting" without intending to, simply because their normal appetite and taste functions are reduced. Emotional factors such as isolation, grief, and depression also contribute to inadequate food intake, and therefore low B_{12} intake. To make matters worse, B_{12} deficiency itself causes further loss of appetite.

Injection or intranasal administration of B_{12} is the recommended method of supplementation because oral absorption can be poor. There is no known toxicity for vitamin B_{12}. A minimum daily therapeutic dose is probably 100 mcg daily, and closer to 1,000 mcg may be more effective. 1,000 mcg sounds like a lot, but it is actually the same as one milligram, which is about one thousandth of a quarter-teaspoon.

Niacin, as Niacinamide

Researchers at the University of California at Irvine gave the human dose equivalent of 2,000 to 3,000 mg of niacinamide (vitamin B_3) to mice with Alzheimer's.[1] It worked. Kim Green, one of the researchers, is quoted as saying, "Cognitively, they were cured. They performed as if they'd never developed the disease." Niacinamide is further discussed in Hoffer A, Saul AW, and Foster HD: *Niacin: The Real Story*. Basic Health Pub., 2012.

Choline

Choline, related to the B vitamins, has repeatedly shown value in treating Alzheimer's disease. Why does it work? Alzheimer's patients have a deficiency of the neurotransmitter acetylcholine because they are deficient in the enzyme choline acetyltransferase, needed to make it. But there is a way around this: increasing dietary choline raises blood and brain levels of acetylcholine. Choline is readily available in cheap, nonprescription lecithin.

Back in 1979, lecithin was successfully employed as a therapy to combat memory loss. (Can drugs improve memory? Kent S. [1979]. *Geriatrics* 34(7):77, 80, 83 passim.) Then, studies at MIT showed increases in both choline and the vital neurotransmitter acetylcholine in the brains of animals after just one lecithin meal. (Magil, S. G., Zeisel, S. H. & Wurtman, R. J. [1981]. Effects of ingesting soy or egg lecithins on serum choline, brain choline and brain acetylcholine. *J. Nutr.* Ill:166–170.)

Then it gets *really* interesting. Animals that actually already *have* dementia improve when fed phosphatidyl choline, a major component of lecithin. (Shu-Ying Chung, Tomoe Moriyama, Eiko Uezu, et al. [1995]. Administration of Phosphatidylcholine Increases Brain Acetylcholine Concentration and Improves Memory in Mice with Dementia. *J. Nutr.* 25(6):1484–1489.)

The same goes for people. A double-blind, placebo-controlled study showed that Alzheimer's patients improve when given choline alfoscerate, a form of choline. (De Jesus Moreno Moreno M. [2003]. Cognitive improvement in mild to moderate Alzheimer's dementia after treatment with the acetylcholine precursor choline alfoscerate: a multicenter, double-blind, randomized, placebo-controlled trial. *Clin Ther.* 25(1):178–93.] Another double-blind, placebo-controlled study indicated that plain lecithin works too. (Little, et al. [1985]. A double-blind, placebo controlled trial of high dose lecithin in Alzheimer's disease. *J Neurology, Neurosurgery and Psychiatry*, 48: 736–742.)

I regularly take lechithin by the tablespoon because I want to remember all my great-grandchildren's middle names and sweater sizes someday. You might want to try it. Notice anything? You can feel the almost caffeine-like increase in your awareness. That is probably the effect of an acetylcholine boost. Think what this might do for an Alzheimer's patient. Lecithin is a very safe substance: it is difficult to hurt yourself with essential fatty acids and choline. Try lecithin granules in yogurt, in a fruit smoothie, or, if you are really new to all this, on ice cream.

Remember, a large quantity of choline (from lecithin) is necessary for clinical results. Lecithin is nontoxic. Start with at least a heaping tablespoon daily, working up to a goal of three or even four tablespoons each day.

Tyrosine

Increasing the body's level of the neurotransmitter norepinephrine may also help Alzheimer's patients. Norepinephrine is made from the amino acid tyrosine, which is made from phenylalanine. We get plenty of phenylalanine from protein in our diets if we eat protein foods, but the conversion to tyrosine and ultimately norepinephrine may not take place if there is a deficiency of another coenzyme: vitamin C, which is necessary for norepinephrine production. Vitamin C may therefore be of special value in the treatment of Alzheimer's.

Vitamin C

Recent research has shown that vitamin C dissolves toxic protein buildup in the brains of mice with Alzheimer's disease (AD). Amyloid plaques, which are made up of misfolded protein aggregates, are fatal to nerve cells. Memory cells frequently are the first to go. However, researchers said, when they used vitamin C to treat brain tissue from AD mice, the toxic protein aggregates were dissolved.[3]

Vitamin E

Alzheimer's patients tend to have abnormally low levels of vitain E in their bodies. This could simply be because they don't eat well, or because the disease increases their nutrient need, or both. But the bottom line is this: Alzheimer's patients who take 2,000 IU of vitamin E per day live longer.[3] Between 400 and 600 IU is a reasonable daily starting dose, with a gradual "test increase" to higher levels.

Other Vitamins

Folic acid may also play a significant role in combating Alzheimer's disease. For a more detailed discussion of recent vitamin research and Alzheimer's, I recommend *What Really Causes Alzheimer's Disease* (Foster, H. D.).

Deficiencies of thiamin, riboflavin, vitamin C, and pyridoxine (B_6) are frequently seen in the elderly, even among individuals using supplements. This indicates that the RDA levels for these vitamins need to be raised. Consider a five-times-a-day dose of a high potency B-complex supplement, with at least 500 to 1,000 mg of vitamin C on the hour.

Aluminum Toxicity

Unintentional intake of aluminum, a known neurotoxin, may increase the risk of Alzheimer's as well. Aluminum cookware, aluminum foil, antacids, douches, buffered aspirin, and even antiperspirant deodorants may contribute to the problem. A single aluminum coffeepot was shown to have invisibly added more than 1600 mcg aluminum per liter of water. (Jackson, J. A.; Riordan, H. D,. and Poling, C. M. (1989). Aluminum from a coffee pot. *Lancet*, I(8641) 781–782, April 8).

This is *thirty-two times* the World Health Organization's set goal of 50 mcg per liter. Aluminum is known to build up in the body tissues of people with Alzheimer's disease, Parkinson's disease, and amyotrophic lateral sclerosis. Aluminum is also a component of so-called "silver" amalgam dental fillings. Composite (white) fillings do not contain aluminum (or mercury, for that matter). Most baking powders contain aluminum. "Rumford" brand baking powder does not, however. Neither does baking soda, which is a different substance entirely.

Artificial kidney dialysis has been known to produce "dialysis dementia," a state of confusion and disorientation caused by excess aluminum in the blood stream. Animals injected with aluminum compounds will also develop nervous system disorders. Conversely, Alzheimer's disease can be treated with metal bonding (chelating) agents, such as desferrioxamine, which remove aluminum from the bloodstream. In appropriately high doses, vitamin C is also an effective (and nonprescription) chelating agent.

Calcium and magnesium significantly slow down aluminum absorption, and that's good. Supplementation with 800 mg of calcium and 400 mg of magnesium every day may be therapeutic for Alzheimer's patients. The citrate forms of these minerals are well absorbed and relatively inexpensive.

There have been a number of studies on the relationship of aluminum toxicity to Alzheimer's disease. A Medline search will promptly uncover a large number of references on the subject. Some examples include:

Martyn, C. N.; Barker, D. J.; Osmond, C.; Harris, E. C.; Edwardson, J. A.; and Lacey, R. F. (1989). Geographical relation between Alzheimer's disease and aluminum in drinking water. *Lancet* I(8629): 59–62.

McLachlan, D. R.; Kruck, T. P., and Lukiw, W. J. (1991). Would decreased aluminum ingestion reduce the incidence of Alzheimer's disease? *Can Med Assn J,* Oct 1.

Garrison Jr., Robert H. and Somer, Elizabeth (1990). *The Nutrition Desk Reference*. New Canaan, CT: Keats, pp. 78–79; 106; 210–211.

Weiner, Michael A. (1990). Aluminum and dietary factors in Alzheimer's disease. *J Orthomolecular Med* 5(2):74–78.

Lead Toxicity

Lead has adverse effects on brain development and function, even at very low levels of exposure. Erin E. Dooley, author of *Linking Lead to Alzheimer's Disease* (Environmental Health Perspectives 10810 October 2000), writes: "Scientists from Case Western Reserve University and University Hospitals presented evidence at the April 2000 annual meeting of the American Academy of Neurology that people who have held jobs with high levels of lead exposure have a 3.4 times greater likelihood of developing Alzheimer disease."

Lead, unfortunately, permeates our environment because of decades of adding it to gasoline. In 1926, the U.S. Surgeon General declared leaded gasoline to be safe. Phasing out leaded gasoline began in the mid-1970s. However, it was not until 1996—after 70 years of use—that the U.S. banned the sale of leaded gasoline.

People can be exposed to lead on the job either by breathing in lead dust or through direct skin contact.

The good news is that very high doses of vitamin C are known to help the body rapidly excrete lead. Dr. Erik Paterson, of British Columbia, reports that:

When I was a consulting physician for a center for the mentally challenged, a patient showing behavioral changes was found to have blood lead some ten times higher than the acceptable levels. I administered vitamin C at a dose of 4,000 mg/day. I anticipated a slow response. The following year I rechecked his blood lead level. It had gone up, much to my initial dismay. But then I thought that perhaps what was happening was that the vitamin

41

C was mobilizing the lead from his tissues. So we persisted. The next year, on rechecking, the lead levels had markedly dropped to well below the initial result. As the years went by, the levels became almost undetectable, and his behavior was markedly improved. (Vitamin supplements help protect children from heavy metals, reduce behavioral disorders. Ortho-molecular Medicine News Service, October 8, 2007.)

Reference

1. Green KN, Steffan JS, Martinez-Coria H, Sun X, Schreiber SS, Thompson LM, & LaFerla FM. (2008). Nicotinamide restores cognition in Alzheimer's disease transgenic mice via a mechanism involving sirtuin inhibition and selective reduction of Thr231-phospho-tau. *J Neurosci.* 28(45):11500–10.

2. F. Cheng, R. Cappai, G. D. Ciccotosto, G. Svensson, G. Multhaup, L.-A. Fransson, & K. Mani. (2011). Suppression of Amyloid beta A11 Antibody Immunoreactivity by Vitamin C: Possible Role of Heparan Sulfate Oligosaccharides Derived from Glypican-1 by Ascorbate-induced, Nitric Oxide (NO)-catalyzed Degradation. *Journal of Biological Chemistry* 286(31): 27559.

3. Pavlik VN, Doody RS, Rountree SD, & Darby EJ. (2000). Vitamin E use is associated with improved survival in an Alzheimer's disease cohort. *Dement Geriatr Cogn Disord.* 28(6):536–40. See also: Grundman M. (200). Vitamin E and Alzheimer disease: the basis for additional clinical trials. *Am J Clin Nutr.* 71(2):630S–636S.

Recommended Reading

Alzheimer's disease and neurotransmitters. *Let's Live* (May 1983): 18.

Balch JF and Balch PA. *Prescription for Nutritional Healing.* Garden City Park, NY: Avery Publishing, 1990, 87–90.

Carper J. Your food pharmacy. [syndicated column] (1 November 1995).

Dommisse J. Organic mania induced by phenytoin. *Can J Psychiatry* 35 (June 1990).

Dommisse J. Subtle vitamin B$_{12}$ deficiency and psychiatry: a largely unnoticed but devastating relationship? *Med Hypotheses* 34 (1991): 131–140.

Dooley E. Linking lead to Alzheimer's disease. *Environmental Health Perspectives* 108 (October 2000).

Fisher and Lachance. Nutrition evaluation of published weight reducing diets. *J Amer Dietetic Assn* 85 (1985): 450–54.

Garrison RH and Somer E. *The Nutrition Desk Reference.* New Canaan, CT: Keats, 1990, 78–79, 106, 210–211.

Goldberg D. *Newsletter* 33 (September 1985).

Hoffer A. A case of Alzheimer's treated with nutrients. *J of Orthomolecular Medicine* 8:43–44, 1993.

Hoffer, A: Alzheimer's—An Anecdote (letter). Townsend Letter for Doctors and Patients, No.179, 107–109, 1998

Jackson JA, Riordan HD, and Poling CM. Aluminum from a coffee pot. *Lancet* 8641 (8 April 1989): 781–782.

Kushnir SL, Ratner JT, and Gregoire PA. Multiple nutrients in the treatment of Alzheimer's disease. *Amer Geriatrics Soc J* 35 (May 1987): 476–477.

Little, et al. A double-blind, placebo controlled trial of high dose lecithin in Alzheimer's disease. *J Neurology, Neurosurgery and Psychiatry* 48 (1985): 736–742.

Martyn CN, et al. Geographical relation between Alzheimer's disease and aluminum in drinking water. *Lancet* 8629 (14 Jan 1989): 59–62.

McLachlan DR, Kruck TP, and Lukiw WJ. Would decreased aluminum ingestion reduce the incidence of Alzheimer's disease? *Can Med Assn J* (1 Oct 1991).

Murray F. A B$_{12}$ deficiency may cause mental problems. *Better Nutrition for Today's Living* (July 1991): 10–11.

Weiner MA. Aluminum and dietary factors in Alzheimer's disease. *J Orthomolecular Med* 5 (1990):74–78.

Williams SR. *Nutrition and Diet Therapy,* 6th ed., St. Louis: Mosby, 1989, 250.

"Men who achieve greatness do not work more complexly than the average man, but more simply."
—THE MAYO BROTHERS

It was a bit odd to have a conversation with my sixty-seven-year-old father about his sex life.

"I'm on this medicine, Andrew," he said. "It's for angina. My doctor sent me to a heart specialist, and they both agreed I have to take it. The problem is that it causes impotence." I let that image sink in as he continued. "Are there any of your natural remedies that can replace the angina medicine?"

Now, it was an unusual event for my dad to ask my view about anything. One of his mottoes is, "If I want your opinion, I'll give it to you." So I was duly impressed with the gravity of the situation.

"Vitamin E, Pa, " I said. "High doses of vitamin E have been used to treat angina since the early fifties. Wilfrid and Evan Shute, who were brothers and cardiologists, gave patients somewhere between 1,600 and 2,000 international units of vitamin E daily and it eliminated angina symptoms in hundreds and hundreds of documented cases."

I fully expected him to ridicule the idea, and I was surprised and not a little gratified when he thoughtfully nodded his head. "Okay," he said, and we eagerly moved on to another topic.

My dad started at about 400 IU a day, gradually working up to 1,600 IU over a period of a few weeks. I've always maintained that the body likes gradual change. This goes for decreasing drugs as well as for increasing vitamins. Pa's general practitioner was an open-minded man, quite British and quite willing to offer my father a dosage-reduction schedule for his medication.

And that is all it took.

Pa called a couple of weeks later. "Is it all right to take this much vitamin E?" he asked.

"How much are you up to?"

"Uh, 1,200 a day."

"How do you feel?"

"Pretty fair," he said. "I'm practically off the medication now."

"Any symptoms?" I asked.

"No."

"Why don't you go to 1,600 with no drugs," I said.

The subject did not come up again for months. What can I say? This is how our family does things.

"So, Pa, how's that angina?" I asked one day.

"What angina?" he said.

"*Your* angina, Pa."

"I don't have angina."

"Well, you did. Maybe a year ago."

"I never had any angina," he said.

"Two doctors said you did, Pa. They had you on medication, remember?"

"Oh, that. I haven't had any sign of that since I took the vitamin E."

"OK. Keep taking the E, Pa."

"I do. 1,600 every day."

And that was that. He never had angina symptoms again.

Usually the fur really flies when you bring up the Shute brothers' vitamin E treatment for cardiovascular disease. This has been a controversial area of medicine for sixty years. Most textbooks state that "E" is of no value here. Textbooks have said for years that vitamin E is a quack's cure in search of a disease. But there is considerable evidence that the texts are wrong and the Shutes were right.

Consider intermittent claudication, which is calf-muscle pain upon walking. Even conventional nutrition textbooks acknowledge scientific proof of this successful treatment with vitamin E. "This therapy helps reduce the arterial blockage," says Williams in *Nutrition and Diet Therapy,* a standard dietetics work. Is there something so special about the arteries between the knee and the ankle? What about "reducing the blockage" in other arteries? This is the whole idea of using vitamin E for circulatory diseases.

WHY YOU ARE SICK IF YOU WANT TO EAT RIGHT
(But It's Perfectly Normal to Treat Angina with Pressure Pants?)

First of all, I am not making this up. "Healthy food obsession sparks rise in new eating disorder: Fixation with healthy eating can be sign of serious psychological disorder" was an actual recent article headline from UK's *The Observer,* founded 1791, the world's oldest Sunday newspaper.

And now, eating right has an official disease name, too: ***orthorexia nervosa.***[1] Oooh! Tell us more!

Symptoms evidently include "refusing to touch sugar, salt, caffeine, alcohol, wheat, gluten, yeast, soya, corn, and dairy foods (and) any foods that have come into contact with pesticides, herbicides or contain artificial additives." Also, "sufferers tend to be aged over 30, middle-class and well-educated" and "solely concerned with the quality of the food they put in their bodies."[2]

Comic strip artist Morrie Brickman once quipped, "I don't know if the world is full of smart men bluffing, or imbeciles who mean it." But orthorexia nervosa is not a prank.

Neither is this:

In Britain, angina patients were actually being treated with vibrating pants. Yes, the vibrating trousers were supposed to increase blood flow to the heart. Treatment was an hour every weekday, for seven weeks . . . at a total cost of (are you ready for this?) 10,500 pounds sterling. That's well over fifteen grand American money. And "most private health insurers will pay for the course, says Vasogenics, the company that makes the vibrating trousers."[3]

You used to be able to watch an American-market sales video at www.vasogenics.com/, and an illustrated patient's guide was available for downloading. By March 2012, neither were accessible.

Monty Python devotees recall the troupe's "Trim Jeans" inflatable reducing pants send-up from 1972 (series 3, episode 2). There are those who might opine that the British equivalent of over $2,000 a week (which works out to $400 per hour) to have your calves squeezed is not comedy. At least, not intentionally.

The inflatable pants (ECP or EECP) therapy may provide symptomatic relief. Or, as Blue-

Cross/BlueShield claims, they actually may not.[4] But either way, it is significant that in all the discussion there is not a breath of mention of vitamin E. Vitamin E is the safest, cheapest, and most effective solution to angina.[5]

And let's be very clear: a "fixation with healthy eating" is, well, healthy. After all, if you are not a health nut, then just what kind of a nut are you?

References

1. Donini LM, Marsili D, Graziani MP, Imbriale M, Cannella C. Orthorexia nervosa: a preliminary study with a proposal for diagnosis and an attempt to measure the dimension of the phenomenon. *Eat Weight Disord.* 2004 Jun;9(2):151–7. See also this mildly critical 2008 article from the *Turkish Journal of Psychiatry:* www.turkpsikiyatri.com/en/default.aspx?modul=article&id=638

2. www.guardian.co.uk/society/2009/aug/16/orthorexia-mental-health-eating-disorder *The Observer,* August 16, 2009, News section, p 12.

3. www.medicalnewstoday.com/articles/14414.php, Oct 4, 2004.

4. English T. "Inflatable-pants" heart failure therapy lacks supporting evidence. Health Behavior News Service. www.sciencedaily.com/releases/2006/02/060221235310.htm or http://seniorjournal.com/NEWS/Alerts/6-02–21-InflatablePantsHeart.htm or Putnam KG, et al. External counterpulsation for treatment of chronic stable angina pectoris and chronic heart failure. (Review). Technology Evaluation Center Assessment Program Vol. 20, No. 12. December 2005. Background: www.bcbs.com/blueresources/tec/what-is-tec.html

5. www.doctoryourself.com/estory.htm *Journal of Orthomolecular Medicine,* Vol. 17, No. 3, Third Quarter, 2002, p 179–181.

Medical doctors Wilfrid and Evan Shute of London, Ontario, successfully treated well over 30,000 cardiovascular disease patients with up to 3,200 IU of vitamin E daily. They were rewarded for that achievement by being ostracized from their medical society. Here are the principles of the therapy:

1. Vitamin E has an oxygen-sparing effect on the heart, enabling the heart to do more work on less oxygen. The benefit for recovering heart-attack patients is considerable. 1,200 to 2,000 IU daily relieves angina very well.

2. Vitamin E moderately prolongs prothrombin clotting time, and has a limited Coumadin/ warfarin effect, "thinning" the blood but, unlike the drugs, not doing so beyond normal limits. This is the reason behind the Shutes' using vitamin E for thrombophlebitis and related conditions. Their dose? About 1,000 to 2,000 IU daily.

3. Vitamin E dilates and promotes collateral circulation and benefits diabetes patients or anyone threatened with gangrene. Dose: tailored to patient; 800 IU daily or more.

4. Vitamin E strengthens and regulates heartbeat like digitalis (foxglove) and its derivatives at a dose adjusted between 800 to 3,000 IU daily.

5. Vitamin E reduces scarring when frequently applied topically to burns or sites of lacerations or surgical incisions along with a daily oral dose of 800 IU.

6. Vitamin E helps gradually break down clots at a maintained daily dose of between 800 IU and 3,000 IU.

7. Vitamin E is vastly safer than drugs, as doses of up to 56,000 IU per day fail to harm adult humans. Gradual dosage increase is advised, and patients with congestive heart failure, rheumatic hearts, or high blood pressure need careful medical supervision.

So why hasn't vitamin E been more highly regarded in medicine? Ambiguous results from a rather small number of highly publicized, poorly controlled studies, that's why. The most common reason for irreproducibility of successful vitamin E cures is either a failure to use enough or a failure to use the natural d-alpha (as opposed to dl-alpha) form, or both. Such studies must be weighed against the Shutes' 30,000 cured patients and their four books: *Complete Updated Vitamin E Book, Health Preserver, Vitamin E for Ailing and Healthy Hearts,* and *Your Child and Vitamin E.*

In less healthy people, there are some valid cautions in giving large doses of vitamin E. Among hypertensive patients, sudden large vitamin E increases cause temporary increases in blood pressure. The solution is to increase the vitamin gradually, with proper monitoring (which hypertensive patients should have anyway). To avoid any possible risks of an asymmetric heart contraction, patients with rheumatic hearts or congestive heart failure need small doses (around 75 IU) and increases under medical supervision. It is best to inquire about all of these conditions when taking or submitting a patient history. For additional information, it is most worthwhile to contact the Shute Institute in London, Ontario, or to read any books by Wilfrid or Evan Shute.

IGNORING VITAMIN E

The Shutes found that vitamin E was the best way to treat heart disease. One might think that the only possible professional response to such important discoveries would be grateful acceptance and widespread journal publication. Just the opposite occurred. Dr. Evan Shute's frustration with an unnaturally stubborn medical profession was justified. The American Medical Association refused to let the Shutes present their findings at national medical conventions. In the early 1960s, the United States Post Office successfully prevented even the *mailing* of vitamin E.[1]

In 1985, Linus Pauling wrote:

"The failure of the medical establishment during the last forty years to recognize the value of vitamin E in controlling heart disease is responsible for a tremendous amount of unnecessary suffering and for many early deaths. The interesting story of the efforts to suppress the Shute discoveries about vitamin E illustrates the shocking bias of organized medicine against nutritional measures for achieving improved health."[2]

It is not overly easy to see how the promise of vitamin E could be ignored for so long. But it was.

References

1. *The Vitamin E Story* by Evan Shute, M.D., James C. M. Shute, editor. Foreword by Linus Pauling. (Burlington, Ontario: Welch Publishing, 1985. This book may be out of print. You might try an Internet bookseller search.

2. Ibid.

Why supplement with vitamin E? Our need for vitamin E increases with advanced age, exposure to toxins (smoking, air pollution, chemical oxidants), pregnancy, and lactation. Even an increased consumption of polyunsaturated fats requires more vitamin E to protect the unsaturated fatty acids from free-radical attack. For most healthy adults, an optimum daily amount of vitamin E would probably be about 600 IU. It must certainly be higher than the RDA of only about 10 or 15 IU.

True, many foods contain vitamin E, including dairy products, eggs, meat, fish, whole-grain cereals and whole-grain breads, wheat germ, and leafy vegetables. However, only very small quantities of the vitamin are present in these foods. Americans do not get enough vitamin E in their diet, and it is impossible to get even 100 IU per day from the finest of diets. This is at least partly due to the widespread refining of flour since the start of the twentieth century. Heart disease has also been on a steep increase since 1900. Very likely there is a connection here.

The New England Journal of Medicine published two papers in the May 20, 1993, issue (vol. 328, pp. 1444–1456) that supported vitamin E megadoses, reporting an approximate 40 percent reduction in cardiovascular disease. Nearly 40,000 men and 87,000 women took part in the study. The more vitamin E they took, and the longer they took it, the less cardiovascular disease they experienced.

And the Shute brothers, those "quacks," pointed it out first—sixty years ago. They said, "We didn't make vitamin E this versatile. God did. Ignore it at your peril."

I am not about to let it be ignored any longer. We will continue discussing details of vitamin E therapy, especially dosage, safety and effectiveness later in this book in the Vitamin E chapter.

But until then, keep this in mind: the very same issue of *The New England Journal of Medicine* that carried the two favorable vitamin E studies included another piece on this amazing vitamin: an editorial, advising doctors not to use it. One can only wonder why.

"Warning: keep this medicine out of the reach of everybody! Use vitamin C instead!"
—LINUS PAULING, TWO-TIME RECIPIENT OF THE NOBEL PRIZE

Any physician who gives twelve courses of antibiotics to an infant is a real quack. I know more than one doctor who does.

Ray, a health professional himself, brought his eleven-month-old son Robbie to me. The child was very sick, and had been so for over a week. No one, and I mean no one, in their family had had any sleep in a long time. They were up night after night with this child, who had a high fever, glazed watery eyes, tons of thick mucus, and labored breathing. The poor child could not sleep and did little else but cry. Day and night, night and day.

Robbie was under the care of a pediatrician who had been prescribing some very serious antibiotics all along. Antibiotics were clearly not working. This was all too apparent to Ray. "Twelve rounds of antibiotics for a baby under a year old, and all the doctor wants to do is give more?" he said. "That makes no sense at all."

"Ray, antibiotics are their knee-jerk answer to a lot of things. When the only tool you have is a hammer, you tend to see every problem as a nail."

"Well, we've thoroughly tried the medical route, and cooperated one hundred percent with the pediatrician. At this point, Robbie is worse, not better. We've got to do something ourselves, and we are going to. My wife is just as emphatic about that as I am." (She was home, taking care of the other children.)

I promptly acquainted Ray with the work of the vitamin C doctors. He agreed to give Robbie as much vitamin C as he could hold without having loose bowels.

So now I have a new case history record to offer: 20,000 mg of vitamin C daily for a twenty-pound baby of eleven months of age. That's how much it took to cure Ray's baby of severe congestion, fever, and listlessness. That is 1,000 mg of vitamin C per pound per day; nearly twice what Dr. Frederick Robert Klenner customarily ordered for patients. And even at that huge amount, the baby never had diarrhea!

You have to marvel at where it all went. More marvelous is how quickly it worked.

"Robbie was noticeably improved in under twelve hours, and slept through the first night," Ray told me two days later. "He was completely well in forty-eight hours. Symptom-free. Completely well!"

Even without considering the harmful side effects of massive antibiotic therapy, we can look at the futility of all those repeated doses. Antibiotics are either going to work with the first or second round, or they are not going to work at all, period. There is no point in emptying twelve fire extinguishers filled with water on an electrical fire. More of the wrong thing is just more wrong. And in a baby, just plain stupid.

The vitamin C posse (Linus Pauling, Frederick Klenner, Emanuel Cheraskin, William J. McCormick, Irwin Stone, Thomas E. Levy, Robert F. Cathcart III, and, ah, me) will tell you that you have a genuine option: use vitamin C as your first choice antibiotic. Taking enough C results in the three Cs: patient comfort, low cost, and parental control.

Because of the medical profession's customarily paternalistic, condescending attitude toward self-care, your choosing vitamin C therapy will be decried and denounced as irresponsible. It takes some real strength for a parent to stand firm and say, "This is what I am going to

48

do: I am going to follow the Klenner/Cathcart vitamin C protocol." Knowing that all you risk is derision from the medical community makes it a little easier.

When I was a kid, everybody got miracle drugs. From sulfa to Physohex, we followed the crowd from waiting room to prescription counter. Our parents gave us "safe" children's aspirin. Oops, not so safe for high fevers, it was discovered. So then it was children's Tylenol (acetaminophen) for everybody. Hmm . . . turns out there's some liver and kidney side effects with that, too. All drugs carry side effects; you just choose your poison carefully. Vitamins are vastly safer.

Antibiotics cause 700,000 emergency room visits per year, just in the United States alone (*Associated Press,* Oct. 17, 2006).

Law: The number one side effect of vitamins is failure to take enough of them.

If you do choose to employ antibiotic drugs, bear in mind that they interfere with normal digestion by killing off beneficial colon bacteria. These are the very bacteria that make vitamin K and the B vitamins cobalamin and biotin, and that help us digest many plant and dairy foods, strengthen the immune system, and repress the overgrowth of pathogenic microorganisms. After antibiotic therapy, all persons should take yogurt and an acidophilus supplement for a month or two to help restore a normal, healthy bowel environment. I have found shamefully few doctors who tell this to their patients.

And this is not just about antibiotics. In the 1980 *Physicians' Desk Reference,* prednisone didn't even have the diamond symbol of a frequently prescribed drug next to its listing. Now it is used almost indiscriminately. For instance, I know a sixteen-year-old girl who had a lousy diet, innumerable colds, and chronic bronchitis. After bucketfuls of antibiotics, the HMO doctors put her on prednisone. Prednisone is a drug of desperation. When they pull out the corticosteroids, they don't know what else to do. Prednisone can cause the following nutritional problems, among others: sodium and fluid retention, potassium loss, osteoporosis, carbohydrate intolerance and increased insulin requirement, and a variety of gastrointestinal complications. Why subject a teenage kid to this?

On the other hand, I have in my possession two *United States Pharmacopoeia* statements on vitamin C for injection asserting that "there are no contraindications for the use of ascorbic acid (vitamin C)." Not to mention the fact that it works. Intelligently employing vitamins can eliminate many dangerous side effects that come from over-reliance on over-the-counter and prescription drugs.

Vitamin C as an Antiviral: It's All about Dose

One of the most frequent questions readers have is, "Just how much vitamin C should I take?"

Our bodies cannot make vitamin C (ascorbate), although most animals can. We must get it from our food and from supplements. But how much do we really need? Persistent arguments on this question may be settled by looking at how much vitamin C animals manufacture in their bodies. The answer is: quite a lot. Most animals make the human body-weight equivalent of 5,000 to 10,000 milligrams a day. It is unlikely that animals would have evolved to make this much vitamin C if they did not need it and use it. Indeed, cells in many human body tissues concentrate vitamin C by 25-fold or more over blood concentration.

Each person's need for vitamin C differs because of differences in genetics and individual biochemistry.[1,2,3] Further, our bodies undergo different stresses, and we certainly eat different foods. Therefore, the daily need for ascorbate to maintain health for an adult varies between 2,000 to 20,000 mg/day. Linus Pauling personally took 18,000 mg of vitamin C daily. Although he was often ridiculed for this, it is interesting to note that Dr. Pauling had two more Nobel prizes than any of his critics. He died at age 93. Abram Hoffer, M.D., a colleague of Pauling's, took megadoses of vitamin C and successfully gave it to thousands of patients over 55 years of medical practice. Dr. Hoffer died at age 91.

When physicians criticized Linus Pauling for advocating vitamin C,
Dr. Pauling wrote a book that became an all-time nutritional bestseller:
Vitamin C and the Common Cold. It won the Phi Beta Kappa Award in Science.

Pauling L. (1970).*Vitamin C, the Common Cold, and the Flu.*
San Francisco: W. H. Freeman. Revised edition, 1976.

Antiviral Function

When we are challenged with a viral infection, our need for vitamin C can rise dramatically, depending on the body's immune function, level of injury, infection, or environmental toxicity such as cigarette smoke.[4,5] Ascorbate at sufficiently high doses can prevent viral disease and greatly speed recovery from an acute viral infection. Surprising to some, this was originally observed by physicians in the 1940s and has been verified and reverified over the last sixty years by doctors who achieved quick and complete recovery in their patients with ascorbate megadoses[5]. The effective therapeutic dose is based on clinical observation and bowel tolerance. Clinical observation is essentially "taking enough C to be symptom free, whatever that amount may be." Bowel tolerance means exactly what you think it means: the amount that can be absorbed from the gut without causing loose stools.[5,6] Very high doses, 30,000 to 200,000 mg, divided up throughout the day, are remarkably nontoxic and have been documented by physicians as curing viral diseases as various as the common cold, flu, hepatitis, viral pneumonia, and even polio.[4,5,7] On first reading this may sound incredible. We invite interested persons to read further, starting with the references listed below, and especially Dr. Lendon Smith's *Clinical Guide to the Use of Vitamin C.* This short book is posted in its entirety at www.seanet.com/~alexs/ascorbate/198x/smith-lh-clinical_guide_1988.htm.

Mechanism for Ascorbate Antiviral Effect

Several mechanisms for vitamin C's antiviral effect are known or suggested from studies.[4,8] The antioxidant property of ascorbate promotes a reducing (electron-abundant) biochemical environment in the bloodstream and tissues, enhancing the body's response to oxidative stress from inflammation,[9] thereby helping to fight microbes and viruses that propagate in stressful conditions.[10] Ascorbate has been shown to have specific antiviral effects in which it inactivates the RNA or DNA of viruses,[11,12,13] or the assembly of the virus.[14]

Vitamin C is also involved in enhancing several functions of the immune system. Ascorbate can enhance the production of interferon, which helps prevent cells from being infected by a virus.[15,16] Ascorbate stimulates the activity of antibodies,[17] and in megadoses seems to have a role in mitochondrial energy production.[18] It can enhance phagocyte function, which is the body's mechanism for removing viral particles and other unwanted debris.[4] White blood cells, involved in the body's defense against infections of all types, concentrate ascorbate up to 80 times plasma levels, which, if you take enough vitamin C, allows them to bring huge amounts of ascorbate to the site of the infection.[4] Many different components of the immune response, B-cells, T-cells, NK cells, and also cytokine production, all with important roles in the immune response, are enhanced by ascorbate.[19–23] Additionally, ascorbate improves the immune response from vaccination.[24,25]

Summary

Vitamin C at high doses is effective in preventing viral infection and enhancing recovery. Several mechanisms are known, including specific viral anti-replication processes and enhancement of many components of the body's cellular immune system. When taken at an appropriate dose in a timely manner, ascorbate is our best tool for curing acute viral illness.

References

1. Williams RJ, Deason G. (1967). *Proc Natl Acad Sci USA*. 57:1638–1641. Individuality in vitamin C needs.

2. Pauling L. (1986; revised ed. 2006). *How to Live Longer and Feel Better*. Corvallis, OR: Oregon State University Press.

3. Hoffer A, Saul AW. (2009). *Orthomolecular Medicine for Everyone: Megavitamin Therapeutics for Families and Physicians*.

4. Levy TE (2002). *Curing the Incurable: Vitamin C, Infectious Diseases, and Toxins*.

5. Hickey S, Saul AW. (2008). *Vitamin C: The Real Story, the Remarkable and Controversial Healing Factor*.

6. Cathcart RF. (1981). Vitamin C, titrating to bowel tolerance, anascorbemia, and acute induced scurvy. *Med Hypotheses*. 7: 1359–1376.

7. Klenner FR. (1979). The significance of high daily intake of ascorbic acid in preventive medicine, in: *Physician's Handbook on Orthomolecular Medicine*, Third Edition, 1979, Roger Williams, PhD, ed., p 51–59.

8. Webb AL, Villamor E. (2007). Update: Effects of antioxidant and non-antioxidant vitamin supplementation on immune function. *Nutrition Reviews* 65:181–217.

9. Wintergerst ES, Maggini S, Hornig DH. (2006). Immune-enhancing role of vitamin C and zinc and effect on clinical conditions. *Ann Nutr Metab*. 50:85–94.

10. Kastenbauer S, Koedel U, Becker BF, Pfister HW. (2002). Oxidative stress in bacterial meningitis in humans. *Neurology*. 58:186–191.

11. Murata A, Oyadomari R, Ohashi T, Kitagawa K. (1975). Mechanism of inactivation of bacteriophage delta A containing single-stranded DNA by ascorbic acid. *J Nutr Sci Vitaminol* (Tokyo). 21:261–269.

12. Harakeh S, Jariwalla RJ, Pauling L. (1990). Suppression of human immunodeficiency virus replication by ascorbate in chronically and acutely infected cells. *Proc Natl Acad Sci* USA. 87:7245–7249.

13. White LA, Freeman CY, Forrester BD, Chappell WA. (1986). In vitro effect of ascorbic acid on infectivity of herpesviruses and paramyxoviruses. *J Clin Microbiol*. 24:527–531.

14. Furuya A, Uozaki M, Yamasaki H, Arakawa T, Arita M, Koyama AH. (2008). Antiviral effects of ascorbic and dehydroascorbic acids in vitro. *Int J Mol Med*. 22:541–545.

15. Gerber, WF. (1975). Effect of ascorbic acid, sodium salicylate and caffeine on the serum interferon level in response to viral infection. *Pharmacology*, 13: 228.

16. Karpinska T, Kawecki Z, Kandefer-Szerszen M. (1982). The influence of ultraviolet irradiation, L-ascorbic acid and calcium chloride on the induction of interferon in human embryo fibroblasts. *Arch Immunol Ther Exp* (Warsz). 30:33–37.

17. Anderson R, Dittrich OC. (1979). Effects of ascorbate on leucocytes: Part IV. Increased neutrophil function and clinical improvement after oral ascorbate in 2 patients with chronic granulomatous disease. *S Afr Med J*. 1;56476–80.

18. Gonz lez MJ, Miranda JR, Riordan HD. (2005). Vitamin C as an Ergogenic Aid. *J Orthomolecular Med* 20:100–102.

19. Kennes B, Dumont I, Brohee D, Hubert C, Neve P. (1983.) Effect of vitamin C supplements on cell-mediated immunity in old people. Gerontology. 29:305–310.

20. Siegel BV, Morton JI. (1984). Vitamin C and immunity: influence of ascorbate on prostaglandin E2 synthesis and implications for natural killer cell activity. *Int J Vitam Nutr Res.* 54:339–342.

21. Jeng KC, Yang CS, Siu WY, Tsai YS, Liao WJ, Kuo JS. (1996). Supplementation with vitamins C and E enhances cytokine production by peripheral blood mononuclear cells in healthy adults. *Am J Clin Nutr.* 64:960–965.

22. Campbell JD, Cole M, Bunditrutavorn B, Vella AT. (1999). Ascorbic acid is a potent inhibitor of various forms of T cell apoptosis. *Cell Immunol.* 194:1–5.

23. Schwager J, Schulze J. (1997). Influence of ascorbic acid on the response to mitogens and interleukin production of porcine lymphocytes. *Int J Vitam Nutr Res.* 67:10–16.

24. Banic S. (1982). Immunostimulation by vitamin C. *Int J Vitam Nutr Res* Suppl. 23:49–52.

25. Wu CC, Dorairajan T, Lin TL. (2000). Effect of ascorbic acid supplementation on the immune response of chickens vaccinated and challenged with infectious bursal disease virus. *Vet Immunol Immunopathol.* 74:145–152.

Reprinted with permission from the *Orthomolecular Medicine News Service,* Dec. 3, 2009.

This goes for viruses, too. Right now there are a whole lot of researchers searching for a good antiviral drug. They already have one. The pharmaceutical industry's mercenary scientists and their medical doctor clones will, in fact, try everything but megadoses of vitamin C. I think of them as birds that are willing to land on any branch except one. Too bad, because that one branch is the best on the tree.

To treat infections with vitamin C, follow the guidelines listed in the chapter "Vitamin C Megadose Therapy."

"A patient cured is a customer lost."
—AUTHOR UNKNOWN (AND ABSOLUTELY CORRECT)

If Dracula were an old woman, he would have sounded a lot like Mrs. Kelremor. Just shy of eighty, this Central European immigrant had been a housekeeper for decades. Overweight, worn out, and weighted down with cares, she came to see me primarily because of osteoarthritis.

It was the 1980s: disco was still considered music, and arthritis was still said to have no nutritional connection or cure. For centuries, "health nuts" have known otherwise. Today, more and more, the medical profession is finally catching on. But Mrs. Kelremor couldn't wait for them. She said to me, in her thick Transylvanian accent, "I can't vork. I om avake all night. I om in pain all oof da time."

I vill now drop the accent; you get the picture.

Mrs. Kelremor bowed her gray-haired head as she continued speaking. "Look at my hands. I can't close them anymore. Look at my knees, all swollen. I am sore all over." As if that were not enough, she showed me an assortment of lumps on her arms and legs. Her doctor had told her they were benign. They certainly were not pleasant to behold. "What can I do?" she said. "My husband does not work. I have to work. I have to clean."

I suggested a real dietary overhaul, beginning with vegetable-juice fasting. There is a fine line between irresponsible promises and stimulating encouragement. I attempted to straddle that line by telling her that she had little to risk with vegetables.

She looked up, for the first time during the interview, and slowly said, "I will try anything."

Anything? Even living on raw vegetable juices eight days in a row, followed by very light eating for three days and a raw-food diet for the next ten?

"Yes," she said. "Anything."

The drop-out rate in such a program is high. That is probably the only true drawback of an otherwise venerable, simple, and safe program. To many, juice fasting conjures up images of starvation, electrolyte imbalance, malnutrition, and exhaustion. All false, and for very elementary reasons.

First, vegetables are especially nourishing foods, and a variety of vegetables guarantees more than adequate nutrition. The fact that they are juiced does not change that. Second, you cannot hurt yourself with produce. There is no down side to a vegetable diet, particularly when accompanied with a couple of good multivitamin pills each day. Eventually you'll want to reintroduce some legumes, sprouts, and nuts to your diet, for their protein, but that is after you've cleansed yourself through juicing.

So adequate nutrition—far more than adequate nutrition, really—can be maintained for weeks at a time on veggies alone. "But why juice? Why not just eat the vegetables?" Because you won't, that's why. Juicing guarantees quantity. If you juice, you simply will consume more vegetables. It is quicker and easier to down the juice than to sit and graze a table's worth of produce, so you will consume more. Additionally, the absorption of juiced vegetables is excellent, far superior to what you can get after just using your choppers to chew. Not being ruminants, like cows or giraffes, we get only one chance to masticate our food. A juicer does the job vastly better.

So that's it, then. A safe therapy that is too simple to work.

But it does. And the wretchedly bent-over Mrs. Kelremor was willing to try it.

Not without a fight, however. For weeks, I got her phone calls. "Can I have soup?"

Sure, if it will please you.

"Can I have some sausage?"

No.

"Can I cook some of the vegetables?"

Some vegetables have to be cooked, such as sweet potatoes and, moving away from a strict meaning of the word *vegetable,* lima beans and rice. If some of these foods will keep a person on the program, fine. Vegetable juices should still be the focus and the bulk of every meal.

"Every meal? Even breakfast?"

Look, folks. For breakfast, you drink hot bean extract (coffee) and eat undeveloped bird embryos (eggs) and the ripened ovaries of trees (fruit). You eat the muscles of ground-up pigs (sausage) placed between pulverized seeds fermented with a fungus (rolls), with a slice of curdled cow breast milk (cheese). And if I suggest vegetable juices, I'm the oddball?

So I conceded this and that to insure her compliance. Don't sweat the small stuff. After over thirty-five years in the field, I know people.

Mrs. Kelremor's calls persisted for a while. At least I knew she was on the program. Over time, they were fewer and fewer. She seemed to be doing fine.

A year passed.

One day I was shopping in a friend's health food store. There were a few people at the checkout counter. One was a tallish lady—or, if not tall, she certainly had very good posture. "Remember me?" she said, with the unmistakable voice of Bela Lugosi on estrogen. I recalled only the voice. It did not match this graceful woman, at ease and smiling, buying a counterful of vitamins.

But it was Mrs. Kelremor.

I greeted her, and she wasted no time in telling me, "I can work. I can bend, and reach, and sit and stand, and walk without any pain. I can work! I feel like a new woman." She actually said something more like, "I veel loke new voman," but enough of that.

I couldn't help but notice that the lumps on her arms and legs were gone. It wasn't surgery; a year and a half of juicing and vegetarian diet had apparently eradicated them. Now that was a bit unexpected. And all this progress, past age eighty.

Mrs. Kelremor is not the only person I know who juiced arthritis away. I saw something similar with a woman half her age.

The early forties is a bit young for rheumatoid arthritis, especially arthritis as severe as Cynthia's. Mostly I remember her hands. They were an old lady's hands. Swollen knuckles, fingers tightly drawn together to a point, almost like a paintbrush. Cynthia could hardly move them, and never without pain. The doctors, and there had been many, all told her that nothing could be done. Well, pain killers, but nothing else. Diet, perhaps? she'd asked them. Of course not, they'd told her.

She disbelieved them just enough to come and see me. I suggested that she do the same thing as Mrs. K had done, and hope for the same results. "And you are so much younger than her," I added. "Perhaps you have an advantage there."

At the very least, she complained a lot less. I had just one or two conversations with her on the phone after that. It was about eighteen months later when I actually saw Cynthia again in person. She had scheduled a follow-up appointment and breezed through the door into my office.

"Hi!" she said.

"Hello!" I answered. But who *are* you? is what I thought. Now I do not have a good head for names or faces to begin with, but this was extraordinary. I really thought there had been a mistake. I had gotten my appointment book messed up. This could not be Cynthia. I was expecting someone else, someone with at least some signs of arthritis.

This woman had none.

"Look!" she said. "Look what I can do!"

She flexed and turned her wrists and opened and closed all her fingers, effortlessly. I'm no orthopedist, but anyone could see that there was nearly complete range of motion.

"Wow!" I said. "What have you been doing?"

She looked at me as if I asked an odd question. "What we talked about," she answered. "I've been juicing every day, and fasting on juices every other week. For the last year and a half! And look at my complexion!"

Cynthia, or whoever this person really was, had almost no wrinkles. Her skin tone was perfect, perhaps a bit on the carotene-orange side. *USA Today* has described this harmless megajuicing side effect as looking like "an artificial sun tan." True. The doctors' *Merck Manual* describes hypercarotenosis as "harmless." Also true.

I describe it as "effective." There is more to juicing than just carotenes. The complex carbohydrates, raw food enzymes, minerals and vitamins, soluble fibers, and other vegetable nutrients makes for the perfect antidote to the protein-dominated, fat-heavy, sugar-laden, arthritis-causing Standard American Diet.

Once my own mother had arthritis. She was just entering her sixties. The symptoms were not severe, but they were getting worse each year. Then she started taking vitamins, juicing, and, most notably, eating lentil sprouts. Mom was a unique person, a "strange bird" as our old hardware-store man used to say. She will stick to an idea, even an untenable one, for a long time. This time, her talents for stubbornness were put to good use.

Every morning, Mom would have a large bowlful of sprouted lentils. Lentils look like brown split peas. To sprout them, she soaked dry lentils overnight in tap water. The next morning, she poured off the soaking water, then rinsed and drained them. Later that day, she rinsed and drained the lentils once more. They were ready for breakfast the next day. This may already sound pretty funky, but she went one step further: she topped them with molasses and ate them with a spoon.

Yum.

Now where does an otherwise intelligent person pick up ideas like this?

Guilty as charged. *C'est moi.*

I will stand on the results, though. I knew this lady and her hands especially well. It was considerably less than a year and my mom had no trace of arthritis. The raw sprout program worked. Juicing worked for Cynthia and Mrs. Kelremor. It all sounds quacky, because it is.

But that's how arthritis was eradicated from three sets of hands. To try it for yourself, start on "Saul's Super Remedy," as outlined in Part 2 of this book.

*"The person who says it cannot be done
should not interrupt the person doing it."*
—CHINESE PROVERB

Some illnesses are perceived as much harder to treat than they really are. Asthma, surprisingly, is a good example. The rule to remember is: Always consider the easiest and safest options first.

Seven Ways to Avoid an Asthma Attack

1. **Take more C**. Low levels of vitamin C may cause asthma. High doses of vitamin C relieve asthma. "Decreased preference for foods containing vitamin C and decreased concentrations of vitamin C in blood plasma are also associated with asthma," says the *American Journal of Clinical Nutrition.*

Robert Cathcart, M.D., recommends a daily vitamin C dosage of between 15,000 to 50,000 mg, divided into eight doses. He writes, "Asthma is most often relieved by bowel-tolerance doses of ascorbate. A child regularly having asthmatic attacks following exercise is usually relieved of these attacks by large doses of ascorbate. So far all of my patients having asthmatic attacks associated with the onset of viral diseases have been ameliorated by this treatment." I have seen this work again and again. See my chapter "Vitamin C Megadose Therapy" for guidelines.

When consumed in regular, frequent, near-saturation-doses, vitamin C is a powerful antihistamine. More on this in my chapter on allergies.

2. **Stop smoking**. Smoking around asthmatics is assault, and smoking around children is child abuse. Smoking, or simply breathing second-hand tobacco smoke, destroys vitamin C. Don't smoke! And do not allow asthmatics near smokers. This goes double for children. It will not surprise anyone to learn that many scientific studies confirm the link between exposure to tobacco smoke and increased incidence of asthma.

3. **Reduce stress**. Stress reduction greatly helps asthmatics. See my chapter "Stress Reduction."

4. **Keep your back in line**. For you, this may mean regular visits to a good chiropractor. For me, it means yoga stretches and exercise nearly every day. Explanations and instructions can be found in the backache chapter.

5. **Avoid dairy products and meat**. Eat a lot of fresh, raw foods such as salads and fresh fruit. This is a tried-and-true naturopathic protocol.

6. **Look into homeopathic remedies**. I'd start with *aconitum napthallus,* a microdilution of the monkshood herb. It is good first aid for an asthma attack. Taking lots of vitamin C will negate your need for even this natural remedy, however.

7. **In addition to vitamin C, eat carotene-rich vegetables**. Why? Because research has shown that vitamin C and carotene intakes are particularly low in males with severe asthma.[1] Another study concluded that children with low vitamin C and carotene intakes have greater asthma risk.[2]

References

1. Misso NL, Brooks-Wildhaber J, Ray S, Vally H, Thompson PJ. (2005). Plasma concentrations of dietary and nondietary antioxidants are low in severe asthma. *Eur Respir J.* 2005 26(2):257–64.

2. Harik-Khan RI, Muller DC, Wise RA. (2004). Serum vitamin levels and the risk of asthma in children. *Am J Epidemiol.* 159(4):351–.

Recommended Reading

Browne GE, et al. Improved mental and physical health and decreased use of prescribed and non-prescribed drugs through the Transcendental Meditation program. Age of Enlightenment Medical Council, Christchurch, New Zealand; Heylen Research Centre, Auckland, New Zealand; and Dunedin Hospital, Dunedin, New Zealand (1983).

Cathcart RF. Vitamin C, titrating to bowel tolerance, anascorbemia, and acute induced scurvy. *Medical Hypotheses* 7 (1981):1359–1376. (This paper is available to read in its entirety at www.orthomed.com.)

Graf D and Pfisterer G. Der Nutzen der Technik der Transzendentalen Meditation für die ärztliche Praxis. *Erfahrungsheilkunde* 9 (1978): 594–596.

Honsberger RW and Wilson AF. The effect of Transcendental Meditation upon bronchial asthma. *Clinical Research* 21 (1973): 278 (abstract).

Honsberger RW and Wilson AF. Transcendental Meditation in treating asthma. *Respiratory Therapy: The Journal of Inhalation Technology* 3 (1973): 79–80.

Kirtane L. Transcendental Meditation: A multipurpose tool in clinical practice. General medical practice, Poona, Maharashtra, India (1980).

Stone I. *The Healing Factor.* New York: Grosset and Dunlap, 1972.

Wilson AF, Honsberger RW, Chiu JT, and Novey HS. Transcendental Meditation and asthma. *Respiration* 32 (1975): 74–80.

Backache First Aid

> *"We're all ignorant, just on different subjects."*
>
> —WILL ROGERS

One of the handiest techniques for putting annoyingly out-of-place vertebrae back into line (or "putting your back in") is called "spontaneous release by positioning." The technique was developed by Lawrence Hugh Jones, a Canadian doctor of osteopathy (D.O.). Dr. Jones published his technique in *The D.O.,* January 1964, pages 109–16. It is a very effective, noninvasive procedure that most anyone can learn and use.

Important caution: Common sense dictates the need of genuine care in dealing with any back problem. Consult a medical, osteopathic, or chiropractic doctor before proceeding with this or any other self-care approach.

Ironically, the very first time I had occasion to require spontaneous release was while I was taking a short course in how to do it. I really wasn't at all convinced of the value of the technique until it was used on me. This is so often the way, isn't it? One day I stepped off the curb to cross a street and suddenly felt my back give way and my leg get weak. I must have moved just right—or should I say, just wrong—and it threw my lower back out severely. I tried assorted exercises at home to try to correct it, but none worked. It was painful in the big muscles of the lower back, the lumbar area, and I couldn't do anything about it. So the next class, I asked the instructor to use me as the example of the day.

I was told to relax, and was rolled up into a ball with my leg up under my chest in an odd but strangely comfortable position. I knew that the teacher was pressing a trigger point beside my lower vertebra, but I only knew he was pressing the point because he told me he was. I felt no pain at all in this position—and believe me, that was amazing after my recent discomfort. A couple of minutes of relaxation passed, and he brought my posture back to normal. The pain was gone, and it did not return. I rested a moment and got up and about again. I've been successfully employing spontaneous release ever since because it is gentle and it works so well.

"Spontaneous release" is another phrase for "nature cured it," applied to your back. Occasionally a slightly displaced vertebra will slip back into place on its own. An unusual sleeping position or a chance movement can return a vertebra to its place, though not quite as easily as it can be put "out." This spontaneous realignment of the spine is not to be confused with "learning to live with it" or any other mere toleration of the aches or pains resulting from misplaced bones. It is one thing for the body to compensate for a problem, and quite another for the body to actually correct the problem.

So why is a technique needed at all if the body corrects itself? First of all, spontaneous release rarely occurs on its own. It would be nice if it did, but legions of backache patients prove otherwise. It seems easier for a bone to go out than to go in, in the same manner that it's easier to break a watch than fix it, or easier to scramble an egg than to put it back together again. Entropy rules, at least in this universe. When a bone goes out, the surrounding muscles also are affected. Dr. Jones explains this well in his paper. It seems that once the bone is out, the tendency of the muscles is to hold this new position. It's only through a unique position coupled with muscle relaxation that the bone can slip back into place almost unnoticed.

This is precisely what "spontaneous release by positioning" seeks to accomplish: this technique recreates the body's posture or position that put the vertebra out in the first place, to encourage it to replace itself of its own accord. It's like retracing your steps looking for your lost car keys.

By carefully positioning the arms or legs up or down, back turned this way or that, hips or neck pivoted right or left, a patient with even severe back pain will all at once find a comfortable position, a position where there is no pain, or almost no pain. It may be quite an odd-looking position, but the discomfort is eased or completely gone. This is the posture that encouraged the bone to go out in the first place; now we'll use the same position to encourage the bone to return. You can always tell when you've discovered the correct position because the patient will be comfortable, even if previously she was barely able to sit or stand. The very posture that put the initial strain on the back is now taking the strain off the back. Says Dr. Jones:

> *Even the severest lesions will readily tolerate being returned to the position in which lesion formation originally occurred, and only to this position. When the joint is returned to this position, the muscles promptly and gratefully relax. These joints do not cause distress because they are crooked; they are paining because they are being forced to be too straight. This is the mechanism of strain.* (p. 110. Reprinted with permission of the American Osteopathic Association.)

In other words, the muscles are "used" to the strain, and contract to hold the bone out of place. When the person tries to straighten up, the bones won't, because the muscles won't let them. And the muscles won't relax because the bones are out of alignment. That is why heating pads, rubs, medicines, and "learn to live with it" do not solve the problem. Because those approaches do not reposition the bone, the muscle cannot relax to normal. That's why there's pain.

How to eliminate the pain? Reposition the bone back to normal. How? Return the person's body to the extreme but now comfortable posture so the muscles will relax. Then hold the person in that position, as the person relaxes, for ninety seconds. Then, keeping the person relaxed, bring him back around slowly to a normal posture. The bone that was out will have returned with the rest of the spine to the normal position.

To better find exactly which vertebrae are out, and also to demonstrate to yourself that the bones do in fact realign and pain does disappear, it may be helpful to utilize what are called "trigger points" along the spine. Looking at the back, one can see the spinal column as a stack of bumps. To either side of each bump will be a trigger point. The distance out from the bump will be about one to two inches. Dr. Jones describes specific trigger locations in detail in his paper, and tells how to use them individually.

Each vertebra has side projections, like wings. If a given vertebra is misaligned, the tissue on one or both sides of that bone will be tender. This is because the bone's somewhat twisted condition strains the musculature and may even put pressure on the nerve emerging to each side of it. If you press there, it may hurt quite a bit. That's how you can tell which bones are out. Gently go up and down the spine and press lightly about one inch out to either side of each vertebral bump. Where there's pain, that's where the nerve is under pressure, where the muscle is locking, and where the bone is out. And that's the trigger point for that bone.

Generally you'll find one side of the vertebra to be more tender than the other. In that case, keep pressing lightly on the tender spot while repositioning the person. When the correct position is reached, the person will say that he no longer feels pain even though pressure is still being applied on the trigger point. This is positive proof that you've found the right trigger point and the right position. Then make sure the person is relaxing, hold the position while pressing the trigger point for at least ninety seconds, and then bring the person back to normal posture while continuing to press the trigger point. If you've corrected the problem, the person will not feel discomfort, and will not feel pain even though you continue to press the trigger point that hurt him before you started.

Summary of the steps of spontaneous release by positioning:

1. Find the right trigger point by gently pressing to each side of each vertebra. Pain indicates the trigger point.

2. While pressing that point, begin to reposition the person, asking him to tell you when the pain stops.

3. When a comfortable position is reached, continue pressing the trigger point while holding the person in that unusual position.

4. Be sure the person is relaxed if you want this to be successful. You, not the patient, must hold the position. If the patient holds the position, he is using the very muscles that you are seeking to relax.

5. After ninety seconds or more, return the person to a normal posture while continuing to press the spot.

6. If the person feels better and the trigger point pressure no longer hurts, then the bone is back in its proper place.

Step-by-step suggestions:

Step 1. The person's back should be uncovered. Some people will feel pain with only the lightest pressure to the trigger point. With other cases, you may have to press fairly hard to find the spot. Very muscular persons often require more pressure. Persons in great pain can require but a touch. I once worked on a relative whose back was in such excruciating pain that just a washcloth's pressure when taking a bath hurt him greatly. After half an hour of spontaneous release by positioning he was so much improved that I could press those same spots on his back until my fingernails were white. That is real relief!

Step 2. Be sure to ask the person to tell you if a given trial position is better, worse, or the same. Some people won't tell you if you're helping or hurting, so ask! Ask constantly, "Better, worse, or the same? Better, worse, or the same?" If you're working on the neck, the person may begin in a sitting position. If you are working on the upper or middle back, the person might sit, or it may be easier to lie face down. For the lower back, the person may lie down on their side or face down. Start symmetrically and end symmetrically; that is, the patient should sit or lie straight to begin, and always end up straight with no crossed legs or slouching.

Step 3. The only comfortable position for the patient may be very unusual or extreme, and that's to be expected. The person may be in no pain at all only when rolled up like a ball, or twisted one leg over the other, or with their head pointed out and up with the chin in the air, or with their arm bent back over their shoulder! You just have to try any position until you get the sure sign that you've found the right one: no more pain.

Step 4. Dr. Jones mentions that "patients will try to help you. Don't let them." This is because spontaneous release by positioning must remain totally passive on the part of the patient; all he or she can do to help is to say when the pain is gone, and relax. That is it. After the procedure, the patient should rest for a while, and later endeavor to keep good posture while resting or working. This is important, because the bone replaced is most likely to slip back out of place if again offered the extreme position that did it before.

Step 5. The length of time that you have to hold the position will vary with each situation, from ninety seconds to as much as five minutes. Generally, the tenser the patient, the longer the hold time. Experience best shows how you can be the judge.

Step 6. With spontaneous release by positioning, as with math, you can always check your work. The trigger point that hurt when you pressed it showed you which vertebra was out; the trigger point when pressed with the person in the correct posture no longer hurt, so it showed you the correct position; the trigger point when pressed throughout the rotation of the person back to normal position no longer hurts, either, and shows you that the release was accomplished.

You cannot practice spontaneous release by positioning on yourself. You cannot have relaxed muscles if you are using them. You must exert force to position your limbs, or to press trigger points. You can either relax a muscle or use a muscle; you cannot do both together. This is why it is good to teach family members this technique: you may be the one needing it some day. If everyone learns, then you can help each other. When I did farm work, with much reaching, lifting, pulling, and carrying, my wife practiced spontaneous release by positioning on me almost every day. But she had her turn: when she was pregnant, particularly during the eighth and ninth months, I had to put her back in as much as twice a day. This prevented the considerable back discomfort that so many women complain of during pregnancy due to the extra weight applied to the back in carrying a child. (Gentlemen, you just try strapping one or two large bags of dog food around your middle and see how it feels!) All that new extra weight must be supported by the same bones.

Spontaneous release by positioning is my preferred way to relieve backache, and warm-up stretches or yoga postures are my preferred ways to prevent backache. See the next chapter for directions on how to do those.

It still takes me aback (good pun) that there isn't more interest in spontaneous release by positioning from chiropractors or osteopaths. Maybe it is because the name is too long. Maybe it is because it takes more time than busy practitioners want to spend. Maybe it is because wellness self-reliance cuts into the profit of fee-per-visit professionals.

In other words, perhaps it is because the procedure works too well. This is a great technique. Help me spread the word.

Backache Prevention

"I've got a weak back."
"Since when?"
"Oh, about a week back."
—FROM AN OLD VAUDEVILLE ROUTINE

There is nothing like comfortably walking straight as a ramrod, proud to be bipedal. If you have back problems, there are two ways to achieve this. One is via a visit to a good chiropractor. The other is to use the techniques below. (*Important caution: common sense dictates the need of genuine care in dealing with any back problem. Consult a medical, osteopathic, or chiropractic doctor before proceeding with these, or any other, self-care approaches.*)

1. First, you can try some **bed stretches**. There are two ways to do them:

Method One: Sit in the middle of the bed, legs straight out in front of you. Then, from the hips up, bend to the right as far as you reasonably can. Now lie back. You should be shaped like a boomerang, mate. And you will feel a profound "pulling" sensation in your lower back, hip, and upper leg. Relax and stay in that position for five minutes. Repeat the process to the left.

Method Two: Lie across the bed face-down. Put your feet over the edge and grab the mattress with your toes. You can do this even if you are not an orangutan. While keeping your feet together, bend your upper body to the right as far as comfortable. You now will look like the other side of a boomerang. Using your arms, give it an extra stretch further to the right and hold it for a minute or two. Relax, and repeat for the left side.

Both of these techniques work best if done first thing in the morning and last thing before going to sleep at night.

2. When you sleep, do so on a good, **firm (but not hard) mattress**. If you cannot afford a good mattress, consider asking Santa for a futon (a thick floor mat). You can also try putting a board under your lousy mattress for the time being.

3. Do back-healthy **exercises**. Try regular (or even irregular) practice of hatha yoga postures. Especially helpful are the Plow and the Hurdle Stretch.

The Plow begins with a shoulder-stand on a well-carpeted floor. That's like a headstand, only your weight is on your shoulders, with your head tucked in and your bent arms propping up your back. I cannot do a real headstand, but I can do this. From the shoulder-stand, let the weight of your legs pull your feet to the ground directly behind your head. You will look and feel like a number 6 tipping over. Hold for the count of twenty, then do it again. And once more. This is a terrific before-you-hit-the-hay exercise.

Hurdle Stretches are easy to do. Sit cross-legged wearing loose clothing. Extend one leg out at a natural 45-degree angle from your hips. Reach down along that leg as far as you are able, drop your head, and reach a bit further. If you manage to reach your ankles, grab them and relax. If you can't, grab what part of your leg you can and relax. Hold with a slight stretch for the count of twenty-five. Repeat with the other leg. Repeat this several times, morning and evening, for best results.

Really want to feel great? Do some back-building, soreness-squelching exercises:

Shrugs. These are as easy as they sound. Simply shrug your shoulders—with a dumbbell in each hand. You can usually use quite a lot of weight for this. Beginners may want to start with five or eight pounds per hand. I use twenty-five-pounders, but then I've been doing this for a while. Your basic up-and-down shrugs can be complemented with shoulder rotations forward together and then backward together. Also, try alternate-shoulder up and down shrugs. These moves really loosen up the neck, shoulders, and upper back.

Flys. Use a *much* lighter weight for these. A "fly" is like a theatrical, expansive yawn with weights in your hands. Another way to describe flys is you look like a large bird stretching its wings, or Batman displaying his entire cape. Stand where you have a lot of free airspace around you and try some. By varying positions (one arm reaching up, the other down; both up or both down; reaching behind you backhanded; etc) you can de-stress the entire upper half of your body to an extent you might not have thought possible. Start with a few and work up to either a larger number of repetitions or to larger weights. You can also hold heavier weights close to your body, with arms bent like a chicken dancing, and repeatedly stick your elbows back as far as they will happily go. Hey, this book is called "Doctor Yourself," not "Look Cool Doing It."

Side-crunches. Lie down on a carpeted floor in the good old "knee bent for sit-ups" position. But there's a twist: let both your knees fall to one side and do your crunches side-saddle. Do an equal number with your knees to the other side, of course. By bringing your knees nearly up to your chin, or extending your bent legs to one side or the other, you will feel a lower back benefit in addition to that most satisfying spare-tire-reduction that crunches are known for.

If you do a set of yoga postures or warm-up exercises first thing in the morning and again at bedtime, you will work better, sleep better, and feel better. Do this every day, and you will notice that you are able to reach further and touch those toes again. My high school phys ed teacher told me a long time ago that the single, simplest test of a person's physical fitness is to see if they can touch their toes. Can you? If not, do stretches. If you can touch them, continue doing stretches.

You can read even more on exercise in my chapter "Evading Exercise."

4. **Lose excess weight**. If you are twenty-two pounds overweight, that is like carrying a big economy-size bag of dog food around with you all day. Forty-four pounds is two big bags of dog food. All that weight pulls on your back and sits on your sacroiliac. Be realistic; it has to go. If you cut down your daily calorie intake by just 120 calories (a puny amount and you know it), you will lose a pound a month. If you do any exercise at all, you will triple the loss easily. Do not scoff at a monthly three-pound weight loss. That's thirty-six pounds in a year.

5. **Fast, Totally Free, Utterly Effortless, Back-Friendly Advice:**

Ladies, stop wearing high heels. Nothing wrecks your posture and all the muscles and bones associated with it like walking around on your toes all day.

Lift, shovel, or rake with your "other" side. This really works. I learned it watching my dad, who one day picked up a large TV set with his left hand. His back went out and he was in considerable discomfort until he reached down and picked up the same TV with the other hand—and put his back "in" again. I used to get a backache after snow shoveling, a common event around these parts (I live just south of Canada). Then, I started shoveling backward. By this, I mean that I reversed the position of my hands on the shovel, dug to the other side, and threw with the other shoulder. This was weird at first, and I could only move a quarter of my usual load. But practice makes perfect, and now I have forgotten which side is my "other" side. I can move a ton of snow (literally) without injury. If you have no snow to move (you lucky person you), may I mention that this technique applies to shoveling dirt, concrete, manure, or anything else you have to toss about.

Wear that purse or backpack on the "other" shoulder. Same idea as above.

Make a point to periodically **notice your sitting posture**, whether working, reading, or watching TV. Can you improve it? Of course you can, once you become aware of it.

I know an unusually large number of chiropractors. This may be because I used to teach at a chiropractic college. One of my very best friends, Kenneth Hack, is an excellent chiropractor. He has "straightened out" my whole family for many years and he is great at it. But Ken lives too far from me for quick visits every time my back bugs me. So I have learned how to take care of it myself. I don't care much for exercise, but I exercise anyhow. Ken told me I have to, and I found out he was right. Good chiropractors teach you how to not need them. So now I do all the stuff I discussed above almost daily, because when I'm done, I feel terrific.

You can take this considerably further if you want to. Thirty-five years ago, I learned a gentle first-aid technique, "spontaneous release by positioning," developed by Lawrence Hugh Jones, D.O. Step-by-step instructions are provided in the previous chapter.

Backache is a common ailment, one of the most common of all chronic health problems. It is certainly one of the chief on-the-job time-loss injuries. Most people will suffer backache at least some time in their lives. But the procedures described above are powerful steps you can take to prevent, and to relieve, backache.

I used to have back trouble. Now I don't.

*"This guy's doctor told him he had six months to live.
The guy said he couldn't pay his bill.
The doctor gave him another six months."*

—HENNY YOUNGMAN

How do bedsores seem to just "happen"?

They don't. They are allowed to happen, and lousy hospital and nursing home food is the major culprit.

No, it's not the mattress. It is malnutrition.

I think bedsores might better be termed "scurvy sores," and in centuries past they often were. Like bleeding gums on a large scale, they are a development of spontaneous pinpoint hemorrhaging. The pressure of brushing the teeth, or lying on a mattress, is enough to break blood vessels grossly weakened by a lack of vitamin C.

Look into this for yourself and see. When you do, you will note that the symptoms of scurvy include poor healing, weak capillaries, easy bruising, open wounds that suppurate (discharge pus), and spontaneous bleeding and internal hemorrhage, often from very minor trauma. Such describes the development of a bedsore.

Bedsores have been associated with necrotizing ulcerative stomatitis (severe inflammation and destruction of soft tissue and bone). Both share a number of symptoms, both occur in malnourished patients, and both are treatable with nutritional supplementation. (Buchanan, JAG, et al. [2006] .Necrotizing stomatitis in the developed world. *Clinical and Experimental Dermatology* 31[3], 372–374.)

Pellagra, a deficiency of niacin (vitamin B_3), causes bedsores as well. This has been known for nearly a hundred years. (*Pellagra: History, Distribution, Diagnosis, Prognosis, Treatment,* etc. by Stewart Ralph Roberts, p 104. http://books.google.com/books?id=XCxQAWDWAh4C&printsec=titlepage). Also see "The Nursing Care of Pellagra," by Lillian Cumbee. *The American Journal of Nursing,* Vol. 31, No. 3 (Mar., 1931), p 272–274

The cure, the only cure, for pellagra is niacin. Not surprisingly, niacin also helps heal bedsores. (Gernand, K. [1951]. Therapy of ulcus cruris and decubitus. *Dtsch Gesundheitspolit.* 6[48]:1388–9. PMID: 14905956.)

So does the mineral **zinc**. Even the medically orthodox *Merck Manual* says that "supplemental vitamin C and zinc may help with healing as well." I would recommend at least 50 mg day, and 150 would be better, divided into three separate doses. Zinc gluconate is readily available, cheap, and well-absorbed.

Vitamins A, B_1 (thiamine), B_2 (riboflavin), and E are probably also helpful. Vitamin A and the B vitamins are in any multivitamin preparation. Vitamin E from capsules may be dripped directly onto a bedsore, painlessly. The benefits are more rapid healing, less discomfort, and reduced risk of infection and scarring.

Conservative treatment is always best, and vitamin supplementation is about as conservative as it gets. Remember what vitamin-discoverer Dr. Roger J. Williams said: "When in doubt, use nutrition first."

Patients given optimally large amounts of these nutrients will be more comfortable in days, and although healing will take weeks, you can expect to see real improvement.   Recon-structive surgery is the last resort. Think about this: if a patient cannot keep their normal skin well, how are they going to recover from a skin graft? Do not subject a patient, especially an elderly patient, to such pain and trauma if you can possibly avoid it.

And yes, you *can* possibly avoid it. But you will not know if nutrition works until you try it.

I have seen this with my own eyes, so don't try to tell me differently: hospitals are not trying nutrition first. My aunt, an activist registered nurse, is campaigning to end elder abuse. Good. Here is an excellent opportunity for you to join her. Don't let your loved one suffer from a bedsore. *Demand oral and intravenous high-potency multiple and B-complex vitamin therapy. Demand oral and intravenous vitamin C as well.*

Let the hospital and doctors tell you it is unsafe if they must. If they try to do so, they have not read their own journals. Here is some of the evidence:

• "Most patients with chronic skin ulcers suffered micronutrient status alterations, and bor-derline malnutrition. Meals did not cover energy requirements, while oral supplements cov-ered basic micronutrient requirements and compensated for insufficient oral energy and protein intakes, justifying their use in hospitalized elderly patients." (Raffoul W, Far MS, Cayeux MC, and Berger MM. [2006]. Nutritional status and food intake in nine patients with chronic low-limb ulcers and pressure ulcers: importance of oral supplements. *Nutrition* 22[1]:82–8.)

• "In the group treated with ascorbic acid there was a mean reduction in pressure-sore area of 84% after one month compared with 42.7% in the placebo group. These findings are statisti-cally significant (P less than 0.005) and suggest that ascorbic acid may accelerate the healing of pressure-sores." (Taylor TV, Rimmer S, Day B, Butcher J, Dymock IW. [1974]. Ascorbic acid supplementation in the treatment of pressure-sores. *Lancet* 2[7880]:544–6. See also: Ascorbic acid and pressure sores. [1971]. *Br Med J* 2[5762]:604–5.)

• "Only patients receiving additional arginine, vitamin C and zinc demonstrated a clinically significant improvement in pressure ulcer healing (9.4+/–1.2 vs. 2.6+/–0.6; baseline and week 3, respectively."(Desneves KJ, Todorovic BE, Cassar A, Crowe TC. [2005]. Treatment with sup-plementary arginine, vitamin C and zinc in patients with pressure ulcers: a randomised con-trolled trial. *Clin Nutr.* 24[6]:979–87.)

• "(O)ral nutritional supplement(ation) resulted in a significant reduction in wound area and an improvement in wound condition in patients with grade III and IV pressure ulcers within three weeks. . . Median healing of wound area was 0.34 cm . . . 2 per day, taking approximately two days to heal 1 cm . . . the amount of exudate in infected ulcers (p = 0.012) and the incidence of necrotic tissue (p = 0.001) reduced significantly." (Frías Soriano L, Lage Vázquez MA, Maristany CP, Xandri Graupera JM, Wouters-Wesseling W, Wagenaar L. [2004]. The effectiveness of oral nutritional supplementation in the healing of pressure ulcers. *J Wound Care.* 13[8]:319–22.)

Note: The recommended dietary allowance (RDA)/Dietary Reference Intake (DRI) is not enough: "Refeeding of pressure sore patients who often are catabolic and have increased needs for protein and energy, should include micronutrients not only to cover recommended dietary allowances, but sufficient to reach normal nutritional status for the individual micronutrient."

(Selvaag E, Bøhmer T, Benkestock K. [2002]. Reduced serum concentrations of riboflavine and ascorbic acid, and blood thiamine pyrophosphate and pyridoxal-5-phosphate in geriatric patients with and without pressure sores. *J Nutr Health Aging* 6[1]:75–7. See also Powers JS, Zimmer J, Meurer K, Manske E, Collins JC, Greene HL. Direct assay of vitamins B1, B2, and B6 in hospitalized patients: relationship to level of intake. *J Parenter Enteral Nutr.* 117[4]:315–6.)

Also note: 1,000 mg of vitamin C is not enough. (ter Riet, G, Kessels AG, Knipschild PG. [1995]. Randomized clinical trial of ascorbic acid in the treatment of pressure ulcers. *J Clin Epidemiol.* 48[12]:1453–60.)

For more information on administering vitamin C by IV, please refer to this book's later chapter "How to Get Intravenous Vitamin C Given to a Hospitalized Patient."

Don't forget to try a topical application of aloe vera gel, squeezed fresh from the plant's thick leaves. It is soothing and healing.

And get those vitamin supplements going before bedsores can develop.

"It is common sense to take a method and try it. If it fails, admit it frankly and try another. But above all, try something."

—FRANKLIN DELANO ROOSEVELT

Joe had terminal lung cancer, and no mistake. He was coughing up so much blood that he had a mostly red handkerchief in his hand all the while I talked with him in the living room of his small suburban home. Joe was too sick to come in to my office. In fact, he was too sick to get out of his recliner. It was in this chair that his life played out, day and night. He could not walk. He was in too much pain to even lie down. He spent the night in his chair. He did not want to eat. But he did still want to live, and he was willing to try even vitamins if they would help him feel any better.

It was October and the leaves, orange and yellow, were falling outside the picture window as we talked. The TV was on, and some of the family was visiting. It is never easy to work with the dying. As a student, twenty years ago, I'd seen enough of them at the Brigham Hospital in Boston. Then, I had listened and watched. Now, I listened and watched and suggested vitamin C.

"How much?" Joe croaked.

"As much as humanly possible under the circumstances," I replied. I explained bowel tolerance to him, and answered the usual questions from the family. Most centered on how well it would work. Some were understandably skeptical; others were in overly optimistic denial. "If I had the sure cure for cancer, I'd be on the cover of *Time* magazine," I cautioned. "I can't promise anything, but vitamin C is very much worth trying, considering how sick Joe is."

All agreed that Joe had nothing to lose.

Here is what happened. Within days, Joe stopped coughing up the blood. If the C had done nothing else, this alone would have been more than enough benefit. But there was more good news within the week.

"Joe's appetite is back," said his wife. "And he is able to lie down in the bed now. He says he is sleeping much better and in much less pain."

Wonderful news, especially if you were Joe. Over and over I have seen profound pain relief and dramatic improvement in sleeping for terminal patients who take huge doses of C. Again, if the C did nothing else, these benefits would be indisputable arguments for using it.

A week or so later, I heard still more news. "Joe is able to walk around the house with a cane. He's even walking around the yard!" His wife was quite emotional as she spoke. She knew, at some level, as we all did, that Joe was not likely to survive such severe cancer. And, in the end, he didn't. But he extended his life, and the quality of that life was extraordinarily enhanced by the vitamin C. He never did all the other stuff I will recommend in this chapter; he couldn't. But he was determined to manage taking the C, and he did.

Oh, yes: how much did he take? About 4,000 mg every half hour he was awake, day or night. That is approaching 100,000 mg a day. He had a big jug of water, a big spoon, a big glass, and a big bottle of vitamin C crystals on the table right next to his recliner. And he never got diarrhea.

You may not believe vitamin C was responsible for the dramatic changes in Joe. I don't blame you—how could you, when you never hear about this stuff from your M.D.s? Rather, you tend to hear about natural treatments for cancer from sources dismissed as quacks, don't you?

Therein lies the problem.

For years, I've asked, "Who are the real quacks?" I've strongly implied, to say the least, that they are the conventional, tunnel-visioned sycophants of the medical, dietetic, and pharmaceutical professions. Not alone in this criticism, I quote endocrinologist Deepak Chopra, author of many a best-selling health book: "More people live off cancer than die from it." There is no profit in prevention, but plenty of money in disease. Like the firemen in Ray Bradbury's *Fahrenheit 451,* medical science encourages fires and then glamorizes their bungled attempts to put them out. By ignoring the evidence they don't like (and dismissing it as anecdotal or nonscientific), doctors and dietitians have closed the mausoleum door on millions.

According to peer-reviewed research, conventional chemotherapy contributes only 2.1 percent to five-year cancer survival in the USA.

Morgan, Ward, and Barton. (2004). *Clinical Oncology* 16:549–560.

Laetrile is a good case in point. This controversial anticancer agent, derived from almonds and apricot pits, has erroneously been called "vitamin B_{17}," but it is not a vitamin. Rather, Laetrile is amygdalin, a cyanide-containing substance. The cyanide is the active ingredient that somewhat selectively kills cancer cells—an action not unlike that of chemotherapy agents (which explains both the need for caution and the stringent rejection it has received from the medical powers that be). The imperious medical monarchy, which includes the AMA, FDA, and their ensuing laws, has made Laetrile therapy strikingly difficult to obtain inside United States borders.

Chapters 8 and 9 of Ralph Moss's *The Cancer Syndrome* disclose nitty-gritty details of some tantalizingly successful Laetrile research at Memorial Sloan-Kettering Cancer Center in New York City. It seems that experienced cancer researcher Dr. Kanematsu Sugiura repeatedly obtained lengthened survival time in mice with spontaneous mammary tumors. He also prevented tumors from spreading to the lungs and obtained temporary stoppage of small tumor growth. The problem is, he did all of this using Laetrile.

Dr. Sugiura's work constitutes limited, but nonetheless significant, findings. Sloan-Kettering's brass wanted him to shut up about the whole thing, and declared in press conferences that Laetrile had no value in cancer treatment. Once, Dr. Sugiura was personally addressed by a reporter, and he most expressly contradicted his bosses. How did author Ralph Moss know about all this? He was the number-two Sloan-Kettering PR man, that's how.

My personal view is that Laetrile is probably a palliative treatment, relieving suffering without necessarily obliterating the disease. Still, the fact that so many orthodox cancer foundations want it kept quiet is in itself sufficient reason to look into it more.

As the Laetrile example shows, there most certainly is a wider range of cancer treatment alternatives than conventional medical sources will allow. Worthy adjuncts and alternatives to chemotherapy, radiation, and surgical treatments are unpopular with organized medicine, yet are employed by far-thinking physicians and self-reliant persons around the world. Why is this? Because all possibilities need to be considered in undertaking the treatment of such a serious disease for which there are far too few survivors. In this chapter I will let you in on some of the evidence that has accumulated and provide a natural protocol for adjunctive cancer treatment and prevention.

Vitamin C Therapy Benefits Cancer Patients

Decades of research repeatedly shows that cancer patients taking supplemental vitamins achieve significantly longer life and vastly improved quality of life. Vitamin C reduces the side-effects of chemotherapy, surgery, and radiation therapy. Patients on a strong nutritional program have far less nausea, and often experience little or no hair loss during chemo. They experience reduced pain and swelling following radiation. They have faster, uncomplicated healing after surgery. Even at very high doses, vitamin C is an unusually safe substance. Given intravenously it kills cancer cells without harming healthy cells.

The blood work of unsupplemented cancer patients will invariably show that they have abnormally low levels of vitamin C. Still, the number of cancer patients who have ever had their doctor recommend a therapeutic trial of truly large quantities of vitamin C remains small.

A patient's therapeutic response is the highest of all guiding principles in medicine. If it works, do it. If it seems to work, do it. If it does no harm, do it. Remember: If there were a sure cure for cancer, you would have heard about it. There isn't. But this just makes it all the more important for patients to demand adjunctive vitamin C therapy from their physicians.

Linus Pauling, Ph.D., megadose vitamin C advocate, died in 1994 from prostate cancer. Dr. Pauling was 93 years old. Charles G. Moertel, M.D., critic of Pauling and vitamin C, also died in 1994 and also from cancer (lymphoma). Dr. Moertel was 66 years old.

One needs to make up one's own mind as to whether this does or does not indicate benefit from vitamin C.

Cancer and Vitamin C

Back in the 1970s, Nobel–prize-winning scientist Linus Pauling, along with Ewan Cameron, a Scottish cancer surgeon, demonstrated the effectiveness of 10,000 mg of intravenous vitamin C a day in reversing terminal cancer in 13 out of 100 patients. These patients were given up as lost by medical authorities. Thirteen out of 100 may not seem like a high percentage of success, but keep in mind that those thirteen were considered beyond hope and then became free of the disease as far as could be determined. Thirteen is infinitely greater than zero. Vitamin C–treated patients lived, on average, five times as long as controls who did not receive vitamin C. Do not be misled by false media hype against vitamin C. A pair of politically motivated Mayo Clinic studies condemning the vitamin were seriously flawed. How? They gave vitamin C orally, not intravenously. And they stopped it too soon. You will want to refer to Cameron and Pauling's seminal book, *Cancer and Vitamin C,* for the full story. There is no substitute for the truth, and there is a good chance you have not heard it.

"After breakfast, I visited Linus Pauling, who was staying in the room next to mine. When I walked in he was busy with a hand calculator. I told him that on the basis of my fifty patients I had concluded that he and Dr. Cameron were right, that vitamin C in large doses did improve enormously the outcome of treatment for cancer."

—ABRAM HOFFER, M.D.

Today, orthomolecular (nutritional) physicians use considerably higher doses than 10,000 mg of vitamin C a day. Such doses are greatly more than what the federal government maintains an average person needs. A reading of *The Healing Factor: Vitamin C Against Disease,* by biochemist Irwin Stone, will explain to you why we need so very much vitamin C, why it should indeed be normal to consume many grams of the vitamin a day, and why the lack of C is responsible for our species' present state of illness. You can find this book posted online in its entirety (see References below). Irwin Stone, by the way, is the person who got Dr. Pauling interested in vitamin C in the first place. For improved quality and length of life, the key is sufficient quantities of C. More orange juice just won't do it.

Scientists have long studied the effects of megadoses of vitamin C to treat a wide variety of illnesses and diseases. Research documents vitamin C as one of the best antiviral agents available. Vitamin C has been shown to neutralize and eliminate a wide range of toxins, and to enhance host resistance, greatly augmenting the immune system's ability to neutralize bacterial and fungal infections. Most importantly, there is extensive published research demonstrating vitamin C's anticancer properties.[1]

Hugh D. Riordan, M.D., and colleagues began in the 1960s to study the underlying causes of cancer and ways to treat cancer in a nontoxic fashion. From this research came the Riordan Intravenous Vitamin C Protocol for Cancer.[2] This protocol is widely recognized in the integrative and orthomolecular medicine community and is commonly used as an effective adjunct to conventional oncologic therapy.

Oncologist Victor Marcial, M.D., has recent experience using it. He says: "We studied patients with advanced cancer (stage 4). 40 patients received 40,000–75,000 mg intravenously several times a week. . . In addition, they received a diet and other supplements. The initial tumor response rate was achieved in 75% of patients, defined as a 50% reduction or more in tumor size . . . As a radiation oncologist, I also give radiation therapy. Vitamin C has two effects. It increases the beneficial effects of radiation and chemotherapy and decreases the adverse effects. But this is not a subtle effect, (it) is not 15–20%, it's a dramatic effect. Once you start using IV vitamin C, the effect is so dramatic that it is difficult to go back to not using it."[3]

In 2009 and 2010, Riordan IV-C and Cancer Symposiums brought together medical professionals, researchers, and IV-C practitioners from the United States and abroad. The latest advancements in intravenous vitamin C cancer therapy were presented in detail, recorded on video, and are now available for free access at www.riordanclinic.org/education/symposium/2009.shtml (twelve lectures) and www.riordanclinic.org/education/symposium/2010.shtml (nine lectures).

Readers are urged to have their physicians (especially oncologists) watch these important presentations.

References

1. Free access to full text papers at www.riordanclinic.org/research/journal-articles.shtml and also at http://orthomolecular.org/library/jom/

2. Download the Riordan protocol free of charge at www.doctoryourself.com/RiordanIVC.pdf or at www.riordanclinic.org/ research/vitaminc/protocol.shtml

3. Presentation at the Medical Sciences Campus, University of Puerto Rico, April 12, 2010.

Opponents of vitamin C therapy would do well to acknowledge that Pauling and Cameron's work has been confirmed, perhaps most notably at Japan's Saga University by Murata and others (see "Recommended Reading" at the end of this chapter). Dr. Murata administered more than 30,000 mg per day and had even better results with terminally ill cancer patients. In the words of Dr. Louis Lasagna of the University of Rochester Medical School, "It seems indefensible not to at least try substantial doses of vitamin C in these patients."

There are many good reasons to give large quantities of vitamin C to a cancer patient. Ascorbic acid strengthens the collagen "glue" that holds healthy cells together and retards the spread of an existing tumor. The vitamin also greatly strengthens the immune system and provides a surprising level of pain relief.

But there is more. As mentioned above, vitamin C has been shown to be preferentially toxic to tumor cells. Laboratory and clinical studies indicate that, in high enough doses, one can maintain blood plasma concentrations of ascorbic acid high enough to selectively kill tumor cells. If you have not heard about this, it is probably because most of the best-publicized (but worst designed) vitamin C and cancer studies simply have not utilized high enough doses. Now, however, Hugh Riordan, M.D., and colleagues have treatment data which "demonstrate the ability to sustain plasma levels of ascorbic acid in humans above levels which are toxic to tumor cells in vitro and suggests the feasibility of using AA as a cytotoxic chemotherapeutic agent." Please see "Recommended Reading" for three of Dr. Riordan's studies.

HALF TRUTH IS NO TRUTH AT ALL

An Internet search for "orthomolecular medicine" can bring up some remarkably official-looking misinformation. A prime example is the American Cancer Society's webpage on orthomolecular medicine, which is incomplete, negative, and fallacious. (www.cancer.org/ Treatment/TreatmentsandSideEffects/ComplementaryandAlternativeMedicine/HerbsVitamins andMinerals/orthomolecular-medicine; accessed June 2012)

Carefully search that same ACS webpage for the word *intravenous*. The word is not even there, even though the U.S. National Institutes of Health sponsored research that clearly showed that intravenous vitamin C selectively kills malignant cells. The study concluded that "Vitamin C at high concentrations is toxic to cancer cells in vitro."[1] *In vitro* refers to a laboratory culture. For a real-world test, the same team then gave IV vitamin C to cancer patients, and it worked very well.[2] You would think that the American Cancer Society would find this at least a little intriguing, and maybe even mention it. But no: no mention at all.

On the other hand, the American Cancer Society is blatantly bullish on chemotherapy. Odd, really, since a peer-reviewed study showed that conventional chemotherapy contributes only 2.1 percent to five-year cancer survival in the United States.[3] As of this writing, the ACS webpage indicates that it has not been updated since 2008, yet all three of these studies were published well before then. Perhaps readers may be able to help ACS modernize and improve the accuracy of their presentation. You can send a message to the American Cancer Society at www.cancer.org/Aboutus/ HowWeHelpYou/app/contact-us.aspx.

References

1. Padayatty SJ, Sun H, Wang Y, Riordan HD, Hewitt SM, Katz A, Wesley RA, & Levine M. (2004). Vitamin C pharmacokinetics: implications for oral and intravenous use. *Ann Intern Med.* 140(7):533–537. Full text free download: www.annals.org/content/140/7/533.full.pdf

2. Padayatty SJ, Riordan HD, Hewitt SM, Katz A, Hoffer LJ, & Levine M. (2006). Intravenously administered vitamin C as cancer therapy: three cases. *CMAJ.* 174(7):937–942. Free full text: www.ncbi.nlm.nih.gov/pmc/articles/PMC1405876/ ?tool=pubmed

3. Morgan G, Ward R, & Barton M. (2004). The contribution of cytotoxic chemotherapy to 5-year survival in adult malignancies. *Clin Oncol (R Coll Radiol)* 16:549–560.

Abstract: www.ncbi.nlm.nih.gov/pubmed?term=Morgan%20G%2C%20Ward%20R%2C%20Barton%20M.%20The%20contribution%20of%20cytotoxic%20chemotherapy

These and many additional C-versus-cancer references may be obtained through your local library. A site search at my doctoryourself.com website will also turn up a bevy of them. You will want to request your librarian's assistance in locating some of the pioneering papers, such as those from the 1940s and 50s by William McCormick. His excellent "Have We Forgotten the Lesson of Scurvy?" and "Ascorbic Acid as a Chemotherapeutic Agent" are worth the search. Dr. McCormick shows that cancer symptoms and vitamin C deficiency symptoms overlap. The similarity between scurvy, which is obvious vitamin C deficiency, and cancer (particularly some forms of leukemia) is so great that it is incredible that many billions of dollars of cancer research in the United States has failed to notice this.

Residential treatment for cancer by nutritional means has, for some time now, been readily available in Mexico, just south of the U.S. border. Odd, isn't it, that Americans have to flee the land of the free and home of the brave to get freedom of choice in cancer therapy? That's free trade for you.

Precious few hospital-based megavitamin programs are available anywhere in the United States. Government, medical society, and insurance company pressure on doctors who advocate nutritional therapy is high, research evidence notwithstanding. This will change, however, if citizens voice their views to the FDA, the AMA, the American Cancer Society, the National Cancer Institute, their lawmakers in Congress and state capitals, their own insurance companies, and their family doctors, and insist on unrestricted freedom of access to all options, including the unorthodox therapies, for cancer patients in this country.

While I'm at it, a caution. Beware of wolves in sheep's clothing: hospitals and other providers that offer so-called "holistic," "nutrition-based," "integrated," or "comprehensive" therapeutic programs. The majority of them are only paying lip-service to consumers' requests for alternative cancer treatments, just to get them in the door. Their main approaches still tend to be chemo, radiation, and surgery. As a benchmark, first ask them if they give intravenous vitamin C, 30,000 to 100,000 mg every other day. That'll settle out the mud in a hurry.

VITAMIN C SLOWS CANCER DOWN AND CAN REVERSE IT

The BBC reported on Aug 4, 2008, that "Vitamin C slows cancer growth. An injection of a high dose of vitamin C may be able to hold back the advance of cancers, US scientists claim. The vitamin may start a destructive chain reaction within the cancer cell." The injection "halved the size" of tumors. Researchers said that vitamin C treatment "significantly decreased growth rates" of ovarian, pancreatic, and malignant brain tumors in mice. These particular forms of cancer are among the most difficult to treat. And yet, such high, cancer-stopping levels of vitamin C can be "readily achieved in humans given ascorbate intravenously."[1] This is very good news.

Here's more: there have actually been **many** well-designed clinical studies that show that large doses of vitamin C and other nutrients improve both quality and length of life for cancer patients. The key is to employ sufficiently high quantities, appropriately administered. More orange juice just won't do it.

Vitamin C has been successfully used as an adjunctive cancer therapy for decades. Over thirty years ago, a review of cancer research concluded that "Many factors involved in host resistance to neoplasia are significantly dependent upon the availability of ascorbate."[2] Beginning in the 1970s, a number of well-designed studies show that very large doses of vitamin C improve both quality and length of life for cancer patients since they invariably are "significantly depleted of ascorbic acid." When given intravenous vitamin C, "The mean survival time is more than 4.2

times as great for the ascorbate subjects . . . This simple and safe form of medication is of definite value in the treatment of patients with advanced cancer."[3] Additional clinical trials have confirmed this over the past several decades.[4]

Even more importantly, recent research indicates that in high doses, vitamin C is selectively toxic to cancer cells. That means vitamin C can function very much like chemotherapy is supposed to, but without the severe side effects of chemotherapy. "A regimen of daily pharmacologic ascorbate treatment significantly decreased growth rates of ovarian, pancreatic, and glioblastoma tumors established in mice. Similar pharmacologic concentrations were readily achieved in humans given ascorbate intravenously."[5]

References

1. Chen Q, Espey MG, Sun AY, Pooput C, Kirk KL, Krishna MC, Khosh DB, Drisko J, & Levine M. (2008). Pharmacologic doses of ascorbate act as a prooxidant and decrease growth of aggressive tumor xenografts in mice. *PNAS* 105(32):11105–9.

2. Cameron E, Pauling L, & Leibovitz B. (1979). Ascorbic acid and cancer: a review. Cancer Res. 39(3):663–81.

3. Cameron E, & Pauling L. (1976). Supplemental ascorbate in the supportive treatment of cancer: Prolongation of survival times in terminal human cancer. *PNAS* 73(10):3685–9. Read the original paper at http://profiles.nlm.nih.gov/MM/B/B/K/ Z/_/ mmbbkz.pdf

4. Murata A, Morishige F, & Yamaguchi H. (1982). Prolongation of survival times of terminal cancer patients by administration of large doses of ascorbate. *International Journal of Vitamin and Nutrition Research,* Suppl. 23:103–113; Null G, Robins H, Tanenbaum, M, & Jennings P. (1997). Vitamin C and the treatment of cancer: abstracts and commentary from the scientific literature. *Townsend Letter for Doctors & Patients;* Vitamin C and cancer revisited. (2008). *PNAS* (32):11037–8; Riordan HD, Riordan NH, Jackson JA, et al. (2004). Intravenous vitamin C as a chemotherapy agent: a report on clinical cases. Puerto Rico Health Sciences J 23(2):115–118.

5. Chen Q, Espey MG, Sun AY, et al. (2008). Pharmacologic doses of ascorbate act as a prooxidant and decrease growth of aggressive tumor xenografts in mice. *PNAS* 105(32):11105–9. See also: Chen Q, Espey MG, Sun AY, et al. (2007). Ascorbate in pharmacologic concentrations selectively generates ascorbate radical and hydrogen peroxide in extracellular fluid in vivo. *PNAS* 104(21):8749–54. Also: Riordan NH, et al. (1995). Intravenous ascorbate as a tumor cytotoxic chemotherapeutic agent. *Medical Hypotheses* 44(3): 207–213.

VITAMIN C AS CANCER TREATMENT: A TIMELINE

2012

Vitamin C shown to prevent and treat radiation-damaged DNA.

Workers with severe radiation exposure at the Fukushima nuclear plant had major reduction in cancer risk when supplemented with vitamin C and other antioxidative nutrients. Sixteen men aged between 32 and 59 years worked five to six weeks in a radiation-contaminated area, collecting contaminated water, measuring radiation levels, operating heavy machinery, and removing debris. Blood samples were obtained to measure whole blood counts and blood chemistry, plasma levels of free DNA, and 47 cancer-related gene expressions. Four workers who took intravenous vitamin C (25,000 mg) therapy before they went in, and continuously took antioxidative supplements during the working period, had no significant change in both free DNA and overall cancer risk.

Three workers that did not have preventive intravenous vitamin C had an increase in calculated cancer risk. After two months of treatment with intravenous vitamin C and oral antioxidative nutritional supplements, free DNA returned to normal level and cancer-risk score was significantly decreased.[1]

These findings, by Atsuo Yanagisawa, M.D., Ph.D., and colleagues, are important clinical demonstrations confirming research done nearly twenty years ago showing that pretreatment with vitamin C, by oral intake or injection, increased cell survival after the injection of radioactive Iodine-131 in mice.[2] Oral intake of alpha-lipoic acid and vitamin E reduced urinary radioactivity and oxidative stress in irradiated children in Chernobyl.[3] Furthermore, there have been numerous scientific studies about the radio-protective effects of other vitamins, minerals, and antioxidative nutrients.

2008

Korean doctors report that intravenous vitamin C "plays a crucial role in the suppression of proliferation of several types of cancer," notably melanoma.[4]

2006

Canadian doctors report intravenous vitamin C is successful in treating cancer.[5]

2005

Research sponsored by the US National Institutes of Health shows that high levels of vitamin C kill cancer cells without harming normal cells.[6]

2004

Doctors in America and Puerto Rico publish clinical cases of vitamin C successes against cancer.[7]

1990

American doctors successfully use vitamin C to treat kidney cancer[8], and in 1995 and 1996, other cancers.[9] Using 30,000 mg of intravenous vitamin C twice per week, they found that "metastatic lesions in the lung and liver of a man with a primary renal cell carcinoma disappeared in a matter of weeks . . . We subsequently reported a case of resolution of bone metastases in a patient with primary breast cancer [1A] using infusions of 100 grams, once or twice per week."[10]

1982

Japanese doctors show that vitamin C greatly prolonged the lives of terminal cancer patients.[11]

1976

Physicians in Scotland show that intravenous vitamin C improved quality and length of life in terminal cancer patients.[12]

We could actually take this timeline all the way back to 1954. That was the year William McCormick, M.D., reported that there was clinical evidence that cancer patients tested for vitamin C were seriously deficient, often by as much as 4,500 mg.[13,14,15] When the RDA for C is 90 mg, is it any wonder?

References

1. Yanagisawa, A. Effect of vitamin C and anti-oxidative nutrition on radiation-induced gene expression in Fukushima nuclear plant workers. Free download of full presentation at www.doctoryourself.com/Radiation_VitC.pptx.pdf.

2. Venkat, R. Narra, Roger W. Howell, Kandula S. R. Sastry, and Dandamudi V. Rao. *J Nucl Med,* 1993. Vol. 34, No. 4, pp. 637–640. See http://jnm.snmjournals.org/content/34/4/637.long.

3. Korkina, L., et al. Antioxidant therapy in children affected by irradiation from the Chernobyl nuclear accident. *Biochem Soc Trans,* 1993. 21:314S. PMID: 8224459. See www.ncbi.nlm.nih.gov/pubmed?term=8224459.

4. Lee SK, Kang JS, Jung da J, et al. Vitamin C suppresses proliferation of the human melanoma cell SK-MEL-2 through the inhibition of cyclooxygenase-2 (COX-2) expression and the modulation of insulin-like growth factor II (IGF-II) production. *J Cell Physiol.,* 2008. 216(1):180–8.

5. Padayatty, et al. Intravenously administered vitamin C as cancer therapy: three cases. *Canadian Medical Association Journal,* 2006. 174(7):937–942. www.cmaj.ca/cgi/reprint/174/7/937.

6. Chen Q, Espey MG, Krishna MC, et al. Pharmacologic ascorbic acid concentrations selectively kill cancer cells: action as a pro-drug to deliver hydrogen peroxide to tissues. *PNAS,* 2005. 102(38):13604–9.

7. Riordan HD, Riordan NH, Jackson JA, Casciari, JJ., Hunninghake, R, Gonzalez MJ, Mora, EM, Miranda-Massari, JR, Rosario, N, and Rivera, A. Intravenous Vitamin C as a Chemotherapy Agent: a Report on Clinical Cases. *Puerto Rico Health Sciences J,* 2004. 23(2):115–118.

8. Riordan HD, Jackson JA, Schultz M. Case study: high-dose intravenous vitamin C in the treatment of a patient with adenocarcinoma of the kidney. *J Ortho Med,* 1990. 5: 5–7.

9. Riordan NH, Jackson JA, and Riordan HD. Intravenous vitamin C in a terminal cancer patient. *J Ortho Med,* 1996. 11:80–82. Also: Riordan, NH, et al. (1995). Intravenous ascorbate as a tumor cytotoxic chemotherapeutic agent. *Medical Hypotheses* 44(3):207–213.

10. Riordan NH, Riordan HD, Hunninghake RE. Intravenous ascorbate as a chemotherapeutic and biologic response modifying agent. www.doctoryourself.com/riordan1.html and www.canceraction.org.gg/recnac.htm. Additional papers may be read at http://brightspot.org/cresearch/index.shtml.

11. Murata A, Morishige F and Yamaguchi H. Prolongation of survival times of terminal cancer patients by administration of large doses of ascorbate. *International Journal of Vitamin and Nutrition Research,* 1982. Suppl. 23 :103–113. (Also in Hanck, A., ed. 1982. Vitamin C: New Clinical Applications. Bern: Huber, 103–113.)

12. Cameron E and Pauling L. Supplemental ascorbate in the supportive treatment of cancer: prolongation of survival times in terminal human cancer. PNAS, 1976. 73:3685–3689. Also: Cameron E and Pauling L. Supplemental ascorbate in the supportive treatment of cancer: Reevaluation of prolongation of survival times in terminal human cancer. *PNAS,* 1978. 75:4538–4542. And: Cameron E and Pauling L. Survival times of terminal lung cancer patients treated with ascorbate. *J. Intern. Acad. Prev. Med.,* 1981. 6: 21–27.

13. McCormick, WJ. (1954) Cancer: The preconditioning factor in pathogenesis. *Archives of Pediatrics of New York,* 1954. 71:313.

14. McCormick, WJ. (1959). Cancer: A collagen disease, secondary to a nutritional deficiency? *Arch. Pediat.,* 1959. 76:166.

15. McCormick, WJ. (1962) Have we forgotten the lesson of scurvy? *Journal of Applied Nutrition,* 1962. 15(1,2):4–12.

For Further Information

Cameron E and Pauling L. 1993. *Cancer and Vitamin C,* revised edition. Philadelphia: Camino Books.

Hoffer A. High doses of antioxidants including vitamin C do not decrease the efficacy of chemotherapy. Townsend Letter for Doctors and Patients. July 2000. #204, p.120–21. www.doctoryourself.com/chemo.html .

Hoffer A and Pauling L. 1999/ Vitamin C and Cancer: Discovery, Recovery, Controversy. Quarry Press, Kingston, ON. Reviewed at www.doctoryourself.com/hoffer_vitc_can.html .

Moss RW. 2000. Antioxidants against Cancer. Brooklyn, NY: Equinox Press. Also: Moss RW. 1995. Questioning Chemotherapy. Brooklyn, NY:: Equinox Press.

Riordan HD, Hunninghake, RE, Riordan NH, Jackson, JJ, Meng, XL, Taylor, P, Casciari, JJ, Gonzalez MJ, Miranda-Massari, JR, Mora, EM, Norberto, R, and Rivera, A. Intravenous Ascorbic Acid: Protocol for its Application and Use. *Puerto Rico Health Sciences Journal,* 2003. 22:3.

WHAT INTRAVENOUS VITAMIN C DID FOR TERESA

Teresa was a seventy-two-year-old lady with liver and colon cancer. Talk about a tough combination. She was in pain, tired, depressed, and had no appetite. Her daughter Alice, bless her heart, refused to take "there's nothing else we can do" as an answer. No sooner were they out the oncologist's door that Alice decided to look into intravenous vitamin C therapy. She downloaded a free copy of Dr. Hugh Riordan's detailed intravenous vitamin C treatment protocol (http://www.doctoryourself.com/RiordanIVC.pdf), and then searched the Internet for a physician that would administer it. Alice had to take her weak and ailing mother for over an hour-long drive to get to him, but she did it. Teresa had a several-hour IV session and received over 30,000 mg of vitamin C.

And here's what happened next.

On the drive home, the mother asked to stop for lunch . . .because she was hungry. And, she was cheerful, optimistic, and comfortable. Imagine: one IV-C treatment and appetite and energy came back immediately. Not weeks; not days. But hours. This is as much about quality of life as it is about stopping cancer.

A MESSAGE TO ONCOLOGISTS READING THIS BOOK

Victor Marcial, M.D., *is an oncologist in Puerto Rico. Here he speaks of his experiences using intravenous vitamin C as an adjunctive cancer treatment:*

"We studied patients with advanced cancer (stage 4). 40 patients received 40,000–75,000 mg intravenously several times a week. These are patients that have not responded to other treatments. Phase 1 of the study is to assess safety and response. In addition, they received a diet and other supplements. The initial tumor response rate was achieved in 75% of patients, defined as a 50% reduction or more in tumor size. In the majority of the patients the tumors grew back when patients stopped the treatment. These interventions have to be continued for a prolonged time, sometimes forever. More studies are needed to have a better understanding on this.

"Our second collaboration is the use of vitamin C during radiation and chemotherapy.As a radiation oncologist, I also give radiation therapy. Vitamin C has two effects. It increases the beneficial effects of radiation and chemotherapy and decreases the adverse effects. But this is not a subtle effect, is not 15–20%, it's a dramatic effect. Once you start using IV vitamin C, the effect is so dramatic that it is difficult to go back to not using it. That is what happened to me.

"Physicians need to gain knowledge in those areas that are not covered in medical school and continuing medical education. We are now seeing a new medicine." (Presented at the Medical Sciences Campus, University of Puerto Rico, April 12, 2010)

In 2009 and 2010, Riordan IV-C and Cancer Symposiums brought together medical professionals, researchers and IV-C practitioners from the United States and abroad. The advancements in intravenous vitamin C cancer therapy were presented in detail, recorded on video, and are now available for free access at http://www.riordanclinic.org/education/symposium/s2009 (twelve lectures) and http://www.riordanclinic.org/education/symposium/s2010 (nine lectures)

For further reading:

Padayatty, et al. (2006). Intravenously administered vitamin C as cancer therapy: three cases. *Canadian Medical Association Journal* 174(7):937–942. www.cmaj.ca/cgi/reprint/174/7/937

OTHER VITAMINS

Beta-carotene

To hear the way media often report about it,[1] carotene somehow causes cancer! Carotene? The orange pigment in carrots? Oh no: just the carotene in vitamin tablets. In one study, the authors actually concluded that "high-dose beta-carotene supplementation appears to increase the risk of lung cancer among current smokers."[2] The "high doses" they say are harmful are only 20–30 milligrams (mg) per day. A milligram is a thousandth of a gram, and a gram is a fourth of a teaspoon. That's a mighty small bit. It is not a "high dose"; it is too low a dose. Antioxidants are consumed in trying to protect smokers from tobacco smoke. Tobacco smoke is loaded with literally dozens of toxins. Studies with smokers reporting failure or claiming actual harm are flawed: low doses of antioxidants are ineffective.[3,4]

Carotene in high doses strengthens the immune system by helping the body to make more helper T cells.[5] One well-controlled study used far more carotene and got very good results: the dose employed was 180 milligrams of beta-carotene per day. This is the equivalent of nearly three dozen carrots.

"Numerous animal and laboratory studies have substantiated beta-carotene's ability to inhibit tumor cell growth and the progression of carcinogenesis," said the authors of a comprehensive review of antioxidant research.[6] Another study showed that men consuming the beta-carotene equivalent of just one carrot each day, over 25 years, had a 28 percent lower risk of death from all causes compared with men eating less.[7] *USA Today* commented that you should "keep eating beta-carotene-rich foods. Nobody disputes that the beta-carotene in food is healthful and safe."[8]

Safe in food, but perhaps not safe in supplements? Whether carotene comes from pills or your plate should not matter, unless synthetic beta-carotene is less effective than natural food-source beta-carotene. And that is a distinct possibility.[7] This is why I recommend carrot juice, and lots of it. More on that later in the juicing chapter.

Nine out of ten Americans do not meet the (rather low) US RDA minimum of five servings a day of fruit or vegetables. One-quarter of Americans do not eat even one single serving of a fruit or vegetable in a given day.

Everywhere you look you see cancer-fighting recommendations for all of us to eat more green and yellow vegetables. For smokers, the stakes are higher. For them, six carrots, or their supplemental equivalent of 20–30 mg of carotene a day is too little, too late. Indeed, cigarette smoking is "significantly related to lower beta-carotene concentrations (even) after supplementation."[9] Smokers need more carotene, not less. And they need it any way they can get it.

Smokers can start by eating their vegetables. (An even better start would be to stop smoking.) Beta-carotene is abundant in orange fruits and vegetables, such as pumpkin, squash, and apricots, as well as dark green leafy vegetables like spinach. One medium carrot has only about 30 calories. It has zero cholesterol. It has zero fat. It is an excellent source of potassium and fiber. A single medium sweet potato contains about 10 milligrams of beta-carotene. Do you really think that two or three sweet potatoes a day is harmful? Do you really think that six carrots a day are bad for you? Smoking is what is harmful to smokers. Carrots are good for you. Cigarettes aren't.

One might say that the recent analysis actually shows that smoking probably destroys at least 20–30 mg of beta-carotene a day. To conclude that smokers need less seems a bit odd, doesn't it? What other antioxidant nutrients do smokers need less of? Certainly they cannot do with less vitamin C. Nearly fifty-five years ago, William J. McCormick, M.D., wrote that smoking just one single cigarette neutralizes in the body approximately 25 mg of ascorbic acid. That is 500 mg of vitamin C deficit per pack. The doctor wrote: "The ability of the heavy smoker to maintain normal vitamin C status from dietary sources is obviously questionable."[10] This was quite a statement in 1954, at a time when physicians were literally endorsing their favorite cigarette in magazines and on television commercials.

At 6 to 7 mg of beta-carotene per typical carrot, the study is saying that the amount of beta-carotene equivalent to four carrots per day is potentially dangerous to smokers. That is a bit counterintuitive. Where are all these carrot-eating corpses? Where are the bodies? If you search decades of the medical literature, and also search the American Association of Poison Control Centers' collected data,[11] you will find there have been no deaths whatsoever from beta-carotene. None. Zip. Nada. Zero. Evidently it must be singularly difficult to kill yourself with carrots. Or with carotene supplements.

Excess carotene causes the skin to turn slightly orange, once succinctly described as resembling an artificial suntan. The medical name for this condition is "hypercarotenosis" or just "carotenosis." "Hypercarotenemia" refers to elevated blood levels of carotene, and is also called just "carotenemia." Both are harmless.

In performing their limited four-study review, the authors said that they looked at many "national brands" of carotene-containing vitamin supplements. The "national brands" they should have been looking at are Marlboro, Winston, and Camel. The authors are finding fault with the wrong plant. It's not carrots that hurt smokers; it's tobacco.

Given all this, it is no surprise that the study found that ex-smokers were not at all negatively affected by beta-carotene. Why? Because they stopped smoking, that's why. The preeminent danger is smoking itself. Stop today, and go have plenty of carotene.

References

1. Harding A. Vision vitamins may be harmful for smokers. Reuters, Thu Jul 10, 2008. www.reuters.com/article/healthNews/idUS-COL06955420080710.

2. Tanvetyanon T, Bepler G. Beta-carotene in multivitamins and the possible risk of lung cancer among smokers versus former smokers: a meta-analysis and evaluation of national brands. *Cancer*. 2008 Jul 1;113(1):150–7.

3. Heinonen OP et al. The effect of vitamin E and beta-carotene on the incidence of lung cancer and other cancers in male smokers. *New England J of Med* 330:1029–1035, 1994.

4. Vivekananthan DP, Penn MS, Sapp SK, Hsu A, Topol EJ. Use of antioxidant vitamins for the prevention of cardiovascular disease: meta-analysis of randomised trials. Lancet. 2003 Jun 14;361(9374):2017–23. Also: Goran Bjelakovic, Dimitrinka Nikolova, Rosa G Simonetti, Christian Gluud. Antioxidant supplements for prevention of gastrointestinal cancers: a systematic review and meta-analysis. *Lancet* 2004; 364: 1219–28.

5. Alexander, M et al. Oral beta-carotene can increase the number of OKT4 cells in human blood, *Immunology Letters*, 9:221–224, 1985.

6. Patrick L. Beta-Carotene: The Controversy Continues. Alternative Medicine Review, Dec, 2000. http://findarticles.com/p/articles/mi_m0FDN/is_6_5/ai_68727251/print?tag=artBody;col1 (This article contains a thorough discussion of natural vs. synthetic beta-carotene.)

7. Pandey DK, Shekelle R, Selwyn BJ, Tangney C, Stamler J. Dietary vitamin C and beta-carotene and risk of death in middle-aged men. The Western Electric Study. *Am J Epidemiol*. 1995 Dec 15;142(12):1269–78.

8. www.usaweekend.com/food/carper_archive/960407carper_eatsmart.html

9. McLarty JW, Holiday DB, Girard WM, Yanagihara RH, Kummet TD, Greenberg SD. Beta-Carotene, vitamin A, and lung cancer chemoprevention: results of an intermediate endpoint study. *Am J Clin Nutr*. 1995 Dec;62(6 Suppl):1431S-1438S.

10. Saul AW. Taking the Cure: The pioneering work of William J. McCormick, M.D. *J Orthomolecular Med*, 2003. Vol 18, No 2, p 93–96. www.doctoryourself.com/mccormick.html

11. www.aapcc.org/dnn/NPDS/AnnualReports/tabid/125/Default.aspx

B-Complex Vitamins

B-complex vitamins (as well as vitamin C) are water-soluble, easily-lost-under-stress vitamins. There is ever-growing evidence that stress itself is a major factor in cancer—which makes sense, since stress depletes the body of B and C vitamins. Only in theory does the "balanced diet" that all of us are supposed to be getting every day supply ample quantities of these and all other vitamins. But no realistic allowance is made for the very real psychological and physiological demands that each person is daily subjected to. This is all the more true for a cancer patient.

In America, vitamin deficiency is the rule, not the exception. We are vitamin-deficient throughout our youth and even during gestation. According to *Nutrition Action Healthletter*, November 1993, researchers at the Children's Hospital of Philadelphia found that the mothers of children with cancer were less likely to have eaten fruits and vegetables, and were less likely to have taken multivitamins during the first six weeks of their pregnancy than mothers of healthy children. This resulting insufficient intake of folate, one of the B vitamins, appears to be a major cause of what are called primitive neuroectodermal tumors.

Vitamin B$_6$ (Pyridoxine)

Vitamin B$_6$ has been found to be as effective, at least, as the drug usually used to treat recurrent bladder cancer, says *American Family Physician*. Many bladder cancer patients are deficient in B$_6$. And they're not alone: 99 percent of adults nineteen and older get less than the RDA of B$_6$.

Vitamin B$_6$ Reduces Colon Cancer

A study of almost 5,000 persons has shown that consuming more vitamin B$_6$ means less colon cancer.[1] The researchers wrote that the effect was "moderately strong," and with cancer, that is very important. Previous studies have indicated the same thing: B$_6$ substantially reduces colon cancer risk.[2,3]

Inadequate intake of B$_6$ is common everywhere in the United States. "Across the study population," said the authors, "we noticed participants with inadequate vitamin B$_6$ status even though they reported consuming more than the Recommended Daily Allowance of vitamin B$_6$, which is less than 2 milligrams per day." Most women using oral contraceptives are vitamin B$_6$ deficient unless they also take vitamin B$_6$ supplements. Smokers and the elderly are also likely to be low. Many of those who take B$_6$ supplements are *still* getting too little.[4]

Many people do not take adequate doses of B$_6$ because they have been cautioned against supplementing with this vitamin. An unelected committee assembled by the National Academy of Sciences' Institute of Medicine's Food and Nutrition Board has created an arbitrary "Safe Upper Limit" of 100 mg.[5] That is nonsense. Alan Gaby, M.D., wrote that B$_6$ (pyridoxine) side effects were found in a few people taking "2,000 mg/day or more of pyridoxine, although some were taking only 500 mg/day. There is a single case report of a neuropathy occurring in a person taking 200 mg/day of pyridoxine, but the reliability of that case report is unclear. The individual in question was never examined, but was merely interviewed by telephone after responding to a local television report that publicized pyridoxine-induced neuropathy." Dr. Gaby stated that there have been no reports of adverse B$_6$ effects at under 200 mg/day.[6]

A hearty serving of beef liver contains only 1.2 mg of B_6. Supplementation appears to make more and more sense.

References

1. Theodoratou E, Farrington SM, Tenesa A, et al. Dietary vitamin B_6 intake and the risk of colorectal cancer. *Cancer Epidemiol Biomarkers Prev.,* 2008, 17(1):171–82.

2. Matsubara K, Komatsu S, Oka T, and Kato N. Vitamin B_6-mediated suppression of colon tumorigenesis, cell proliferation, and angiogenesis (review). *J Nutr Biochem.,* 2003. 14(5):246–50. See also: Komatsu S, Yanaka N, Matsubara K, and Kato N. Antitumor effect of vitamin B_6 and its mechanisms. *Biochim Biophys Acta.,* 2003, 1647(1–2):127–30 ("Epidemiological studies have reported an inverse association between vitamin B(6) intake and colon cancer risk"). See www.ncbi.nlm.nih.gov/pubmed/12686121.

3. Zhang SM, et al. Folate, vitamin B6, multivitamin supplements, and colorectal cancer risk in women. *Am J Epidemiol.,* 2006,163(2): 108–115. See http://aje.oxfordjournals.org/cgi/content/full/163/2/108.

4. Morris MS, Picciano MF, Jacques PF, and Selhub J. Plasma pyridoxal 5'-phosphate in the US population: the National Health and Nutrition Examination Survey, 2003–2004. *Am J Clin Nutr.,* 2008, 87(5):1446–54. See also: www.lef.org/whatshot/ 2008_05. htm#Vitamin-B6-RDA-questioned.

5. See www.iom.edu/CMS/3788/3971.aspx.

6. Gaby AR. "Safe Upper Limits" for nutritional supplements: one giant step backward. *J Orthomolecular Med,* 2003, 18(3,4):126–130. See http://findarticles.com/p/articles/mi_m0ISW/is_243/ai_109946551 and www.iahf.com/20040127.html.

Nonvitamin Factors

Chlorophyll, the substance in plants that makes them green, may help control cancer by inhibiting cell mutations. Sprouts and the live food factors within them, such as enzymes and chlorophyll, have been extensively used by Dr. Ann Wigmore in nutritional programs to shrink or reduce tumors. The world's foremost authority on the anticancer properties of sprouts, wheat grass juice, fasting, and raw foods, Dr. Wigmore's lessons on the subject began with her Lithuanian grandmother and culminated with her self-cure of colon cancer using living foods. Her books include *Why Suffer?, Be Your Own Doctor,* and *Recipes for Longer Life.*

Zinc may also play a role in the prevention and treatment of certain forms of cancer. A study at MIT showed that animals fed a low-zinc diet are more likely to get cancer than those with normal diets. The majority of Americans do not get adequate zinc in their diets, either. There is almost certainly a link between selenium intake and cancer. Parts of the country with selenium-rich soils have less cancer than selenium-poor-soil populations.

Of course, all these vitamin and mineral deficiencies are just aspects of the big problem: the overcooked, sugar-laden, meat-heavy diet we eat that got us into trouble in the first place. These "foods"—and other processed, worthless stomach fillers—are not good sources of what we need to live in health. Our national cancer epidemic is not a mystery. You don't have to just wait in line for a terminal disease with your name on it. There is much more to cancer prevention and therapy than the "food groups" and chemotherapy, radiation, or surgery. As much as these may help, there is at least as much good scientific evidence that nutritional alternative approaches to cancer work just as well or better. The essential cause of cancer most likely is many years of deficient diets.

It Takes a Team to Win the Game

Our population-wide but medically disavowed vitamin deficiency that is almost certainly the single most overlooked predisposing cause of cancer. It would be a tragic mistake to center any discussion of cancer on a single nutrient, or only on nutrients. Research will continue to confirm that all nutrients, and most certainly all the vitamins, are required to prevent and to stop cancer. After all, which wheel on your car can you afford to do without? Which wing on your airplane can we leave off next time you fly?

There are other factors, such as stress, that increase risk of virtually all diseases including cancer. Stress causes vitamin washout. We can either decrease stress or increase our vitamin supplementation, or preferably do both. Transcendental Meditation has been demonstrated to be clinically effective in both stress reduction and disease prevention. There have literally been hundreds of scientific papers discussing this important effect.[1] Even critics concede that about fifty rigorous research studies provide strong, statistically significant confirmation. One example: Dr. David Orme-Johnson has shown that hospital admissions for benign and malignant tumors are less than half as common for long-time meditators.[2] If there were a drug that reduced tumor incidence by 50 percent, you would have heard it proclaimed from the rooftops. Simple and natural tools are greatly underrated.

References

1. Scientific Research on Maharishi's Transcendental Meditation and TM-Sidhi Program: Collected Papers, Vols. 1–5. Maharishi Intl Univ of Management, Fairfield Iowa, 1989. http://www.mum.edu/tm_research/bibliography.html

2. Orme-Johnson, D.W. Medical care utilization and the Transcendental Meditation program. *Psychosomatic Medicine* 49: 493–507, 1987. See also: Orme-Johnson, D.W. and Herron, R.E. An innovative approach to reducing medical care utilization and expenditures. *The American Journal of Managed Care* 3: 135–144, 1997.

DAILY ASPIRIN USE LINKED WITH PANCREATIC CANCER

Research has indicated that women who take just one aspirin a day, "which millions do to prevent heart attack and stroke as well as to treat headaches—may raise their risk of getting deadly pancreatic cancer. . . . Pancreatic cancer affects only 31,000 Americans a year, but it kills virtually all its victims within three years. The study of 88,000 nurses found that those who took two or more aspirins a week for 20 years or more had a 58 percent higher risk of pancreatic cancer."[1] *Women who took two or more aspirin tablets per day had an alarming 86 percent greater risk of pancreatic cancer.*

Study author Dr. Eva Schernhammer of Harvard Medical School was quoted as saying: "Apart from smoking, this is one of the few risk factors that have been identified for pancreatic cancer. Initially we expected that aspirin would protect against pancreatic cancer."

Reference

1. Fox M. Daily aspirin use linked with pancreatic cancer. Reuters, Oct 27, 2003.

The time to turn it all around is now, whether you have cancer or not. There is no need to wait for AMA, FDA, *New York Times,* American Cancer Society, or anyone else's approval. The safety margin with nutrients is enormous. Deficiency is what's dangerous. A determined patient, some good references and reading, an open-minded doctor, and the nutritional facts can do wonders. You may experience some difficulty in coming up with the open-minded doctor, but the rest is completely within your power. The following guide can help get you started. *Before embarking on any anticancer program you should consult your health care provider.*

Nutritional Support for Cancer Patients: A Naturopathic Approach

A. Digestive enzyme tablets Two or more multiple digestive enzyme tablets per meal. The theory is that in cancer patients, the liver produces insufficient enzymes. Cancer patients eat and eat and eat but don't get the good stuff out of their food. They appear to be starving to death. Enzymes break down food so you can get the nourishment in it. A "multiple digestive enzyme" preparation is most efficient.

B. Kelp 5–8 kelp tablets per day. Kelp tablets are an iodine supplement. They have been reported to help resist healthy cell damage from radiation treatments.

C. Carrot juice Begin by drinking at least one pint of carrot juice per day. Goal: up to two quarts (eight glasses). Raw food has lots of enzymes, and carrots are loaded with anticancer carotenes. About two pounds of carrots make one pint of juice. If possible, buy organic and buy in bulk. Look for economical twenty-five-pound bags because carrots keep fairly well. Select only fresh produce to get good-tasting juice. Yellow sprouts on carrots mean they are old. Brush or scrape the carrots to clean them; there's no need to peel.

D. Green drink Drink one glass (8 oz) green drink per day. Green drink is the freshly made juice of any green vegetable: celery, cucumber (peel to remove wax), green peppers, cabbage, broccoli, kale, lettuce (leaf, like romaine), whatever you find easiest to get down. Green drink is raw liquid chlorophyll, and chlorophyll and hemoglobin have curiously similar molecular structures. For green drink do not use spinach, rhubarb, or asparagus. They contain oxalic acid.

E. B_{12} treatments Either of the following will insure B_{12} absorption: intranasal B_{12} gel, paste, or spray, three times weekly; or weekly injections of 1,000 mcg. Ask for a prescription for the injections, or make your own intranasal B_{12} and save a fortune. See my chapter on B_{12} for directions.

F. Potassium Potassium is in most fruits and vegetables. Carefully read the potassium chart ("K" stands for potassium) in Max Gerson's *A Cancer Therapy: Results of 50 Cases.* Eat no salt, and eat no "convenience" or canned foods, because they contain lots of salt. Cancerous cells love sodium, according to Dr. Gerson. More on the Gerson therapy in the next chapter.

G. Protein *Meat:* Avoid it, especially red. Try to become a vegetarian. The Gerson diet is vegetarian. If you can't go all the way, fish is an excellent complete protein. Yummy recipe hint: broil or bake fish, or poach it in half an inch of apple juice, simmering a few minutes on each side.

All this talk about avoiding meat and the chemicals it contains is not just hippie health-nut rhetoric.

PASS THE MUSTARD, OR JUST PASS ON THE HOT DOG?

More hot dogs are eaten at the 4th of July holiday than at any other time of the year. The National Hot Dog and Sausage Council (yes, an all-too-real trade organization) says that "during the Independence Day weekend, 155 million will be gobbled up" and that Americans will consume more than seven billion hot dogs over the summer. "Every year," they proudly proclaim, "Americans eat an average of 60 hot dogs each."[1]

That looks to be a modest average of just over one hot dog per week per American. But there are at least 7 million vegetarians in the U.S., and another 20 million who would be inclined to avoid meat.[2]

This means that even if you do not eat any hot dogs at all, someone else is eating your share. But a hot dog or two a week? Big deal!

Maybe it is. Children who eat one hot dog a week double their risk of a brain tumor; two per week triples the risk. Kids eating more than twelve hot dogs a month (three a week) have nearly ten times the risk of leukemia as children who eat none.[3]

And it is not just about kids. Of 190,000 adults studied for seven years, those eating the most processed meat such as deli meats and hot dogs had a 68 percent greater risk of pancreatic cancer than those who ate the least.[4] Pancreatic cancer is especially difficult to treat.

Think twice before you serve up your next tube steak. If your family is going to eat hot dogs, at least take your vitamins. Hot-dog-eating children taking supplemental vitamins were shown to have a reduced risk of cancer.[5] Vitamins C and E prevent the formation of nitrosamines.[6,7] It is curious that, while busy theorizing many "potential" dangers of vitamins, the news media have largely ignored this clear-cut cancer-prevention benefit from supplementation.

May I also suggest that you have your kids chew their hot dogs extra thoroughly. In landfills, "Whole hot dogs have been found, some of them in strata suggesting an age upwards of several decades."[8]

Bon appétit.

References

1. www.hot-dog.org.

2. www.vegetariantimes.com/features/archive_of_editorial/667.

3. Peters JM, Preston-Martin S, London SJ, Bowman JD, Buckley JD, Thomas DC. (1994). Processed meats and risk of childhood leukemia. *Cancer Causes Control* 5(2):195–202.

4. Nothlings U, Wilkens LR, Murphy SP, et al. (2005). Meat and fat intake as risk factors for pancreatic cancer: The Multiethnic Cohort Study. *J Nat Cancer Inst* 97:1458–65.

5. Sarasua S, Savitz DA. (1994). Cured and broiled meat consumption in relation to childhood cancer: Denver, Colorado (United States). *Cancer Causes Control* 5(2):141–8. Comment at www.ralphmoss.com/hotdog.html.

6. Scanlan RA. Nitrosamines and cancer: http://lpi.oregonstate.edu/f-w00/nitrosamine.html.

7. Cass H; English J. (2002). *User's guide to vitamin C*. Basic Health Publications, 64–67.

8. *Smithsonian,* July 1992, p 5.

Tofu: Soy products contain cancer-fighting substances. Cut up some tofu into small pieces and throw it into whatever you are making. It will take on the flavor of the recipe.

Cheese: Natural, with no coloring added. Eat cheese if it will keep you off meat.

Yogurt: Low-fat, plain. Sweeten it yourself with a little fruit or honey.

Nut butters: Delicious and easy to digest. Buy them fresh and keep them in the fridge. Almond butter may inhibit the growth of tumors. Cashew butter is high in the amino acid tryptophan, which helps you sleep. With any nut butter, select the fresh, natural variety without added fat or sugar.

Milk: Speaking as a former dairyman, there is nothing like high-quality raw milk. I raised a family on it from infancy onward. Certified raw milk is inspected daily. Try to find it at a health food store or from a farmer. If not available, sweet acidophilus milk or watered-down yogurt digests better than pasteurized milk.

Sprouts: Eat two jarfuls per day. That is not a misprint. Sprouts are a complete protein, a complete food. A person could survive on a variety of sprouts and nothing else. Buy untreated seed. Alfalfa is a good one to start with, but also go for wheat and lentil. Toss in some mung bean, clover, cabbage, and radish sprouts for added flavor. Each day start two more jars. Harvest alfalfa at the end of 4–7 days; the others may be ready sooner. Wheat and lentil take only a day or two. Eat them in a sandwich or as the base for a salad. Dressings and garnishes are okay. Collect 12–15 wide-mouth quart jars and start farming. Ann Wigmore's books will tell you how to sprout, and why.

H. Fruits Eat as many as you wish, any kind, any time. Before eating, wash them with soapy water and repeatedly rinse.

I. Grains Choose whole-grain breads that are 100 percent whole grain. Read that label! Also choose brown rice and whole-wheat pasta instead of their refined cousins.

J. Special Vegetables Eat all the cauliflower, cabbage, Brussels sprouts, kale, and broccoli that you can. Research confirms that these cruciform vegetables are naturally rich in several phytochemicals that fight tumors. The other exceptionally fine food class is the legumes: peas, beans, and lentils. They are loaded with fiber, protein, minerals, and complex carbohydrates. And they are really cheap. Eat lots.

K. Good Snacks Fresh, unsalted popcorn is very healthy. On it put 2 teaspoons nutritional yeast flakes, which give the popcorn a cheesy taste and additional B vitamins, chromium, and selenium. Raw veggies are the healthiest snack of all. Keep a tray of all your favorites in the center of your fridge, where you can reach it twenty-four hours a day. Celery, carrots, peppers, broccoli, cucumbers, tomatoes, and snap pea pods are all good choices.

L. Beverages Vegetable juices, fresh and raw. (Whenever you cook, bottle, or can anything, the heat destroys its natural enzymes.) Other healthy drinks are fresh fruit juices, spring water or mineral water, herbal teas, and green tea or decaffeinated black tea.

M. Supplements Vitamins are concentrated nutrients. They are not drugs, so the safety margin is excellent.

Vitamin C: Do not be put off this valuable adjunctive therapy by unscientific scare tactics. The only valid controversy remaining is whether vitamin C should be administered orally or intravenously. The answer is yes. In other words, either. Both is better.

Orally: Begin with 1,000 mg at each meal (3,000 mg per day). Your goal is bowel tolerance, which may be anywhere from 20,000 to 120,000 mg per day. It would be ideal to take some vitamin C every half hour you are awake, but that's a real nuisance. Do the best you can to divide the dose for maximum absorption. For stomach comfort at these high levels, buffering your vitamin C is strongly encouraged. Taking a calcium-magnesium supplement (any kind will do for buffering purposes) along with the C is the simplest way to accomplish this.

For economy and a "fewer pills to take" feeling, try using vitamin C powder instead of tablets. Mix the powder in a sweet beverage such as fruit juice. Take the amount of vitamin C needed to feel better, to show improved lab tests, and to get well. Patients in remission should continue taking it for life.

Intravenously: National Institutes of Health scientists confirmed that vitamin C is selectively toxic to cancer cells and that tumor-toxic levels of vitamin C can be attained using intravenous administration.[1]

References

1. Chen Q, Espey MG, Krishna MC, Mitchell JB, Corpe CP, Buettner GR, Shacter E, Levine M. (2005). Pharmacologic ascorbic acid concentrations selectively kill cancer cells: Action as a pro-drug to deliver hydrogen peroxide to tissues. *Proc Natl Acad Sci U S A* 102(38):13604–9. Epub 2005 Sep 12.

2. Cameron E, Pauling L. (1976). Supplemental ascorbate in the supportive treatment of cancer: Prolongation of survival times in terminal human cancer. Proc Natl Acad Sci U S A 73(10):3685–9. The original paper is posted at http://profiles.nlm.nih.gov/ MM/B/ B/K/Z/_/mmbbkz.pdf. See also: Cameron E, Pauling L, Leibovitz B. (1979). Ascorbic acid and cancer: a review. *Cancer Res.* 39(3):663–81.

3. Casciari, J.J., Riordan NH, Schmidt, T.L., Meng, X.L., Jackson JA, Riordan HD. (2001). Cytotoxicity of ascorbate, lipoic acid, and other antioxidants in hollow fibre in vitro tumours. *British J Cancer* 84(11):1544–1550.

Vitamin D

Vitamin D deficiency plays a role in causing at least seventeen varieties of cancer, as well as heart disease, stroke, hypertension, autoimmune diseases, diabetes, depression, chronic pain, osteoarthritis, osteoporosis, muscle weakness, muscle wasting, birth defects, and periodontal disease.[1] This does not mean that vitamin D deficiency is the only cause of these diseases. What it does mean is that vitamin D, and the many ways in which it affects a person's health, must no longer be overlooked.

Here is a very important example: Ample intake of vitamin D (about 2,000 IU/day) can **cut breast cancer incidence by half.**[2] If vitamin D levels were increased worldwide, 600,000 cases of breast and other cancers could be prevented each year. Nearly 150,000 cases of cancer could be prevented in the United States alone.

A four-year study of 1,179 healthy, postmenopausal women showed that taking calcium, along with nearly three times the U.S. government's recommendation of vitamin D showed a dramatic 60 percent or greater reduction in all forms of cancer.[3] Additionally, there is growing evidence that maintaining vitamin D levels in the body during the winter prevents the flu and other viral infections by strengthening the immune system.[4]

How much vitamin D does the average person need? In the summer, those with at least 15 minutes of sun exposure on their skin most days should take 1,000 IU of vitamin D_3 each day. In the winter, those with dark skin, or those who have little sun exposure on their skin, should take up to 4,000 IU each day. Suit your vitamin D_3 supplementation to your lifestyle: those who have darker skin, are older, avoid sun exposure, or live in the northern U.S. should take the higher amounts.

Vitamin D is remarkably safe; there have been no deaths caused by the vitamin.[5] The best way to be sure you are getting the right amount is to have your doctor give you a blood test for 25-hydroxyvitamin D. If your vitamin D intake from all sources is maintaining your blood level at or near 50 ng/ml, you have a good vitamin D status. If it is more than 10 percent below this level, supplemental sources of vitamin D_3 should be increased.

People consuming only government-recommended levels of 200–400 IU/day often have blood levels considerably below 50 ng/ml. This means the government's recommendations are too low, and should be raised immediately.

The great value of vitamin D for cancer patients is further discussed in Part Two.

References

1. The Vitamin D Council, www.vitamindcouncil.com.

2. Garland CF, Gorham ED, Mohr SB, Grant WB, Giovannucci EL, Lipkin M, Newmark H, Holick MF, Garland FC. (2007). Vitamin D and prevention of breast cancer: pooled analysis. *J Steroid Biochem Mol Biol* 103(3–5):708–11.

3. Lappe JM, Travers-Gustafson D, Davies KM, Recker RR, Heaney RP. (2007). Vitamin D and calcium supplementation reduces cancer risk: results of a randomized trial. *Amer J Clin Nutrition* 85(6):1586–1591. www.ajcn.org/cgi/content/abstract/85/6/1586.

4. Cannell JJ, Vieth R, Umhau JC, Holick MF, Grant WB, Madronich S, Garland CF, Giovannucci E. (2006). Epidemic influenza and vitamin D. *Epidemiol Infect* 134(6):1129–40. Epub 2006 Sep 7, http://journals.cambridge.org/action/displayAbstract?fromPage=online&aid=469543.

5. Saul, AW. (2003). Vitamin D: Deficiency, diversity and dosage. *J Orthomolecular Med* 18(3;4):194–204. www.doctoryourself.com/dvitamin.htm.

A study of 3,299 persons indicates that those with higher blood levels of vitamin D cut their risk of dying from cancer in half.[1] Another recent study shows that ample intake of vitamin D, about 2,000 IU per day, can cut breast cancer incidence by half.[2] Research also found that inadequate vitamin D is "associated with high incidence rates of colorectal cancer" and specifically urges that "prompt public health action is needed to increase intake of vitamin D to 1000 IU/day."[3] In 2006, researchers commented that "The evidence suggests that efforts to improve vitamin D status, for example by vitamin D supplementation, could reduce cancer incidence and mortality at low cost, with few or no adverse effects."[4]

Using vitamin D to stop cancer may seem like news, but it is not new news. Physicians have reported that vitamin D stops cancer for decades. In 1951, T. Desmonts reported that vitamin D treatment was effective against Hodgkin's disease (a cancer of the lymphatic system).[5] That same year, over sixty years ago, massive doses of vitamin D were also observed to improve epithelioma.[6] In 1955, skin cancer was again reported as cured with vitamin D treatment.[7] Then, in 1963, there was a promising investigation done on vitamin D and breast cancer.[8] In 1964, vitamin D was found to be effective against lymph nodal reticulosarcoma, a non-Hodgkin's lymphatic cancer.[9]

The Orthmolecular Medicine News Serivce wrote: "The American Cancer Society has been obsessed with finding a drug cure for cancer. Pharmaceutical researchers are not looking for a vitamin cure. And when one is presented, as independent investigators and physicians have continuously been doing since 1951, it is ignored."[9A]

Boston University professor Michael Holick, M.D., has said: "We can reduce cancer risk by 30 to 50% by increasing vitamin D. We gave mice colon cancer, and followed them for 20 days. Tumor growth was markedly reduced simply by having vitamin D in the diet. There was a 40% reduction in tumor size."[10]

It is possible to get too much vitamin D, but it is not easy. "One man took one million IU of vitamin D per day, orally, for six months, "says Dr. Holick. "Of course, he had the symptoms of severe vitamin D intoxication. His treatment was hydration (lots of water), and no more vitamin D or sunshine for a while. He's perfectly happy and healthy. This was published in the *New England Journal of Medicine*.[11] I have no experience of anyone dying from vitamin exposure. In thirty years, I've never seen it."

It is common sense that persons with preexisting conditions should have physician supervision and periodic testing before and while taking very high doses of vitamin D. A dose of 1,000 IU per day is simple and safe . . . and probably too low. Some authorities recommend much more.[12, 13]

References

1. Pilz S, Dobnig H, Winklhofer-Roob B, et al. Low serum levels of 25-hydroxyvitamin D predict fatal cancer in patients referred to coronary angiography. *Cancer Epidemiol Biomarkers Prev.,* 2008, 17(5):1228–33. Epub 2008 May 7.

2. Garland CF, Gorham ED, Mohr SB, et al. Vitamin D and prevention of breast cancer: pooled analysis. *J Steroid Biochem Mol Biol,* 2007, 103(3–5):708–11.

3. Gorham ED, Garland CF, Garland FC, Grant WB, Mohr SB, Lipkin M, Newmark HL, Giovannucci E, Wei M, and Holick MF. Vitamin D and prevention of colorectal cancer. *J Steroid Biochem Mol Biol.*, 2005,97(1–2):179–94.

4. Garland CF, Garland FC, Gorham ED, Lipkin M, Newmark H, Mohr SB, and Holick MF. The role of vitamin D in cancer prevention. *Am J Public Health,* 2006, 96(2):252–61.

5. Desmonts T, Duclos M, and Dalmau. Favorable effect of vitamin D on the evolution of a case of Hodgkin's disease. *Sang.*, 1951, 22(1):74–5. And Desmonts, T. Favorable action of vitamin D in leukemic erythroderma and Hodgkin's disease. *Pathol Gen.*, 1951, 51(326):161–4. Also, Vaccari R. Vitamin D2 and experimental carcinogenesis. *Boll Soc Ital Biol Sper.*, 1952, 28(8–10):1567–9.

6. Sainz de Aja Ea. Case of an epithelioma in a patient treated with massive doses of vitamin D. *Actas Dermosifiliogr.*, 1951,43(2):169–70.

7. Linser P. Spontaneous cure of skin carcinoma by vitamin D treatment. *Dermatol Wochenschr.*, 1955, 132(40):1072–3. German.

8. Gordan GS, and Schachter D. Vitamin D activity of normal and neoplastic human breast tissue. *Proc Soc Exp Biol Med.*, 1963, 113:760–1.

9. Desmonts T, and Blin J.Action of Vitamin D3 on the course of a lymph nodal reticulosarcoma. *Rev Pathol Gen Physiol Clin.*, 1964, 64:137. French.

9A. Vitamin D Stops Cancer; Cuts Risk In Half. American Cancer Society Drags its Feet. Orthomolecular Medicine News Service, Oct 2, 2008.

10. Andrew W. Saul Interviews Michael F. Holick, MD, PhD. www.doctoryourself.com/holick.html.

11. Koutkia P, Chen TC, and Holick MF. Vitamin D intoxication associated with an over-the-counter supplement. *N Engl J Med.*, 2001,345(1):66–7.

12. Vitamin D Boosts Health, Cuts Cancer Risk in Half. Orthomolecular Medicine News Service, October 3, 2007. http://orthomolecular.org/resources/omns/v03n06.shtml.

13. Doctors Say, Raise the RDAs Now. Orthomolecular Medicine News Service, October 30, 2007. http://orthomolecular.org/resources/omns/v03n10.shtml.

For More Information

Saul AW. Vitamin D: Deficiency, diversity and dosage. *J Orthomolecular Med*, 2003, 18(3,4):194–204. www.doctoryourself.com/dvitamin.htm

Online access to free archive of nutritional medicine journal papers: http://orthomolecular.org/library/jom/

Vitamin E Against Cancer

The medical professions have virtually ignored vitamin E's important role as a cancer fighter. Odd, really. For when researchers compared persons taking the most vitamin E with those taking the least, there was a 61 percent reduction in lung cancer risk.[1] Lung cancer is the most common kind of cancer on earth. Well over one million people are diagnosed with it each year, and the outlook is not very cheerful. Lung cancer accounts for 12 percent of all cancers, but 18 percent of all cancer deaths.[2] A 61 percent reduction in lung cancer with vitamin E? How could the news media have missed it?

Then there was another study, this time of colon cancer patients "who received a daily dose of 750 mg of vitamin E during a period of 2 weeks. Short-term supplementation with high doses of dietary vitamin E leads to increased CD4:CD8 ratios and to enhanced capacity by their T cells to produce the T helper 1 cytokines interleukin 2 and IFN-gamma. In 10 of 12 patients, an increase of 10% or more (average, 22%) in the number of T cells producing interleukin 2 was seen after 2 weeks of vitamin E supplementation." The authors concluded that "dietary vitamin E may be used to improve the immune functions in patients with advanced cancer." *Improvement was seen in just two weeks.*[3]

This information did not just fall into my hands off the back of a turnip truck. Searching the US National Library of Medicine via MEDLINE will bring up over 3,000 studies on the subject, some dating back to 1946. By the early 1950s, research clearly supported the use of vitamin E against cancer.[4] Before 1960, vitamin E was shown to reduce the side effects of radiation cancer treatment.[5]

It is high time to press oncologists to get with the program. If your doctor does not recommend supplemental vitamins, it is time to stand up and demand that s/he read the above.

Begin with 200 IU of natural mixed tocopherols and tocotrienols and gradually work up to about 1,000 IU daily. If you are on an anticoagulant drug (such as Coumadin), or if you are on medication for high blood pressure, your vitamin and drug doses probably will need to be tailored over a period of weeks. You can quite easily monitor your blood pressure at home, and your doctor can and should frequently check your prothrombin time for you. Occasionally blood pressure goes up slightly in folks not used to vitamin E. It is usually temporary. Reduce the vitamin E for a while, then resume a leisurely increase. If your "protime" gets too long, have your doctor reduce the drug dose, not the vitamin. Vitamin E greatly reduces the side effects of radiation therapy. Vitamin E is the body's number one antioxidant, very valuable in slowing tumor growth and slowing the spread of malignancies. You will very much want to read *Vitamin E for Ailing and Healthy Hearts,* by Wilfrid Shute, M.D., or any other book by him or his physician brother, Evan. They will walk you through the whole process.

References

1. Mahabir S, Schendel K, Dong YQ, Barrera SL, Spitz MR, and Forman MR. Dietary alpha-, beta-, gamma- and delta-tocopherols in lung cancer risk. *Int J Cancer.,* 2008, 123(5):1173–80.

2. http://info.cancerresearchuk.org/cancerstats/geographic/world/commoncancers/.

3. Malmberg KJ, Lenkei R, Petersson M, et al. A short-term dietary supplementation of high doses of vitamin E increases T helper 1 cytokine production in patients with advanced colorectal cancer. *Clin Cancer Res.,* 2002, 8(6):1772–8.

4. Telford IR. The influence of alpha tocopherol on lung tumors in strain A mice. *Tex Rep Biol Med.,* 1955. 13(3):515–21. And Swick RW, Baumann CA, Miller WL Jr, and Rumsfeld HW Jr. Tocopherol in tumor tissues and effects of tocopherol on the development of liver tumors. *Cancer Res.,* 1951, 11(12):948–53.

5. Fischer W. The protective effect of tocopherol against toxic phenomena connected with the roentgen irradiation of mammary carcinoma. *Munch Med Wochenschr.,* 1959, 101:1487–8. German. Also, Sabatini C, Balli L, and Tagliavini R. Effects of vitamin E and testosterone in comparisons of skin exposed to high doses of roentgen rays administered by semi-contact technic. *Riforma Med.,* 1955, 69(18S):1–4. Italian. See also, Graham JB, and Graham RM. Enhanced effectiveness of radiotherapy in cancer of the uterine cervix. *Surg Forum.,* 1953, (38th Congress):332–8.

Carotenes and Lycopene: Until you get a juicer, eat raw vegetables whenever you can. And don't forget: you can do a lot with conventional cooked vegetables. Eat lots of yams, sweet potatoes, and winter squash. These are all very high in the natural carotenes, not just the best known beta form. Tomatoes, any way you like them, are loaded with lycopene, which is even more valuable than carotene. Cooked tomatoes are very nearly as good for you as raw ones. (Ried K, and Fakler P. Protective effect of lycopene on serum cholesterol and blood pressure: Meta-analyses of intervention trials. *Maturitas,* 2011, 68(4):299–310.)

Do not let anyone keep you from your tomatoes with the old scare story that tomatoes are in the nightshade family and are therefore naughty. Balderdash! Tomatoes are good food. Studies in Italy (of course) showed that men who ate five to ten fresh tomatoes daily had almost no prostate cancer. Red or purple grapes (and other red/yellow/orange fruits and vegetables) are high in many other cancer-fighting antioxidants related to the carotenes.

Iron: If your physician says you need iron, take ferrous gluconate or ferrous fumarate iron tablets, which would substitute for your current prescription of harder-to-handle ferrous sulfate. Chelated iron tablets are better absorbed and, therefore, better utilized by the body. Iron is best absorbed if taken with vitamin C but not at the same time as vitamin E.

Selenium: Only a minuscule amount is needed, generally around 300 mcg. A microgram is a millionth of a gram. Selenium works closely with vitamin E. Avoid excesses; more is not better in this case.

Zinc: The zinc in your multivitamin (perhaps 15 mg?) is low. Take 50 mg of zinc gluconate or preferably zinc monomethionine. Work up to perhaps 100 mg per day. Zinc reduces postsurgical healing time and profoundly strengthens the immune system.

Calcium and Magnesium: Tablets can be used to conveniently buffer between-meal vitamin C doses. 1,500 mg of calcium and 500 mg of magnesium is a good target amount. Divide the doses as much as possible, including snack time and bedtime. Your body will absorb it much more efficiently that way.

Vitamin B Complex: Take one balanced B-50 tablet with each meal. If you are on intense drug therapy or are very fatigued, you can take additional B-complex between meals. Patients on chemotherapy report greatly reduced nausea and much less hair loss when they take their B and C vitamins. You have to try this to believe it.

Suggestions

If you get diarrhea, ease up on the vitamin C or the vegetable juices. If not sure which, decrease one, then the other, to confirm the culprit. Bear in mind that diarrhea may be due to radiation or chemotherapy treatments. Cheese tends to help stop simple diarrhea. Chronic diarrhea requires medical attention.

If you need to sweeten something, try a little honey, sweet molasses, or pure maple syrup.

Give this protocol a full four-month trial, with 100 percent effort, before evaluating its success.

Don't eat anything without reading the label. Don't eat anything unless you know what it is. If you cannot pronounce it, don't eat it.

If your medical doctor is not familiar with orthomolecular (megavitamin) nutrition, hand him books, with the bookmarks stuck throughout, and ask, "Have you read what we've read?" Let Dr. Pauling and Dr. Hoffer and Dr. Riordan and Dr. Gerson and Dr. Cameron do the talking. When you go to battle, don't go without your best soldiers. If you are still unfamiliar with these physicians and their work, you are not ready to fight.

No-Nos

Sugar, smoking, and alcoholic beverages. (Organically produced red wine in moderation is a reasonable compromise. It is best to dilute it with two parts water before drinking. Better yet, drink grape juice.) Avoid artificial colorings and all preservatives. Do not consume aspartame (NutraSweet). Never eat any product containing saccharin, which has been found to cause cancer in laboratory animals. My reading of the literature leads me to believe that there are no truly safe artificial sweeteners.

Who gets the credit (or blame?) for this therapy? Certainly not me, although who wouldn't love to take the bow? But no, this is the collected, derivative work of many researchers. I'm not smart enough to come up with all this. I am just barely smart enough to find out who is getting good results . . . and copy them.

VITAMINS AS PARTNERS WITH CHEMOTHERAPY

by Abram Hoffer, M.D.

Patients suffering from ovarian cancer have a dismal survival record. The authors of a recent study[1] point out that a majority of patients with cancer also seek complementary and alternative therapy with megavitamins and herbs for a variety of reasons, most often without telling their oncologists. The authors write: "In this study, two patients with advanced epithelial ovarian cancer were studied. One patient had Stage IIIC papillary serous adenocarcinoma, and the other had Stage IIIC mixed papillary serous and sero mucinous adenocarcinoma . . . Patient 1 began oral high-dose antioxidant therapy during her first month of therapy. This consisted of oral vitamin C, vitamin E, beta-carotene, and coenzyme Q10 and a multivitamin/mineral complex. In addition to the oral antioxidant therapy, patient 1 added parenteral (intravenous) ascorbic acid as a total dose of 60 grams (60,000 mg) given twice weekly at the end of her chemotherapy, and prior to consolidation paclitaxel/carboplatinum chemotherapy. Patient 2 added oral antioxidants just prior to beginning chemotherapy, including vitamin C, beta-carotene, vitamin E, coenzyme Q10 and a multivitamin/mineral complex. Patient 2 received six cycles of paclitaxel/carboplatinum chemotherapy and refused consolidation chemotherapy despite radiographic evidence of persistent disease. Instead she elected to add intravenous ascorbic acid at 60 grams twice weekly. Both patients gave written consent for the use of their records in this report."

Patient 1's CA-125 was normal after her first cycle of chemotherapy and is still normal 3.5 years later. There is no evidence for recurrence. Patient 2's CA-125 was normal after her first round of chemotherapy but still had residual disease in the pelvis. She refused further chemotherapy and added intravenous ascorbic acid. She is well three years later. Neither patient suffered grade three or four toxicity and were able to complete the six cycles. Both had mild short- lived nausea. Patient 1 had numbness and tingling hands and feet as well as fatigue, shortness of breath and peripheral edema during the first course of chemotherapy but before starting intravenous vitamin C. She was found to have tricuspid and aortic valve regurgitation well controlled on medication. Neither patient had any hematologic toxicity, required colony-stimulating factors, suffered elevated renal or liver enzymes nor febrile neutropenia or infection.

In their discussion they referred to clinical studies which showed high dose ascorbic acid is a potent immunodulator, cytotoxic to cancer cells, and activates natural killer cells in vivo and both B and T cell activity. But there was little toxicity to normal cells. They pointed out that most clinical studies used multiple antioxidants referring to vitamin E, beta- carotene and vitamin A. Their conclusion was that with these two cases the antioxidants improved the efficacy of chemotherapy safely. They questioned the concept that antioxidants are contraindicated during most chemotherapy regimens, stating that such a statement is not valid.

Reference

1. Drisko JA, Chapman J and Hunter VJ. The use of antioxidants with first-line chemotherapy in two cases of ovarian cancer. J American College of Nutrition 222,119- 123, 2002.

Reprinted with permission from the *Doctor Yourself Newsletter* (3:23, Oct 20, 2003)

CONTINUUM OF HEALING

With very sick cancer patients, what we really want is total cure. If we cannot get that, then we'd like to stop the disease from getting any worse. If we can't do that, then we want to slow disease progression down.

Sometimes, we have to settle for increased length of life and improved quality of life. Those are very important, very realistic, and very attainable benefits of nutritional therapy. I say this without hesitation or hedging: every single cancer patient I have worked with for thirty-five years has experienced prompt and obvious quality-of-life improvement. And, the majority have lived considerably longer than their oncologists predicted. However, if I, or anyone else, had the sure cure for cancer, it would mean a photo on the cover of *Time* magazine and being crowned Surgeon General of the Galaxy. Hasn't happened yet. There simply are no guarantees. What we are doing when we fight cancer nutritionally is primarily boosting the patient's immune system and trying to get the body to heal itself. Sometimes vitamins and even foods can selectively kill cancer cells. Laetrile, broccoli, and huge intravenous does of vitamin C have been known to do this. I strongly feel it is worth a therapeutic trial.

For Further Reading

Gonzalez M, Miranda-Massari J, Saul AW. (2009). *I Have Cancer: What Should I Do? Your Orthomolecular Guide for Cancer Management.* Laguna Beach, CA: Basic Health Publications.

Comfrey for Cancer

In an old issue of *Let's Live* (Oct–Dec 1958), H. E. Kirschner, M.D., wrote an almost unbelievable article about several important clinical uses of the comfrey plant (*Symphytum officinale*). Dr. Kirschner used comfrey in his medical practice to promote the healing of ulcers and wounds. He traces the history of comfrey back to 1568 and W. Turner's *Herball* which said "of Comfrey Symphytum, the rootes are good if they be broken and dronken for them that spitte blood, and are bursten. The same, layd to, are good to glewe together freshe woundes. They are good to be layd to inflammation."

He then cites Gerard's 1597 *Herball,* which indicated comfrey for ulcers of the lungs or kidneys, and Parkinson's 1640 *Theatrum Botanicum:* "The rootes of Comfrey, taken fresh, beaten small, spread upon leather, and laid upon any place troubled with the gout, doe presently give ease of the paines and applied in the same manner, giveth ease to pained joynts, and profiteth very much for running and moist ulcers, gangrenes, mortifications and the like."

Most significant is a citation from Tournefort's 1719 *Compleat Herbal,* which tells of one who "cured a certain person of a malignant ulcer, pronounced to be a cancer by the surgeons, and left by them as incurable, by applying twice a day the root of comfrey bruised, having first peeled off the external blackish bark or rind; but the cancer was not above eight or ten weeks standing." Even allowing for a possible misdiagnosis, this account is interesting.

Dr. Kirschner personally observed the powerful anticancer effects of comfrey on a patient of his who was dying from advanced, externalized cancer. He prescribed fresh, crushed-leaf comfrey poultices throughout the day. Much to the surprise of the patient and her family, there was obvious healing within the first two days of treatment, with continued visible improvement over the next few weeks. "What is more," he writes, "much of the dreadful pain that usually accompanies the advanced stages of cancer disappeared," and there was a dramatic decrease in swelling. Dr. Kirschner concludes by regretfully saying that the cancer had already spread to the inner organs "which could not be reached with the comfrey poultices, and the woman died."

Just in terms of quality of life, the degree of healing that *did* occur under the comfrey poultice treatment is of tremendous significance. Here is a "folk" remedy providing, at the very least, significant palliative relief, and to a remarkable extent reversing a cancerous growth. We can ill afford to overlook the full potential of external comfrey-leaf poultices to heal sores and wounds of all types, including burns and gangrene, as well as "tumors both benign and malignant," says Dr. Kirschner.

Taken internally as decoction (boiled root tea), comfrey is described as effective against tuberculosis, internal tumors, and ulcers, and promotes the healing of bone fractures. If it is hard to understand how one simple plant can be so widely useful in healing, remember that penicillin's supporters have made some pretty broad claims for the mold on oranges.

Dr. Kirschner describes in his article how to prepare comfrey leaves and roots for home use. The leaves are for external use, and the root for internal use. Anyone can grow comfrey in their garden. In fact, just try to stop this virtually indestructible perennial. As a young man, I decided to plant comfrey all over my yard. That took about fifteen minutes. It grew so vibrantly that I eventually decided to eradicate the comfrey. It took twenty years to root it all out. Well, most of it. There is still that patch over there on the side. . . . I got my "starter" comfrey from a friend, and now I know why he was smiling so broadly as he handed the huge sack of roots to me.

Comfrey is widely available. Ask around and see who's got some to share. Or try a garden supplier, nursery, or herb store. How to plant comfrey: stick the root under ground and come back in a month or two. To grow: stand back and watch.

To use the leaves, one simply picks them, crushes them into a nice emerald green paste, and applies topically. Although dried leaves are often available in herb and health food stores, it is much better to use fresh-cut leaves right from the garden.

Roots can be prepared by boiling one-half to one ounce of minced or crushed root in two cups of water. I thoroughly brush and wash the root under tap water before slicing it up. Then I place the chunks in the water in a glass or stainless steel pan. Bring it to a boil, continue boiling for five to ten minutes, and let sit until it is cool enough to drink. This *decoction* is much more effective than simply steeping in hot water. Dose: one six-ounce glass, several per day, as required. Fresh root is almost certainly best, but I expect that dried root retains some therapeutic value.

Caution: Herbs may be the most natural of medicines, but they are still medicines. There are potentially harmful side effects if non-boiled comfrey is consumed in appreciable quantity. This warning especially applies to what is sometimes called "comfrey-leaf tea," which I specifically advise you to avoid. In my opinion, pregnant or nursing women should decline to use any medicine. To be comfy with comfrey, consult your doctor and a reliable herbal textbook (such as John B. Lust's *The Herb Book*) before employing this, or any, herbal remedy. It is important to meet potential physician objections with a clear understanding of the "comfrey rule": *fresh leaves externally, boiled root decoction internally.*

Allantoin, a key ingredient found in abundance in comfrey, may be among the reasons comfrey works. Allantoin helps cells to grow and grow together. Since this is precisely what is needed for ulcers, tumors, burns, broken skin, broken bones, and perhaps even malignancy, it is little wonder that comfrey has a respect in folklore and medical practice throughout the world. For a definitive explanation of how, why, and what comfrey heals, with detailed infor-

93

mation on the chemical constitution of allantoin, read a long-forgotten sixty-page work entitled *Narrative of an Investigation Concerning an Ancient Medicinal Remedy and its Modern Utilities* by Charles J. MacAlister, M.D., and A.W. Titherley, D.Sc. It is full of case histories, research, and historical information. Clinical observations, notes on malignancy, and instructions on how to prepare the remedy are included. This 1936 book is even rarer than Dr. Kirchner's article that I cited above. Reprints of either may still be available on microfilm. It is a good idea to ask your public library's interlibrary loan person to help you obtain copies.

Recommended Reading

Cameron E and Pauling L. *Cancer and Vitamin C,* revised edition. Philadelphia: Camino Books, 1993.

Dr. Harold W. Manner: the man who cures cancer. *Mother Earth News* (Nov/Dec 1978): 17–24. This article is about documented Laetrile cures. Your librarian can obtain a copy for you to read.

Hanck A, ed. *Vitamin C: New Clinical Applications.* Bern: Huber, 1982, 103–113.

Hoffer A. *Vitamin C and Cancer: Discovery, Recovery, Controversy.* Kingston, ON: Quarry Press, 1999.

Kulvinskas V. *Survival into the Twenty-First Century.* Wethersfield, CT: Omangod Press, 1975.

Moss R. *The Cancer Syndrome.* New York: Grove Press, 1980.

Moss R. *The Cancer Industry.* New York: Paragon Press, 1989.

Murata A, Morishige F, Yamaguchi H. Prolongation of survival times of terminal cancer patients by administration of large doses of ascorbate. *Int J Vitamin and Nutrition Res Suppl* 23 (1982): 103–113.

Orme-Johnson D. Medical care utilization and the transcendental meditation program. *Psychosom Med* 49 (1987): 493–507.

Pauling L. (1986; revised ed. 2006). *How to Live Longer and Feel Better.* Corvallis, OR: Oregon State University Press.

Riordan HD, Jackson JA, Schultz M. Case study: high-dose intravenous vitamin C in the treatment of a patient with adenocarcinoma of the kidney. *J Ortho Med* 5 (1990): 5–7.

Riordan NH, Riordan HD, Meng X, Li Y, Jackson JA. Intravenous ascorbate as a tumor cytotoxic chemotherapeutic agent. *Medical Hypotheses* 44 (March 1995): 207–213.

Riordan N, Jackson JA, Riordan HD. Intravenous vitamin C in a terminal cancer patient. *J Ortho Med* 11 (1996): 80–82.

Stone I. *The Healing Factor: Vitamin C against Disease.* New York: Grosset and Dunlap, 1972.

Vitamin C and Cancer: What can we conclude? Comments by Andrew W. Saul, Michael J. Gonzalez, Jorge R. Miranda-Massari, Jorge Duconge, and Fernando Cabanillas. http://prhsj.rcm.upr.edu/index.php/prhsj/article/ viewFile/546/384

Wigmore A. *Why Suffer?* New York: Hemisphere Press, 1964.

Wigmore A. *Recipes for Longer Life.* Garden City Park, NY: Avery, 1982. (All her recipes contain no cooking at all!)

Wigmore A. *Be Your Own Doctor.* Garden City Park, NY: Avery, 1983.

Williams RJ, Kalita DK, eds. *A Physician's Handbook on Orthomolecular Medicine.* New Canaan, CT: Keats, 1977.

"Max Gerson was a medical genius who walked among us."

—NOBEL LAUREATE ALBERT SCHWEITZER, M.D.

Max Gerson, M.D., started his professional life as a distinguished physician and ended it condemned as a quack. This highly trained scientist turned his back on conventional medicine and never recanted.

The renegade doctor does not fit the public perception of quack very well. We want our quacks flaming, as Homer Simpson wanted all his gay acquaintances to be. Only a real nut, an utterly uneducated, criminally flamboyant fraud, is repellent enough to be sure to scare patients into the waiting arms of the drug doctors. Max Gerson is therefore a problem from the start, best left ignored. He was entirely too qualified, too experienced, and too radical. You will look long and hard for any positive reference to him in any medical history or textbook. And yet, this man developed the single most successful treatment for cancer in existence—more than sixty years ago.

Gerson was a surgeon in the German army during the first world war. He and other doctors worked MASH-like twenty-hour days, operating on what was left of their countrymen evacuated from the front lines. The British naval blockade of Germany had resulted in a dire shortage of morphine for patients in recovery. The doctors, who drank coffee to stay awake day and night to operate, found that coffee also relieved pain in the wounded. To this day, caffeine is one of the active ingredients in many an extra-strength pain reliever. Some soldiers had so much of their faces, throats, and stomachs shot away that they were fed by rectum—not an uncommon practice in the old days. Desperate nurses were instructed to put coffee in the enema water of these individuals. It worked; any port in a storm.

This was the first reason why Dr. Gerson would later give coffee enemas to cancer patients: pain relief. He later claimed another: rectally administered coffee seemed to stimulate the liver to flush waste from the system. He was neither the first nor the last to believe that "accumulated toxins" are a cause of cancer. It is a persistent and recurrent quacky notion . . . which is also probably quite accurate.

The cancer-preventive aspects of high-fiber diets support this. One study showed that Hispanic women have far lower rates of breast cancer than do black or white women. When all factors were considered, only one difference could be found: Hispanic women eat considerably more beans than black or white women do. The fiber is almost certainly the secret. Other research has pointed to the flip-side conclusion: low-fiber diets are carcinogenic. In a low-fiber diet, any consumed carcinogens have a longer transit time through the body's digestive tract. More time in contact with the lining of the GI tract means more opportunity for carcinogenesis.

Lots of fiber may also help the body excrete excess endogenous chemicals, such as estrogen, thereby lowering the rate of some hormone-dependent cancers. Additionally, soluble fiber removes excess bile acids (by-products of fat digestion) that are also linked with cancer. David Reuben's *Save Your Life Diet* (yes, he was an M.D. as well) discusses fiber's anticancer roles in detail. That book came out in the 1970s; this is not new information. Why isn't it more widely known? Fiber is simply too cheap for any pharmaceutical company to make big bucks off it. There is more money in chemo than Beano.

The goal of the Gerson approach, which makes it the exact opposite of chemotherapy, is its attempt to detoxify the body, focusing on restoring and strengthening liver function. Is this a reasonable focus? Well, weighing in at about four pounds, the liver is the largest gland in the body. It is the body's site of detoxification of alcohol and other drugs, and could very well detoxify a cancer patient. If so, the liver may well be the key organ for cancer therapy.

To build up the body's ability to fight cancer, Dr. Gerson then employed the most damning therapy in the twentieth century: vitamins. On top of that, he was among the pioneers recommending extensive vegetable juicing. There you go: this all would be right at home on a shopping channel at 2 A.M.

Oddly enough, it was because he had chronic, severe migraines that Max Gerson got into vitamins and juicing. He found no help in the drugs of the day. Remember, he was a doctor and he well knew what was available. Nothing worked. So Gerson tried the logic of that great nonperson, Sherlock Holmes: if all reasonable explanations fail, the answer must be some unreasonable one. Immersed in the unreason that only pain can generate, Gerson tried different foods, doing an early version of what was probably much like allergy testing. He found that juiced vegetables, not medicines, were the cure for his headaches. He was as surprised as you would be, perhaps even more so, because he was a drug doctor who had been taught nothing of natural healing, except perhaps contempt for it.

Nothing succeeds like success. Word got around and people started to seek out this doctor who cured migraines when the other doctors failed to. Gerson began to note that many of his migraine patients were also getting cured of assorted conditions that they hadn't even initially told him about. He reasoned that juicing was a "metabolic therapy," nonspecific and broad in nature. If that concept annoys you, think of the diverse sicknesses that are expected to respond to a given antibiotic.

Up until this point, Gerson was not even thinking of treating cancer. When ultimately asked to try, he refused, having no intention of becoming known as another cancer quack. Pressure from suffering patients eventually changed his mind. He hesitatingly began using the metabolic therapy, cleansing and restoring the cancer patient's body, and was curing more than 50 percent of terminal cancer patients. This extraordinary success rate was in part the basis for a 1946 Congressional hearing on cancer therapies. Gerson took fifty of his carefully documented case histories before an investigative committee. Radiation, surgery, and chemotherapy were all approved for the "war on cancer." Vitamins, juices, and Gerson were excluded, by just a handful of votes.

Well, what do you expect? His mistake, and it was a big mistake, was to recommend coffee enemas for cancer patients. The fact that dying patients were recovering was secondary. It all sounded too quacky. The juices and the vitamins just added insult to injury. In the great traditions of Congress, they got it wrong and threw out the baby with the bathwater. Gerson remained a medical outsider for the rest of his life.

For over sixty years, cancer treatment and research has been almost entirely restricted to cut, zap, and drug: surgery, radiation, and chemotherapy. Billions and billions of dollars have been expended investigating every cure *but* a nutritional one. Ridicule, not science, has kept the Gerson therapy away from your local oncologist's office. Try a simple test: ask ten doctors what they think of using the Gerson therapy against cancer. Then ask the same doctors what they *know* of the Gerson therapy. I'll lay good odds that about all they know is that the guy used coffee enemas. "Would you like cream and sugar with that?" a physician once said to me. And you'll likely hear worse.

The best possible summation of Dr. Gerson comes from the great Nobel laureate Albert Schweitzer: "I see in Dr. Max Gerson one of the most eminent geniuses in the history of medicine. He has achieved more than seemed possible under adverse conditions. Many of his basic ideas have been adopted without having his name connected with them. He leaves a legacy which commands attention and which will assure him his due place. Those whom he has cured will attest to the truth of his ideas."

Recommended Reading

Gerson C and Bishop B. *Healing the Gerson Way: Defeating Cancer and Other Chronic Diseases.* Totality Books, 2007.

Gerson C and Walker M. *The Gerson Therapy.* New York: Kensington, 2001.Gerson M. *A Cancer Therapy: Results of Fifty Cases and the Cure of Advanced Cancer.* San Diego, CA: The Gerson Institute, 2000.

Straus H. *Dr. Max Gerson: Healing the Hopeless.* Kingston, ON: Quarry Press, 2002.

"People's minds are changed through observation and not through argument."

—WILL ROGERS

Dysplasia is a study in scurvy. In vitamin C–deficiency disease, there is insufficient production of collagen, the strong, healthy glue that holds your cells together. Whether dysplasia is triggered by a virus, physical irritation, or other cause, the fundamental problem is weak intercellular ground substance due to inadequate ascorbic acid. (Specific vitamin C megadosage instructions are provided in the chapter "Vitamin C Megadose Therapy.")

Chronic dysplasia is often feared to be precancerous. Cervical cancer is the second most common cancer in women, and once it has spread, is very dangerous indeed. A major factor in preventing such an unwanted development is the amino acid L-lysine. I have seen physician reports that women who take several thousand milligrams of L-lysine daily get far less cervical cancer. Research has now confirmed this.[1] This is because you can get lots of lysine by eating lots of beans. Beans, and all the other legumes, are loaded with lysine. Peas are very high in lysine. So are lentils, refried beans, pinto beans, kidney beans, three-bean salad, bean soup, bean burritos, veggie bean-burgers, and even chickpeas. Lima beans are relatively low in lysine; soybeans (and anything made from soy) are unusually high. An effective dose is about 3,000 to 4,000 mg of lysine daily. That is about a can and a half of beans each day.

Reference

1. Roomi MW, Ivanov V, Kalinovsky T, Niedzwiecki A, Rath M. Suppression of human cervical cancer cell lines Hela and DoTc2 4510 by a mixture of lysine, proline, ascorbic acid, and green tea extract. *Int J Gynecol Cancer*. 2006 May–Jun;16(3):1241–7.

Wait! Before you go off singing the "musical fruit" song, hear me out. I know you are going to ask, and I have an answer all ready for you:

Suggestions for Reducing Social Embarrassment after Following Saul's Bean Program

First, drain 'em! Do NOT use the liquid that canned beans are packed in, nor the water that you soak or cook beans in. Such processing liquid is high in raffinose sugars, which are gas-producing par excellence. Why? Because bacteria love them, that's why. Odoriferous gas is produced by bacteria in the large intestine as they munch on incompletely digested food. You will doubtless be pleased to know that most intestinal gas is odorless methane, odorless hydrogen, and odorless carbon dioxide. But then there's hydrogen sulfide (from bacteria eating protein) which the human nose can detect at just *one part per two billion.*

Odor also partly results from amines, which are formed by intestinal bacteria from amino acids (protein again). Eating less protein in general, and less flesh protein in particular, has an olfactory benefit. The stool of a cow is a lot less unpleasant than the stool of a dog. Since the average American eats two to three times more protein a day than is necessary, you need not worry about wasting away from reduced protein consumption.

Did you know that the average person forms 1 to 3 pints of bowel gas each day, with about fourteen emissions?

Did you know that this was one of the most quoted facts students lifted from my Clinical Nutrition lectures?

Okay, now for the "bottom" line.

GAS Rx

ONE: slow down and chew your food very well. Undigested starches are a major culprit in flatulence. The slower you eat and better you digest, the less of a problem you'll have.

TWO: sprout your beans, or cook them thoroughly. Remember: drain off that canning or cooking water!

THREE: allow time for intestinal bacteria to adapt to dietary changes. Most new near-vegetarians have a not-new body, full of stuff from the old days of revelry. Transition can take a while, but I think you will *feel* better right away. As your legume-lovin' bowel bacteria (and other good intestinal flora) begin to really thrive, you will barely notice that you have become a virtual dean of the beans. And that ever worrisome "crowded elevator syndrome" will also decrease dramatically.

FOUR: cut down on sweets. Excess simple carbohydrates are a good culture medium if you want excess bacteria, so put the little beggars on a diet.

Congestive Heart Failure

*"Man is a food-dependent creature. If you don't feed him, he will die.
If you feed him improperly, part of him will die."*
—EMANUEL CHERASKIN, M.D., DMD

In an average lifetime, the human heart will beat two and a half *billion* times. But, as in Vegas, there is no guarantee that the odds will favor anyone. Congestive heart failure (CHF) is the end product of any of a number of cardiovascular diseases that degrade the heart's ability to pump blood efficiently. Much has been written on diagnosing CHF but rather less is known about treating it. This is because broken hearts are tough to fix. A diagnosis of CHF means that it is too late for nutritional prevention. The horse is long gone by the time most people decide to shut the stable door. But nutritional intervention can still greatly help a damaged heart.

In the past, drugs such as digitalis were often given to strengthen and to some extent regulate heartbeat. Vasodilators (blood vessel–opening drugs) are given to improve cardiac output and relieve backed-up blood from blood vessels throughout the body, especially in the lungs. Fluid buildup (edema) is commonly treated with diuretic drugs.

It may be possible to naturally augment, or perhaps substitute for, these pharmaceutical drugs. The following is a protocol that can be tried under the auspices of a qualified health practitioner.

Vitamin E

One of the body's most powerful defenses against free-radical damage is the antioxidant vitamin E. The natural form, d-alpha-tocopherol, can also be cautiously used to strengthen and regulate heartbeat. To avoid any possible risks of an asymmetric heart contraction, patients with CHF need to start small with vitamin E. An initial dose of vitamin E should be only about 50 IU daily. This is roughly equivalent to 50 mg. Doses may be gradually increased under medical supervision. For additional information, it is most worthwhile to read any books by Wilfrid or Evan Shute. Their books are often hard to find, so try an interlibrary loan at any public library.

Thiamin

Some CHF is actually caused by thiamin (vitamin B_1) deficiency. 25–50 mg with each meal will overcome any such deficiency. I think a thiamin-containing 50 mg "balanced B complex" tablet each meal would be even better.

Common Sense

No added salt. No alcohol. No smoking. No extra weight. No kidding.

Herbal Diuretics

It may be possible to use herbal medicines to reduce swelling due to retained fluids. There are no fewer than 180 herbs with diuretic properties listed in John Lust's *The Herb Book*. I am not suggesting that you take 180 herbs. I am suggesting that you read up on your options before committing yourself only to drugs.

Selenium

Selenium deficiency can cause a congestive heart disease called Keshan disease. 100 to 300 mcg of selenium daily will insure against this. In addition, selenium works to help your body recharge and efficiently reuse its vitamin E.

Magnesium

The role of magnesium in normal heart function is tremendous. Profound magnesium deficiency causes muscles to malfunction or not function at all. Several hundred of your body's most important biochemical reactions depend on this mineral, including the synthesis of proteins, DNA, fats, and carbohydrates. Even most, ah, "healthy" adults fail to get the RDA of magnesium, which is about 400 mg. These figures are elemental weights: just the corn, not the can. Most magnesium supplements are compounds of magnesium with something else. The weight of the "something else" is often obscured in dosage recommendations. That is why Melvyn Werbach cites studies that advocate daily dosages of 2,000 mg of magnesium compound per day for CHF in his *Textbook of Nutritional Medicine*. The elemental quantity is significantly lower than that. Green vegetables and whole grains contain quite a bit of magnesium. Pinto beans, almonds, and especially figs are other outstanding food sources.

MAGNESIUM DEFICIENCY IS WIDESPREAD

Over two-thirds of the population do not get the RDA of magnesium.[1] Deficiency can cause a wide variety of symptoms, including osteoporosis, high blood pressure, heart disease, asthma, depression, and diabetes. Magnesium can be purchased in many forms. The most widely available form is magnesium oxide, which is not very effective because it is only about 5 percent absorbed[2]. Magnesium oxide supplements are popular because the pills are smaller—they contain more magnesium, but won't help most people. Better forms of magnesium are magnesium citrate, magnesium malate, and magnesium chloride. It's always good to consult your doctor to determine your ideal intake. Testing may reveal unexpected deficiency.[3]

References

1. King DE, et al. Dietary magnesium and C-reactive protein levels. *J Am Coll Nutr June*, 2005, 24(3):166–171. Free, full text paper at www.jacn.org/content/24/3/166.full.pdf+html (or www.jacn.org/content/24/3/166.long).

2. Dean, C. (2006). *The Magnesium Miracle*. New York: Ballantine Books.

3. www.doctoryourself.com/epilepsy.html.

(Excerpted with permission from the Orthomolecular Medicine News Service, Jan 17, 2012.)

Of the oral supplements, magnesium aspartate or magnesium orotate may have the best chance of getting into cardiac muscle cells. These forms of magnesium are rarely found on store shelves. Your doctor may be able to have them compounded for you by a cooperative pharmacist, or you might find them with an Internet search. Intravenous administration of magnesium may be necessary in more serious cases of CHF. Have a test ordered to check serum magnesium. Most doctors don't. It is even better to check myocardial magnesium. This is because the amount of magnesium in the heart muscle cells may be considerably lower than that in the blood.

Potassium

Potassium deficiency is associated with CHF, and is connected with magnesium deficiency. Low potassium can cause erratic heartbeat (heart arrhythmia). A very safe and very easy way to increase dietary potassium is to eat lots of easily digestible fruits and juiced vegetables. They are loaded with potassium. Nuts, whole grains, and legumes are good, too. Four ounces of almonds contains a whopping 800 mg. Brazil nuts have almost as much.

Coenzyme Q10

Coenzyme Q10 increases energy, probably due to its role in facilitating cellular respiration in the mitochondria of heart muscle cells. One of the best things about Coenzyme Q10 is that it is harmless, having no negative side effects or contraindications of any kind. No physician or hospital can make a case against taking it. The downside is that it is pricey. But then, so are heart transplants. Clinical studies and patient reports that show success with CoQ10 usually use somewhere around 400 mg a day, divided into several doses. 35 or 50 mg per day simply will not work.

I have read physician reports asserting that after regularly taking CoQ10, patients with severe CHF (so severe that they were waiting for a heart transplant) no longer needed the operation. I can't imagine higher praise than this.

Amino Acids

As a rule, I am in favor of getting amino acids through the protein in one's diet. With really sick people, however, a case can be made for amino acid supplementation. Dr. Werbach recommends L-arginine at a daily dose of 5,600–12,600 mg because it opens peripheral blood vessels and raises the heart's output. Patients given the supplement found they could walk longer, due to the improvement in blood flow while exercising. Arginine is normally considered by dietitians to be a "semiessential" amino acid, necessary only for growth. But growth may well include regrowth, strengthening, and repair of cardiac muscle. Eggs, cheese, whole grains, and legumes are good food sources. Peanuts are absolutely loaded with arginine, containing three times as much as meat does. You'd need to consume roughly a twelve-ounce can of peanuts a day to get in the middle of the dose mentioned above. That, or consider supplements. Chew nuts well for best absorption.

Taurine is an amino acid normally made in your body from another amino acid, methionine. Methionine is found in eggs, cheese, beans, nuts, and whole grains. Brazil nuts have over twice as much methionine as meat, ounce for ounce. Extreme stresses to the body (hospital food, perhaps?) can cause taurine deficiency. Taurine appears to help regulate heartbeat. Dr. Werbach recommends a dosage of 4,000–6,000 mg per day.

The amino acid L-carnitine is also made in your body *if* (and, to misquote Ed Sullivan, this is a "really big" if) you consume plenty of the amino acids methionine and lysine, and vitamin B_6, niacin, and vitamin C. Most people, especially the elderly suffering from chronic illness, do not get nearly enough of these vitamins. One study recommends 2,000 mg of L-carnitine daily for CHF.

Large amounts of supplemental creatine, still another amino acid that your body normally produces, may help strengthen heartbeat. As creatine phosphate, it is involved in supplying energy to power muscle tissue, especially cardiac muscle. Dr. Werbach cites studies indicating that persons with CHF have a deficiency of creatine in the heart muscle itself, and that daily doses of 20,000 mg per day improve cardiac function, physical strength, and endurance.

All quantities mentioned above should be divided up into several smaller doses throughout the day. I would add vitamin C, ranging anywhere from 4,000–10,000 mg per day all the way up to bowel tolerance. C is vital because of its antioxidant properties and because of its role in amino acid synthesis. I also suspect that since the heart prefers fatty acids for fuel, a long-standing deficiency of essential fatty acids causes deterioration of heart muscle. Lecithin, fish, and primrose oil are sources of essential fatty acids.

If these natural options do not speak strongly enough to you, bear in mind that

1. There is no drug cure for congestive heart failure;

2. The pharmaceutical drugs given in an attempt to cope with the condition have many side effects; and

3. The National Institutes of Health have issued some rather depressing statistics about CHF. Nearly 5 million Americans have CHF, and half of the patients diagnosed with CHF will be dead within five years. Each year, there are an estimated 400,000 new cases. And CHF is the most common diagnosis in hospital patients age sixty-five and older.

Incidence of CHF is equally frequent in men and women, but survival following diagnosis of congestive heart failure is worse in men. Even in women, only about 20 percent survive much longer than twelve years. The outlook is not much better than for most forms of cancer. The fatality rate for CHF is high, with one in five people dying within only one year. CHF remains a highly lethal condition.

An ideal CHF therapy would be to improve the heart's pumping ability, open clogged arteries, and prevent tissue damage from free radicals, a byproduct of the body's metabolic processes.

Most people appear to have found very little reason to believe that there are serious options for people with this serious disease.

But there are.

Recommended Reading

Data Fact Sheet: Congestive heart failure in the United States: a new epidemic. U.S. Dept of Health and Human Services, Public Health Service, National Institutes of Health, National Heart, Lung, and Blood Institute, September 1996.

Desai TK, et al. Taurine deficiency after intensive chemotherapy and/or radiation. *Am J Clinical Nutrition* 55 (1991): 708.

Ghidini O, Azzurro M, Vita A, Sartori G. Evaluation of the therapeutic efficacy of L-carnitine in congestive heart failure. *Int J Clinical Pharmacology, Therapy and Toxicology* 26 (1988): 217–220.

Roberts H, Hickey S. [Saul AW, series editor] *The Vitamin Cure for Heart Disease.* Laguna Beach, CA: Basic Health Publications, 2011.

Werbach M. *Textbook of Nutritional Medicine.* Tarzana, CA: Third Line Press, 1999, 273–275.

Cuts, Lacerations, and Slivers (Oh My!)

*"I am always doing what I cannot do yet,
in order to learn how to do it."*

—VINCENT VAN GOGH

Ever since I got a letter from a woman who wanted instructions for doing her own thoracic surgery—by correspondence—I have more truly realized the need for absolute clarity in writing a section like this one. So here it is: I am not utterly opposed to using the valid skills of well-trained medical professionals. Get a physician's opinion first, of course. There are limits to what you can do. (By the way, I told the woman to see a surgeon. I considered suggesting that she also see a psychiatrist.) Yet there are many things we can do for ourselves—and arguably better than a harried, hurried, hired practitioner.

I offer for your consideration (as Rod Serling would say) one or two of my more delightful childhood medical dramas, or should I say, traumas.

As kids, we were always building something in the woods behind my parents' house. After we built our tree fort (as differentiated from a mere tree house, mind you), we practically lived there. As work gloves were for sissies, we were prime targets for every splinter in the area, especially our hands.

My first line of treatment was my father. He was, after all, the one who always patched up our old tomcat, Tony. Tony's nocturnal avocations resulted in his coming home with substantial portions of his fur, skin, and ears missing. We went through many a bottle of A&P hydrogen peroxide on that cat, since vets were for rich kids' pets.

For wood splinters in our skin, Pa used the tried-and-true Army approach: sterilize a sewing needle (the bigger the better, it would seem) and unceremoniously dig the splinter out. This form of frontal attack worked, although of course it hurt. Once, however, I had a sliver way up under a fingernail. Even Dad backed away from that one. I was delighted when my folks sent me to our family doctor. There, I was certain, I would receive the adept and painless ministrations of a sympathetic healer.

Wrong.

The doctor sat me on his old-time, all-purpose, leather-covered examination table, and painted my finger orange with lots of mercurochrome (23 percent mercury in a colorful solution). Then he turned to his little white cabinet of goodies and calmly produced a particularly large pair of black-handled office scissors. These are formidable-looking blades to see coming at your little fingertip.

Without a word, and without any anesthetic, the doctor began cutting away my fingernail. I was so surprised I could barely yell . . . for a moment, anyway. In a few agonizing minutes, he had removed over half the fingernail, and the splinter along with it. I decided that the mercurochrome's real role was to hide the color of the blood, which it very nearly did. But surely the pain of a forcibly removed fingernail is more suited to prisoner-of-war torture stories than to a doctor's office.

It was almost immediately afterward that I decided that not only could my father have done as well, I could have done as well myself. After all, we had a pair of ten-inch paper shears at home that were almost as big as the ones the doctor used.

The next time I had an under-the-finger sliver, I had the inspired idea to actively avoid the needle, or scissors, or battle ax, or whatever they might throw at me. I had some experience with "black drawing salve" (I think the brand of the day was Ichthamol). Black drawing salve is so-called because it is black (duh) and because it helps "draw" pus out of a wound or boil. I wondered if it would physically draw out a sliver of wood. So I applied a small glob of it, covered it with gauze, and waited.

The next morning, enough of the splinter was protruding from under my fingernail for me to simply grab it with tweezers and pull it out.

No pain. No blood. No skill needed.

How does this work? I have no idea. But I've seen it happen, time and time again.

Equipment list: black drawing salve (available at any discount drug store), your mother's eyebrow tweezers, and one Band-Aid.

Let's now up the ante somewhat and consider deep cuts and lacerations. How can we close them without stitches? With butterfly bandages, also available at any pharmacy or discount store.

Butterfly bandages look like doll-sized white paper bow ties. They are narrow in the middle, hence the name, and have a strong adhesive on the back. To use them properly, you first must staunch the flow of blood so you can see what you are doing, and ensure that they will stick. Pressure on or above the wound will usually do this. With a clean cloth or gauze, blot and dry the area as best you can. Do not use tissues or toilet paper, as these paper products will disintegrate when dampened and make a mess. Paper towels are okay. Remove the plastic adhesive-protecting strip from one side only of the bandage. This is easiest if you have an assistant help you. Then apply the bandage, like a bridge over troubled tissue, to hold the cut together. *The trick is to put a stretch into it.* To do so, you have to place the first side of the butterfly bandage further away from the cut than you'd think. When you pull it over, it will close the wound. Hold it, remove the adhesive-cover on the remaining side, and press it down to complete the maneuver. You can pre-remove the adhesive-covers from both sides in advance if it works better for you, but this is the way I do it.

Expect to make a schlock job of it the first time. Have at least half a dozen butterfly bandages on hand and do not worry if you have to scrap a few and try again. Keep the wound area as dry as possible, though, and you are likely to get it right on the first few tries.

Even if the first closure works well, I usually apply a second butterfly bandage. I do this even if the wound is a small one. I put the second one on at a slight angle to the first, to contact different skin and increase the likelihood of success. This results in an X shape that impresses children a great deal. Then I cover the X with a one-inch-wide Band-Aid. Or two. This helps lock the butterflies in place and, to a moderate extent, keeps them from getting wet. Wet bandages lose their stick and come off earlier. Better the outer ones than the butterflies, though, for it is easy to slap on a plain Band-Aid or two any time, any place. Ideally, you do not want to remove the butterfly closures for several days to a week, depending on the severity of the cut. This gives the skin a chance to knit together deep down as well as on the surface, and makes it unlikely that the wound will reopen.

On a long laceration, you can repeat the "bridging" process with a series of butterfly-bandage crosses. There is a limit to how far you can go with this, so use uncommon sense and get medical assistance whenever you need it.

Here's a hint: as the skin heals, it will tend to dry and "pull" and itch. Dropping some natural vitamin E onto the wound, simply squeezed from a pricked capsule, will help. Do not

105

do this too early, for not only will the oil in vitamin E capsules completely ruin the bandage adhesive, but applied too soon, vitamin E's modest anticoagulant properties will delay surface clotting. Wait a few days to a week until you can see that the wound is solidly closed and you are ready to let the bandages come off anyway. As a side note, I might mention that if you want to spare your kids the pain of removing a bandage (slow or fast, it sure does hurt if there is hair under there), try this vitamin E technique. You will never hear an ouch again, for the bandages will easily come off on their own, and the kids will get the healing vitamin E benefits to boot.

In addition, healing is likely to be uncomplicated (no infection, scarring, or keloid formation) if you keep putting a tiny bit of vitamin E on the wound twice a day. Again, be sure the wound area is dry. Vitamin E oil and water don't mix. You can apply vitamin E to a conventional line of sutures, too. It overnight reduces soreness and swelling in and around the sutured area.

Bleeding is nature's way of cleaning a wound, so antiseptics and antibiotics are needed only rarely. If the wound is less than perfectly clean, I apply some iodine tincture to it, *but not right away,* because it hurts! Wait until you see slight redness after a couple of days. Iodine tincture is less disruptive of bandage adhesive than is vitamin E oil, and may be applied sooner, but sparingly. (You will need to carefully remove the outer covering of bandages to do this, of course, but you will want to see how the wound is coming anyway.) No need to remove the butterflies; just touch the iodine applicator to the exposed edge of the wound and it will be drawn in by itself. One or two applications is usually enough if you then follow up with the vitamin E treatment as mentioned above.

In summary:

1. Pressure to stop blood flow.

2. Dry the wound.

3. Butterfly bandage(s) applied with a stretch.

4. Cover with Band-Aid(s).

5. Add topical vitamin E after healing is well underway.

I may know how to do all this, but I confess that I still hate buying Band-Aids. This is because as a parent, I know all too well for whom I am buying them. I especially grimace when buying butterfly bandages. The only good thing about them is that they work as well or better than the alternative: stitches. I have only rarely had to use butterfly bandages on each of my children. Once my daughter fell in primary school and cut her chin. She had a Band-Aid on when she got off the bus. When we removed it, we saw that the cut was deep enough to expose yellow-orange fat. That is a deep cut. I very carefully applied a pair of butterfly bandages, which held the skin tightly together. After four or five days we started applying vitamin E to the site. Healing was so successful that you cannot find what surely would have been a scar had we gone the stitches route. When I had a chin laceration of my own some years before, I had stitches (not then knowing the butterfly technique). I have a scar to this day (which I hide nicely under my beard).

I have personally observed children getting stitched up in an emergency room. It is a scene to be avoided. In my daughter's case, it was. A laceration was effectively closed without needles, without the pain they necessarily cause, and without the stress of going to and waiting for assistance. I don't relish the task, but I'd prefer to be the one delivering care to my own kids. I think they greatly prefer it as well.

If it is a question of competence, then we must become competent, for even emergency room personnel might not be. "Many U.S. emergency rooms are staffed by doctors who were never taught how to treat a heart attack, resuscitate a child or treat bleeding," says the Rochester, New York *Democrat and Chronicle*. According to "Dr. L. Thompson Bowles, president of the National Board of Medical Examiners and chairmen of a group of 38 health care authorities who studied the issue . . . many [emergency room doctors] lack training and adequate experience in any aspect of primary health care."

Still, if you really need an ambulance, call one! Major traumatic injuries and some other situations absolutely demand medical technology. Even if the medical residents are not experienced, chances are the nurses and paramedics are. I submit, however, that we can reclaim a significantly larger part of our own health responsibility than most doctors would allow, and by simpler steps than most doctors would admit. I actually learned how to use the butterfly bandage from a friend over the phone, and by reading the directions on the package. It was time well spent to save my little girl from added pain and a facial scar.

ORAL REHYDRATION THERAPY FOR EMERGENCIES

Our bodies contain and exist in a watery environment. When adults lose too much water during illness, it is serious. But when sick young children lose too much water, it can be life-threatening. Dehydration in babies is a medical emergency. Contact your health provider promptly. And, here is a book to keep handy, because it contains the best emergency re-hydration instructions for parents that I have ever seen: David Werner's *Where There Is No Doctor: A Village Health Care Handbook* (Berkeley, CA: Hesperian Foundation, 1977, revised 1992, p 181–190), www. hesperian.org/hespubs.htm. Although allopathic in tone, this book remains a favorite of mine. It includes information on how to make your own butterfly bandages, how to suture a wound, and even how to set fractures. No, I am not even hinting that you should do all those things. Just learn about what you can do, and what you might have to do if you absolutely had to. Like the Scouts say, Be prepared. And like *Doctor Yourself* says, Be informed. In advance.

"When I wrote many papers early in my career, they were considered pretty good as long as they did not say anything, like most psychiatric papers today."

—DR. ABRAM HOFFER

Depression affects close to 20 million American adults. Those of us that have experienced the depths of clinical depression know just how awful it really is. When you are in the bag, it is hard to think out of the bag. But there is a way out. You have already begun. If you are making the effort of reading this, your depression can't be beyond help. Let's put the positive right out front.

> ### A reader says:
>
> "I'm twenty years old now, but my depression started when I was in seventh grade. I went to the doctor at age eighteen, and I was diagnosed with bipolar, depression, and anxiety. I was on lamictal and wellbutrin for two years, and I just wasn't seeing any improvement. I weaned off the medicine and found myself feeling even worse for the next year. Checking *Doctor Yourself* out from the library changed my life. In the past two weeks, I've changed my diet to mostly raw foods and started taking a multivitamin, B_{12} and 300 mg of niacin a day. I feel like the person I've always wanted to be. I went out last week for the first time in a year. I've literally been too scared to leave the house having been bombarded with terrible social anxiety. It's all gone away. I feel more productive and energized then I ever have in my life. I just wish I would have found out sooner, and not had to suffer for the last eight years. Thank you so much for the large wealth of information, and thank you for changing my outlook on life."

Now on with it: what you can you do to help eliminate depression without drugs?

Exercise

You'll rust out faster than you wear out. You probably already know that. So get moving! My "Evading Exercise" chapter is fun to read, contains nudity, and may serve as motivation to get you started. Or start laughing, as the case may be.

Niacin, Thiamin, and B_6

Depression may be caused by a deficiency of all or a deficiency of just one of these vitamins. Ample amounts of B-complex vitamins, especially B_1, B_3 and B_6 (pyridoxine) must be present for your body's normal, depression-fighting chemical reactions to occur. Niacin and thiamin are added to many foods in small quantities, but not nearly enough. The RDA of niacin is under 20 mg. We need several hundred milligrams a day at least. I take 3,000 mg/day, in divided doses. Vitamin B_6 deficiency is very common in Americans, and that "deficiency" is measured against an already ridiculously low U.S. RDA of only two milligrams. The amount of B_6 needed for clinical effectiveness in, say, rabbits, is the human dose equivalent of 75 mg daily. That is over 35 times more than the RDA! The RDA for thiamin is also in the neighborhood of two milligrams, and it too is absurdly low. Instead, 75 mg/day is much more reasonable. Try these numbers and see how it helps you.

> ### Another reader says:
>
> "I am thirty-eight years old and I've suffered from severe anxiety, depression, mood swings, social phobias, and so much more, for most of my life. Three years ago, I was prescribed medication for my depression and another drug for my mood swings. After one month on these medicines I became so manic I couldn't sleep and I suffered from horrible nightmares. I truly felt I was losing my mind and that there was nothing left to do. I have been taking Zoloft and Ativan for the last two years. Then, about a month ago, I looked into nutrition therapy and I figured, why not? So I started off on niacin, vitamin C, and a multivitamin. I can't believe the results. I feel perfectly normal and happy for the first time in my life. I am amazed at how much energy I have and how great I sleep, and I wake up so rested in the mornings! This is truly the best thing that's ever happened to me. Thank you so much for getting this information out there. You have helped give my husband back his wife, my daughter her mother, and me a life."

There are virtually no known side effects with thiamin supplementation. Really enormous doses of B_6 taken alone have produced temporary neurological side effects. It usually takes between 2,000 and 5,000 mg daily for symptoms of numbness or tingling in the extremities. Some side effects have been reported as low as 500 mg daily, but these are very rare indeed. Therapeutic doses between 100 and 500 milligrams daily are commonly prescribed by physicians for PMS relief. A daily total of a few hundred milligrams of individual B_6, especially if taken in addition to the entire B-complex to ensure balance, is very safe indeed.

Niacin characteristically causes a warm "flushing" of cheeks, neck and extremities. It is harmless, but can be annoying. You can select flush-free niacin if you prefer. As for me, I live in the very-Northern US, just across the lake from Canada. For me, warm is good.

Water

Believe it or not, drinking more water can improve mood. (And talk about economical . . .) According to Dr. Hugh Riordan, an expert on depression, "As we get older, one of the major problems is dehydration. When we were young, the ratio of water inside the cell to outside the cell [was] 1.2 to 1. There is more water inside the cell than there is outside. By the time we are 60, the ratio is 0.8 to 1. Even if you are drinking enough water, you are dehydrating all the time. So the goal is to drink sufficient water."

Reference

Overcoming Depression, Hugh D. Riordan, M.D. Health Hunters, February 2003, Vol 17, No. 2, p 1. www.riordanclinic.org/education/newsletter/89025108.pdf.

Omega-3 Fatty Acids (in fish oils)

Japan and Korea have very little incidence of depression. Again, from Dr. Riordan: "Japanese and Koreans eat fish. The omega-3 fat in most fish manipulates brain chemicals in ways that boost mood."

Make Your Own Neurotransmitters

Rather than give a synthetic drug to block or mimic the body's chemical nerve messengers (neurotransmitters), it is possible nutritionally to encourage the body to make its own natural ones. If we are what we eat, then our nerves also depend on what they are fed. Here is tremendous potential for the alleviation of depression and related disorders.

Norepinephrine

A depletion of the neurotransmitter called norepinephrine may result in poor memory, loss of alertness, and clinical depression. The chain of chemical events in the body resulting in this substance is:

L-phenylalanine (from protein foods) $\longrightarrow$ L-tyrosine (made in the liver) $\longrightarrow$ dopa $\longrightarrow$ dopamine $\longrightarrow$ norepinephrine $\longrightarrow$ epinephrine

This process looks complex but actually is readily accomplished, particularly if the body has plenty of vitamin C. Since one's dietary supply of the first ingredient, L-phenylalanine, is usually adequate, it is more likely to be a shortage of vitamin C that limits production of norepinephrine. Physicians giving large doses of vitamin C have had striking success in reversing depression. It is a remarkably safe and inexpensive approach to try.

Dr. Riordan said:

"Many years ago, I had a lady who was a teacher and she was profoundly depressed. She had profound fatigue and was barely able to function at all. Testing revealed she had no detectable vitamin C in her, so we gave her 500 milligrams of vitamin C a day—not very much by our standards. In a couple of weeks, she thought a miracle had occurred. No miracle had occurred. She was low on vitamin C and depression is the natural consequence of that. If you are depressed, vitamin C is worth considering."

Acetylcholine

Acetylcholine is the end neurotransmitter of your parasympathetic nerve system. This means that, among other things, it facilitates good digestion, deeper breathing, and slower heart rate. You may perceive its effect as "relaxation."

Your body will make its own acetylcholine from choline. Choline is available in the diet as phosphatidyl choline, found in lecithin. Lecithin is found to a modest extent in egg yolks. But that is not enough. Three tablespoons daily of soya lecithin granules provide about five grams (5,000 milligrams) of phosphatidyl choline. Long-term use of this amount was favorably mentioned in *The Lancet* (February 9, 1980). Lecithin supplementation has no known harmful effects whatsoever. In fact, your brain by dry weight is almost one-third lecithin! How far can we go with this idea of simply feeding the brain what it is made up of? In *Geriatrics* (July 1979) lecithin was considered as a therapy to combat memory loss. Studies at MIT show increases in both choline and acetylcholine in the brains of animals after just one lecithin meal.

Lecithin is good for you. How good? Each tablespoon (7.5 grams) of lecithin granules contains about 1,700 mg of phosphatidyl choline, 1,000 mg of phosphatidyl inositol, and about 2,200 mg of essential fatty acids as linoleic acid. It also contains the valuable fish-oil-like, omega-3 linolenic acid. It is the rule, not the exception, for one or more of these valuable substances to be undersupplied by our daily diet.

Lecithin tastes crummy. How crummy? Well, the lecithin that is available in capsules is the most popular. These are sold at health food stores and are admittedly convenient, but are also expensive. In order to get even one tablespoon of lecithin, you would have to take eight to twelve capsules! Since a normal supplemental dose is three or more tablespoons daily, that's a lot of capsules to swallow. Much less costly is liquid lecithin. A taste for liquid lecithin has to be acquired, shall we say. It is easier to take if you first coat the spoon with milk or molasses. After taking liquid lecithin, it is wise to have a "chaser" of any dairy product or, again, molasses. Beef and sheep brains are also an excellent source of lecithin, but don't expect me to recommend them.

Probably the best way to get a lot of lecithin easily is to take lecithin *granules*. Stir the granules quickly into juice or milk. They won't dissolve, but rather will drift about as you drink. Lecithin granules can also be used as a topping on any cold food. Ice cream comes to mind. Also, they are not bad if stirred into yogurt. If you put lecithin granules on hot food, they will melt and you will then have liquid lecithin.

If that "brains" comment a while back is still bothering you, please bear in mind that all supplemental forms of lecithin are made from soy beans. An alternate non-soy source is egg yolk. Generally, maximum benefit is obtained when you eat the yolk lightly cooked (such as in a soft-boiled egg).

By the way, the correct pronunciation of "lecithin" is "LESS-A-THIN. This is easy to remember because you are probably less-a-thin than you used-to-a-be.

111

A reader says about panic attacks:

"I have coped for years with regular panic attacks and severe depersonalization episodes. I've done the therapist routine (fifteen different therapists in the course of twenty years). I have found other approaches (acupuncture, meditation) to be of limited value. I definitely wanted to avoid psychotropic drugs, but it was not looking good. For months I went through a period where the attacks were coming every few days and might last for days. Finally, in desperation, I started taking B vitamins(B-100 complex, 2 to 3 times daily), vitamin C to help with the metabolism of tryptophan-rich foods (which I have tended to crave without knowing why), and daily doses of lecithin (2 to 4 tablespoons/day).

"The change feels almost miraculous. I still have episodes, but they are much more manageable. I can maintain some sane perspective and can see them *as* episodes rather than as something unbearable that feels like it will go on forever. I am convinced that it is not only the nutritional substances that are making the difference but also the fact that I managed—with your help—to take agency in my own healing."

Serotonin

Before the FDA removed tryptophan supplements from the market due to a temporary, and now corrected, industrial manufacturing error, millions of people had safely taken regular suppertime doses of this amino acid, usually 500–2,000 mg, to help them sleep. Inside you, tryptophan is broken down into anxiety-reducing, snooze-inducing niacin. Even more important, tryptophan is also made into serotonin, one of your body's most important neurotransmitters. Serotonin is responsible for feelings of well-being and mellowness. It has such a profound effect that Prozac, Paxil, and similar antidepressants artificially keep the body's own serotonin levels high. They are called selective serotonin reuptake inhibitor (SSRI) drugs.

You can accomplish something very similar through your diet. Self-medication with food is not uncommon. You might as well do it right. And no one can tell us that good, natural foods are toxic if you eat a lot of them! Some foods that naturally increase your serotonin levels are beans, avocados, pineapple, eggplant, plums, bananas, walnuts, peas, cheese, nuts, sunflower seeds, and good ol' wheat germ. Any and all of these help enhance how you feel if you are depressed.

People often feel better in general when they've eaten. There are many reasons for this, of course, but here is a reason that is underappreciated. A meal with plenty of carbohydrates helps tryptophan get to where it does the most good: your brain. In order to cross the blood-brain barrier and get in, carbs are required. So cheese and crackers provides a better effect than the cheese standing alone. Cover your ears, animal friends, for I am also about to condone eating the occasional dead bird. Poultry, especially the dark meat, is a rich (yet very cheap) source of tryptophan. Add potatoes or stuffing, and you have the reason everybody is sprawled out and snoring up a storm after a typical Thanksgiving food orgy. But to be able to look your parakeet in the eye after the fourth Thursday in November, you can stay vegetarian and still get tanked up on tryptophan.

Consider that five servings of beans, a few portions of cheese or peanut butter, or several handfuls of cashews provide 1,000–2,000 mg of tryptophan, which will work as well as prescription antidepressants—but don't tell the drug companies. Some skeptics think that the pharmaceutical people already know, and that is why the FDA is less than enthusiastic about tryptophan supplements. Here are two quotes in evidence:

"Pay careful attention to what is happening with dietary supplements in the legislative arena. . . . If these efforts are successful, there could be created a class of products to compete with approved drugs. The establishment of a separate regulatory category for supplements could undercut exclusivity rights enjoyed by the holders of approved drug applications."
—FDA Deputy Commissioner for Policy David Adams, at the Drug Information Association Annual Meeting, July 12, 1993

"The task force considered many issues in its deliberations including to ensure that the existence of dietary supplements on the market does not act as a disincentive for drug development."
—FDA Dietary Task Force Report, released June 15, 1993

Remember that tryptophan is one of the ten essential amino acids you need to stay alive. By law it is added to liquid feedings for the elderly and to all infant formulas. This says a great deal about its safety, as well as its importance.

You can buy L-5-hydroxytryptophan (5-HTP), a nonprescription tryptophan derivative, at health food stores and on the Internet. 5-HTP is quite costly, however. The good news is that plenty of inexpensive vitamin C enables your body to convert dietary tryptophan into your own 5-HTP, and then on into serotonin. And, tryptophan is really quite easy to get directly and cheaply from the good foods listed below.

So go, eat, and be happy!

Foods High in the Amino Acid L-Tryptophan

(In milligrams per 100-gram (3.5 ounce) portion, about the size of a deck of playing cards. That is not a large serving, and in a single meal you might easily double or triple the figures listed here.)

Beans

Lentils 215	Navy 200	Red kidney 215
Dried peas 250	Pinto 210	Soy 525

Nuts and Seeds

Brazil nuts 185	Pumpkin seeds 560
Cashews 470	Sesame seeds 330
Filberts 210	Tahini (ground sesame seeds) 575
Peanuts 340	Sunflower seeds 340
Peanut butter 330 (natural, not commercial)	

Other nuts generally provide at least 130 mg per small serving; usually more.

Grains

Wheat germ 265

Cheese

Cheddar 340	Swiss 375	Parmesan 490

Other cheeses tend to be lower in tryptophan, but are still very good sources.

Eggs 210

Poultry 250

(Note how vegetarian sources are as good as, and often much better than, flesh sources.)

Brewer's Yeast 700

(Source: USDA, Amino Acid Content of Foods)

Meats are generally regarded as a good source of tryptophan, organ meats supposedly being the highest. However, most meats are in the range of 160–260 mg/100 g, with organ meats ranging between 220 and 330. These figures certainly do not compel meat eating. They compel split pea, cheese, and cashew eating!

Another reader says:

"Having discovered that vitamin B complex, vitamin C, and zinc cured my postnatal depression (I was on lots of medication), I decided that this was something the whole world had to know about. Well, needless to say, I have since discovered that the world doesn't want to know or isn't listening properly. My pastor didn't even believe me. Sometimes I get really discouraged, but then sometimes I discover something like this and I feel reinvigorated. One just has to keep on going, never losing faith. I'm working on my sister, who's a psychiatrist. Maybe one day she'll prescribe supplements instead!"

"The best part of a donut is the hole."

—DR. PAUL C. BRAGG, HEALTH CRUSADER AND TEACHER OF JACK LALANNE

One in every sixteen people has diabetes. Nearly three million Americans are on insulin. Many instances of blindness, amputations, and death (more than 160,000 annually) result from the circulatory complications of diabetes. Diabetes mellitus is a group of metabolic disorders in which the body does not produce sufficient insulin, the hormone used to metabolize glucose (blood sugar). When glucose isn't metabolized efficiently, blood sugar levels rise, and this leads to impaired energy, growth, and immune response. Over time, this can cause damage and eventual failure of many organs, including the heart, blood vessels, kidneys, nerves, and eyes.

Diabetes is divided into two prevalent forms. Type 1 diabetes, often called insulin-dependent or juvenile-onset, seems to be an autoimmune disease (where the body's own immune cells attack it) and is the most serious of the two. Type 2 diabetes, often called non-insulin-dependent or maturity-onset, generally occurs later in life, especially in overweight people, and is the result of poor diet and lifestyle habits: faced with a lifelong barrage of simple carbohydrates from sweets and refined starches, the pancreas eventually becomes exhausted and can no longer pump out enough insulin. Even many utterly orthodox medical doctors agree with me that this one can be solved through diet and supplementation.

Five Musts for a Diabetic

1. **Eliminate Sugar**. No one would tell a child with a broken leg to jump off the garage roof. But perhaps we should not even let children *without* broken legs jump off garage roofs. Dietitians would never recommend that diabetics regularly eat lots of sweets. But really, no one should. The vast majority of us overconsume sugar to an alarming degree. Can this not only aggravate diabetes, but actually *cause* it? In the case of type 2, it is almost certainly so. And with type 1, the risk is there. There is no downside to avoiding sugar except, perhaps, putting your local dentist on unemployment. Avoid simple starches too, such as pasta, white rice, and white bread. These are quickly converted into sugars by the body. Instead, choose complex carbohydrates like whole wheat bread and brown rice. These are converted into sugars much more slowly.

2. **Avoid Milk**. Milk consumption in childhood can contribute to the development of type 1 diabetes. Certain proteins in milk resemble molecules on the beta cells of the pancreas that secrete insulin. In some cases, the immune system makes antibodies to the milk protein that mistakenly attack and destroy the beta cells. Even so august an authority on children as the late Dr. Benjamin Spock changed his recommendations in his later years and discouraged giving children milk.

3. **Avoid Fluoride**. Even at only one tenth (0.4 ppm) of the U.S. government's maximum "safe" allowed level, fluoride is known to interfere with kidney function, and impaired ability to normally excrete fluoride has been found in people with diabetes. Fluoride accumulates in living systems—such as, say, your children. And it may accumulate especially fast in persons with

nephrogenic diabetes, because of a polydipsia-polyurea syndrome that results in their increased intake, plus an abnormally high tendency to retain fluoride. Dr. Albert Burgstahler, Emeritus Professor of Chemistry, University of Kansas, says, "Children with nephrogenic diabetes insipidus or untreated pituitary diabetes have been found to develop severe dental fluorosis from drinking water containing only 1 or even 0.5 ppm fluoride" and that diabetics "are especially susceptible to the toxic effects of fluoride." Although fluoride is more poisonous even than lead, the Environmental Protection Agency allows over 250 times as much fluoride in your water as it allows lead in your water (4.0 ppm vs. 0.015 ppm). And the EPA's stated goal is to ultimately reduce lead levels to zero. No such luck with fluoride.

QUESTIONING FLUORIDE

When scientific journals refused to publish studies questioning water fluoridation, the journal *Fluoride* was started to get the research in print.[1] This peer-reviewed journal was first published in 1968 and continues to be published to this day. You have likely never heard of it. Neither has your dentist or doctor.

Someday, you might at least be able to find this journal at the US National Library of Medicine/Medline (NLM). But don't hold your breath. NLM, your taxpayer-supported "largest medical library on earth," censors your access to journals it does not like. Worldwide, as well as in the United States of America, most people feel that such behavior from a public library is reprehensible. If you are among those who do, you can write to NLM and tell them so. Their most up-to-date customer service e-mail address is online and easily found with any Internet search engine. At publication, it was custserv@nlm.nih.gov. Access is also available at www .nlm.nih. gov/contacts/contact.html or http://apps2.nlm.nih.gov/mainweb/siebel/nlm/index.cfm/.

Reference

1. Free access to *Fluoride's archives at www.fluoride-journal.com/ or www.fluorideresearch.org/.*

4. **Avoid Caffeine**. Caffeine is a drug, and can interfere with normal blood sugar levels. Caffeine magnifies the effects of the hormones glucagon and adrenaline, causing more sugar from the liver to be released into the blood stream. This means a raise in blood glucose levels. The more caffeine consumed, the more this is true.

5. **Question Immunization**. Be very cautious of vaccination. Harris Coulter, in *Vaccination and Violent Crime,* writes that diabetes is ten times more common today in the United States than it was in the 1940s. The pertussis vaccine, in particular, has an impact on the insulin-producing centers in the pancreas. Overstimulation, and ultimate exhaustion, of these centers can lead to diabetes. The risk of type 1 diabetes may also be increased if the hepatitis B vaccine is given to babies when they are six weeks old.

B-Complex Vitamins

One of the first nutrition zingers I ever read was Dr. Carlton Fredericks's comment in *Food Facts and Fallacies* that diabetics could be weaned off insulin with extremely high doses of B-complex vitamins. I am a conservative person and I have my sincere doubts if a type 1 diabetic could ever be entirely free of the need to take insulin. On the other hand, I have personally seen such diabetics require significantly less insulin when they take a 100 mg balanced B-complex tablet every two to three hours. The potential benefits are so great that I think diabetics should demand a suitably cautious therapeutic trial of megavitamin therapy *with insulin dosage adjustment made and supervised by their physicians.*

A daily dosage of 1,500 to 2,500 mg of niacin or niacinamide (one of the B-complex vitamins) may improve carbohydrate tolerance in diabetics. People with niacin deficiency may show hypersensitivity to insulin, with their blood sugar decreasing more readily than normal subjects after an injection of insulin. This means that niacin or niacinamide diminishes the requirements of insulin needed to keep the blood sugar of diabetics within normal limits. The dosage can be given in 500 mg amounts three to five times daily at first, then reduced as the blood sugar comes down.

A chiropractor in Pennsylvania wrote to me and said, "I recently had a pharmacist take one of my female diabetic patients off niacin (after an extremely successful course of therapy with niacin that eliminated years of insomnia) because he told her that it would mess up her blood sugar. I had another female diabetic patient who got some decent results with niacin for depression but was told by her pharmacist not to use it with diabetes. Yet I cannot seem to find anything to support *not* using niacin in diabetics."

That is simply because niacin works, and in doing so, creates a management issue. When megadoses of niacin lower the need for insulin, that is success, but an inconvenience (and perhaps an embarrassment) for the pharmophilic (drug-loving) health professional. But the main point must not be missed: a reduction in insulin requirement is good news for the patient. I would like to receive information about studies alleging evidence of any problems with niacin or niacinamide administration in diabetics. Please send it to drsaul@doctoryour self.com.

Vitamin C

In his recent book *Vitamin C: Who Needs It?*, Emanuel Cheraskin says, "What do the experts tell us about a vitamin C connection in the control of sugar metabolism? We turned to five of the leading textbooks dealing with diabetes mellitus published during the last five years. Would you believe? There was not one word indicating any connection or a lack of correlation between ascorbic acid and carbohydrate metabolism? This is even more incomprehensible when one realizes that reviews of the literature as far back as 1940 showed that blood sugar can be predictably reduced with intravenous ascorbate." One case study suggests that for each gram (1,000 mg) of vitamin C taken by mouth, the amount of insulin required could be reduced by two units. Vitamin C may also help to keep capillaries from bursting, a major cause of diabetic complications, by increasing the elasticity of these smallest of blood vessels. Physicians investigated the effect of 600 mg per day of magnesium and 2,000 mg per day of vitamin C on a group of fifty-six non-insulin-dependent diabetics. The vitamin C improved control of blood sugar levels. It also lowered cholesterol and triglyceride levels, and reduced capillary fragility. Additionally, the magnesium lowered blood pressure in the subjects.

Magnesium

Magnesium is unusually important to the diabetic. Magnesium is needed to metabolize carbohydrates, and magnesium has a role in the production and utilization of insulin. Magnesium deficiency can increase insulin resistance, and therefore can worsen a type 2 diabetic's control of blood sugar. To compound the problem, high blood sugar increases urinary loss of magnesium in a person who already does not have enough of it. While there is disagreement as to how important this deficiency actually is for the diabetic, when has a long-term nutrient deficiency ultimately been proven to be beneficial? Taking a supplement providing at least the RDA of magnesium (about 400 mg) is, in my opinion, vital.

Exercise and Weight Control

Just do it! It helps tremendously. Suggestions on how are in my "Evading Exercise" chapter. Type 2 diabetes is clearly associated with overweight persons. Hint, hint.

Stress Reduction and Meditation

Diabetics (and most everyone else) will find that a wide variety of physical and mental benefits are among the advantages of regular, deep relaxation. The best relaxation techniques I have found are described in my chapter on "Stress Reduction."

Chromium

The trace mineral chromium is found in skin, fat, muscle, brain tissue, and adrenal glands. There is only about 6 milligrams in you, but is it ever important! Absorption by way of your intestine is poor, and it is excreted in urine. Chromium is an essential component of glucose tolerance factor (GTF). GTF helps insulin to work better by "bridging" it to cell membranes. Chromium as GTF improves glucose tolerance in diabetics whether they are children or adults.

Far and away the best food source of chromium is brewer's yeast. You can also use nutritional yeast, which is nutritionally similar and better tasting. Brewer's yeast is a by-product of beer-making and tends to be a bit bitter. Nutritional yeast is primarily grown to be a food. Try nutritional yeast flakes on popcorn. It tastes so much like cheese that you may well like it. One Friday night, without telling what was in it, I sprung some of my stealthy, healthy ersatz "cheese popcorn" on some really finicky friends of mine. They happily munched away while trouncing me at euchre.

Aside from teaching them when to lead the left bower, one of the best things you can do is give your family a teaspoon or two of this stuff every day. In addition to chromium, it is a good source of B vitamins. Way too much, by the way, may cause temporary and harmless skin irritation in some especially sensitive people. If you start low and increase slow, this will probably not occur.

Other food sources of chromium include nuts, prunes, mushrooms, most whole grains, and many fermented foods, including beer and wine. Please remember the negative nutritional aspects of alcohol, and instead go for the yeast. If you simply must tip a few, at least try to select additive-free, organically grown beverages and use them in moderation.

If you are a teetotaler, and your interest in yeast is rapidly waning, the best supplements usually combine chromium with niacin, which seems to greatly enhance uptake. An example is chromium polynicotinate, which has been demonstrated to be especially well absorbed and retained. However, almost any chromium supplement will get decent results.

I would *always* supplement with 200–400 mcg of chromium daily if there is any hint of hypoglycemia (and that's most of us). In fact, I take that much every day. The RDA is 50–200 mcg daily. Even traditional diet textbooks admit that the conventional U.S. diet does not reliably

117

supply even this amount. For the diabetic, chromium supplementation is essential . . . unless you are a *huge* fan of yeast.

Fiber

There is a well-established reduction of hyperglycemia in people who consume extra dietary fiber. This means a probable decrease in insulin requirement for type 1 diabetics, and even better news for type 2s. Generally, the more fiber eaten, the less medication needed. Try it and see how much better you feel. Soluble fiber, such as pectin (a thickener used to make jelly), may also help. It appears that even ever-delightful, over-the-counter Kaopectate has been used medically in the treatment of diabetes. Ugh. But the really good news is that fibers like pectin are found in the cell walls of all fruits and vegetables. Diabetics should eat a lot more vegetables.

Vitamin E

Persons with low vitamin E levels have almost four times the risk of type 2 diabetes. Large quantities of vitamin E (1,800 IU daily) restored normal blood flow in the retina of the eyes of type 1 (insulin dependent) diabetics. Patients initially having the worst blood flow were the ones who improved the most. Vitamin E may also reduce the risk for the development of retinopathy or nephropathy in diabetics. Vitamin E's strong protective influence suggests that damage by free radicals may be a cause of these complications of the disease. Further information on vitamin E and diabetes can be found in the books of Evan and Wilfrid Shute, especially *Vitamin E for Ailing and Healthy Hearts.*

118

Vanadium

Some years ago, I had the pleasure of teaching clinical nutrition with Cornell University researcher Wes Canfield, M.D. Trace minerals are Dr. Canfield's special interest, and he believes that vanadate is very important in the prevention and treatment of diabetes, because of its ability to mimic insulin. Do not go belting down megadoses of vanadium just yet, as there are concerns about vanadium's potentially toxic side effects. A free search at the National Library of Medicine website (known as PubMed, www.nlm.nih.gov) will bring up some two hundred papers on the subject.

Iatrogenic (Doctor-Caused) Diabetes

At least some instances of diabetes may be a major side effect of antibiotics and other common pharmaceuticals. Diabetes, usually thought to be largely of genetic or dietary origin, may be increasing so much in recent decades because of the proliferation in the use, and overuse, of medicines. To the extent that this is true, alternative measures need to be fully explored. I consider Melvyn Werbach's *Nutritional Influences on Illness,* and his more recent *Textbook of Nutritional Medicine,* to be must-reads. Werbach provides valuable summaries of research indicating the therapeutic value of various supplemental nutrients, and their specific dosages, for diabetics.

Smoking

Diabetes type 2 is nearly twice as likely to develop in both men and women who smoke. And the more you smoke, the greater the likelihood. You're not really surprised about that, now are you? So stop now, or at the very least, cut *way* down. Save your pancreas, your insulin, your blood sugar, and likely your life. Not to mention a whole lot of money. (Rimm EB, Manson JE, Stampfer MJ et al. Cigarette smoking and the risk of diabetes in women. *Am J Public Health.,* 1993, 83[2]:211–4; Rimm EB, Chan J, Stampfer MJ et al. Prospective study of cigarette smoking, alcohol use, and the risk of diabetes in men. *BMJ.,* 1995, 310[6979]:555–9.)

Recommended Reading

Balch JF and Balch PA. *Prescription for Nutritional Healing.* Garden City Park, NY: Avery Publishing, 1990.

Barnard RJ, et al. Response of non-insulin-dependent diabetic patients to an intensive program of diet and exercise. *Diabetes Care* 5 (1982): 370–74.

Bennett PH, et al. 1979. The role of obesity in the development of diabetes of the Pima Indians. In J. Vague and P.H. Vague, eds. Diabetes and Obesity. *Excerpta Medica,* Amsterdam.

Brighthope I. *The Vitamin Cure for Diabetes.* Laguna Beach, CA: Basic Health Publications, 2012.

Bruckert E, et al. Increased serum levels of Lipoprotein(a) in diabetes mellitus and their reduction with glycemic control. *JAMA* 263 (1990): 35–36.

Cheraskin E. *Vitamin C: Who Needs It?* New York: Arlington Press, 1993.

Cheraskin E, et al. Effect of caffeine versus placebo supplementation on blood glucose concentration. *Lancet* 1 (June 1967):1299–1300.

Cheraskin E and Ringsdorf WM. Blood glucose levels after caffeine. *Lancet* 2 (September 1968): 21.

Classen JB. Childhood immunization and diabetes mellitus. *New Zealand Medical Journal* 195 (May 1996).

Corica F, et al. Effects of oral magnesium supplementation on plasma lipid concentrations in patients with non-insulin-dependent diabetes mellitus. *Magnes. Res.* 7 (1994): 43–46.

Coulter H. "Childhood Vaccinations and Juvenile-Onset (Type-1) Diabetes." Testimony before the Congress of the United States, House of Representatives, Committee on Appropriations, Subcommittee on Labor, Health and Human Services, Education, and Related Agencies, April 16, 1997.

Cunningham JJ, Mearkle PL, and Brown RG. Vitamin C: an aldose reductase inhibitor that normalizes erythrocyte sorbitol in insulin-dependent diabetes mellitus. *J Am Coll Nutr* 13 (August 1994): 344–45.

Dental fluorosis associated with hereditary diabetes insipidus. *Oral Surgery* 40 (1975): 736–41.

Dice JF and Daniel CW. The hypoglycemic effect of ascorbic acid in a juvenile-onset diabetic. *International Research Communications System* 1 (1973): 41.

Eriksson J and Kohvakka A. Magnesium and ascorbic acid supplementation in diabetes mellitus. *Annals of Nutrition and Metabolism* 39 (July/Aug 1995): 217–23.

Garrison RH and Somer E. *The Nutrition Desk Reference.* New Canaan, CT: Keats, 1990 216–22.

Hoffer A. *Vitamin B-3 (Niacin) Update; New Roles For a Key Nutrient in Diabetes, Cancer, Heart Disease and Other Major Health Problems.* New Canaan, CT: Keats,1990.

Hoffer A and Walker M. *Orthomolecular Nutrition.* New Canaan, CT: Keats, 1978, 14, 21–26, and 100–101.

Junco LI, et al. "Renal Failure and Fluorosis," Fluorine and Dental Health. *JAMA* 222 (1972): 783–85.

Kapeghian JC, et al. The effects of glucose on ascorbic acid uptake in heart, endothelial cells: Possible pathogenesis of diabetic angiopathies. *Life Sci* 34 (1984):577.

Mather HM, et al. Hypomagnesemia in diabetes. *Clinical and Chemical Acta* 95 (1979): 235–42.

119

McNair P, et al. Hypomagnesemia, a risk factor in diabetic retinopathy. *Diabetes* 27 (1978): 1075–77.

Pfleger R and Scholl F. Diabetes und vitamin C. *Wiener Archiv für Innere Medizin* 31(1937): 219–30.

Salonen JT, et al. Increased risk of non-insulin dependent diabetes mellitus at low plasma vitamin E concentrations: a four year follow-up study in men. *BMJ* 311 (October 1995):1124–27.

Setyaadmadja ATSH, Cheraskin E, and Ringsdorf WM. Ascorbic acid and carbohydrate metabolism: II. Effect of supervised sucrose drinks upon two-hour postprandial blood glucose in terms of vitamin C state. *Lancet* 87 (January 1967): 18–21.

Sinclair AJ, et al. Low plasma ascorbate levels in patients with type 2 diabetes mellitus consuming adequate dietary vitamin C. *Diabet Med* 11 (November 1994): 893–98.

Snowdon DA and Phillips RL. Does a vegetarian diet reduce the occurrence of diabetes? *Am. J. Public Health* 75 (1985):507–12.

Som S, et al. Ascorbic acid metabolism in diabetes mellitus. *Metabolism* 30 (1981): 572–77.

Stone I. *The Healing Factor: Vitamin C Against Disease.* New York: Grosset & Dunlap, 1972, 146–51.

Timimi FK, et al. Vitamin C improves endothelium-dependent vasodilation in patients with insulin-dependent diabetes mellitus. *J Am Coll Cardiol* 31 (March 1998): 552–57.

Toxicological Profile for Fluorides, Hydrogen Fluoride, and Fluorine (F). Agency for Toxic Substances and Disease Registry, U.S. Dept. of Health and Human Services, April 1993, 112.

Werbach M. *Nutritional Influences on Illness.* New Canaan, CT: Keats Publishing, 1988.

Werbach M. *Textbook of Nutritional Medicine.* With Jeffrey Moss. Tarzana, CA: Third Line Press, 1999.

Williams SR. *Nutrition and Diet Therapy,* 6th edition, chapter 19. St. Louis, MO: Mosby, 1989.

120

*"And we have made of ourselves living cesspools,
and driven doctors to invent names for our diseases."*

—PLATO, THE REPUBLIC

Secretly, I called her my Auntie Mame. She dressed with flair, worked in the big city, drank Manhattans, and was nothing if not outspoken. "Blunt" might be more accurate, but she was also a lot of fun. As a career bank teller, my Aunt Ruth had personally been held up three times. It didn't faze her a bit. Whenever I was upset, she urged me to go do something I liked to do, especially if it involved focus and/or physical exertion. She called it "making aggression cookies."

Only one thing slowed this dynamo down. In her later years, my aunt needed oxygen to put on her socks. A severe case of emphysema, which a lifetime of smoking had failed to cure, was the reason. She was just one of an estimated 16 million Americans suffering from chronic obstructive pulmonary diseases (COPD), all primarily caused by tobacco use.

The fourth leading cause of death, COPD kills over 100,000 annually. That number is increasing; medical research has contributed virtually nothing to stop it. (www.nhlbi.nih.gov/meetings/workshops/copd_wksp.htm).

But you can stop COPD from starting by stopping smoking, and by stopping other people from starting smoking, and by starting smokers stopping. I love good wordplay. Maybe later in the book you'll encounter some. But for now, I'll also add that we need to stop nonsmokers, especially children, from "involuntary smoking," also known as breathing secondhand smoke.

Okay, the lecture is over, and now for the part that you tuned in for: what can be done for the disease itself?

I think the following are worth trying:

1. Vitamin E helps the body, especially the heart, to do more work on less oxygen. This has been known for some fifty years. My suggestions for use and for adjusting dosage are in the Vitamin E chapter in Part Two.

2. Carotene (in orange and green vegetables) and lycopene (in tomatoes) are powerful antioxidants. At least some of the damage of emphysema is caused by oxidants such as free radicals. While vitamin E is your body's number-one antioxidant, vegetable juices will provide a great variety of others.

3. Pricey though it is, I would recommend coenzyme Q10 for COPD sufferers, at least 300 milligrams daily, divided into six 50 mg doses. This is a hospital-friendly supplement, as there are no known negative side effects and therefore no basis to deny it to any patient. My crash course on negotiating with hospitals is provided in "How to Get Intravenous Vitamin C Administered to a Hospitalized Patient" near the end of this book. Extensive, detailed discussion is provided in Hoffer A, Saul, AW, and Hickey S. *Hospitals and Health* (Basic Health Publications, 2011).

4. Some emphysema is due to inflammation. Vitamin C at saturation doses fights chronic inflammation better and more safely than anything else I know. Yet just ask anyone *you* know with

emphysema this simple question: Have you tried it yet? Saturation of vitamin C is easily reached through frequent oral doses, and is described later in the book.

Frederick R. Klenner, M.D., a board-certified chest specialist, had this treatment policy: when in doubt, take a huge amount of vitamin C. Dr. Klenner wrote: "Some physicians would stand by and see their patients die rather than use ascorbic acid. Vitamin C should be given to the patient while the doctors ponder the diagnosis." Very ill patients may need vitamin C intravenously. How to get your doctor to order this is in the section titled "How to Get Intravenous Vitamin C Administered to a Hospitalized Patient."

5. Chiropractic adjustment, while certainly not a cure for emphysema, may help reduce some shortness of breath symptoms.

For more about your "Unsung Lungs," be sure to read the "Asthma" chapter.

> *"She said she could not stop swearing, and smoking and drinking,
> because she had never done those things. So there it was. She had neglected her habits. She was
> a sinking ship, with no freight to throw overboard"*
>
> —MARK TWAIN

Ask any of the 5 million women who have it, and they will tell you just how miserable endometriosis can be. In this chronic disease, tissue (endometrium) that you would expect inside the uterus ends up outside of it, often throughout the pelvic cavity. The monthly menstrual cycle aggravates the problem with (among other things) internal bleeding, inflammation, and considerable pain and discomfort.

Selenium

In cattle, endometriosis can be due to selenium deficiency. Since your cow can't give you any milk without having a baby first, dairymen well know to supplement all cows' feed with selenium. This is usually accomplished with a multimineral tablet the size of a microwave oven. Okay, it's a mineral-fortified salt block that cows can lick any time they want.

Human females should do as well, but they don't.

We go out of our way to supply selenium to cattle, particularly in geographical regions that have selenium-poor soil. Farmers simply must have healthy, fertile, happily pregnant, uncomplicated-delivering Bossys by the herd. It's economics: farmers cannot afford otherwise; a herd with endometriosis would be bankruptcy on the hoof.

Women with endometriosis, on the other hand, mean an economic windfall for doctors, nurses, support staff, surgeons, hospitals, administrators, HMOs, insurance companies, pharmaceutical manufacturers, drug salespeople, and lots of others dependent on unwell people.

A reader says:

"I was diagnosed with endometriosis about six years ago. I was told by my gynecologist to go on birth control and have surgery, which wouldn't be a permanent fix. Knowing that there was no way that I could live my life in chronic pain, and not wanting to have synthetic hormones affecting my body, I searched all over the place for naturopathic treatment or cures. I was on natural hormones, diets, drinks, and so on. I spent hundreds of dollars that I couldn't really afford in an eighteen-month period and I was still in pain. I decided to search your website because I'd already been successfully treating my extreme allergies with vitamin C for longer than I'd known I had endometriosis. You'd written that selenium is one of the least expensive minerals one could purchase. So I tried it, a few hundred micrograms every day. I felt and knew the difference within weeks: less or no pain. I had normal cycles and my hormonal issues were almost completely cured."

The secret to endometriosis is to see it for what it is: an end result of malnutrition. Farmers see this. Physicians do not. Cows are raw-food vegetarians who obtain their minerals from grains, leafy greens, and smart dairymen who provide mineral supplements preventively. Physicians and their ilk try to treat endometriosis 1) after it has occurred, and 2) with drugs.

Endometriosis is not due to a drug deficiency. It may be due to a selenium deficiency. Selenium is probably important in stopping endometriosis because this trace mineral works so closely with vitamin E. Vitamin E has been known to ensure that animals have healthy uterine linings since the 1930s. The research trail on this is as long as your arm. (Bicknell and Prescott, *The Vitamins in Medicine,* 3rd edition.) Therefore, supplementing the diet of a human female with natural vitamin E, 400–1,000 IU daily, plus around 200 mcg selenium, is a good move.

Note that selenium is measured in micrograms. A microgram is a *millionth* of a gram, and a gram is only about a quarter-teaspoon. You do not need a lot of selenium, but you do need it. Dr. Abram Hoffer has prescribed 200 mcg three times a day, totaling 600 mcg. He thought that more than 1,000 mcg per day would be harmful. (www.doctoryourself.com/hoffer _cancer_2. html.)

Folate (Folic Acid)

I suspect folate deficiency as a cause of endometriosis. To some extent I base this opinion, once again, on cows. And I repeat that cows are vegetarians. Raw-food vegetarians.

Folate is named after the dark green leafy vegetables it was first extracted from. *Folium* is Latin for "leaf." Folic acid contains three parts: pteroic acid, glutamic acid, and para-amino-benzoic acid (PABA). Folate is an important coenzyme in your body, helping to move carbon units around, and is necessary for synthesis of the nitrogen-containing purines and pyrimidines essential for the synthesis of nucleotides, which make up your RNA and DNA. Folate is also necessary for making the heme (the iron-containing, nonprotein part of hemoglobin) in your red blood cells.

Too little folate causes megoblastic anemia (that's large, immature red blood cells that can't carry oxygen well). This is especially important during growth situations, such as pregnancy, infancy, and childhood.

Cows get plenty of folate because they eat plenty of foliage (green leafy stuff, like grass). They are also blissfully free from a silent folate-stealer: the birth control pill. Oral contraceptives dramatically increase (at least double) the need for folic acid in women. And disease in general increases need for folic acid.

Adolescents in particular are likely to have insufficient folic acid intake. Why? Because food sources of folate are often quite unpopular. They are:

1. green leafy vegetables (Teens *love* these. Not.)

2. organ meats ("Awesome!")

3. asparagus ("McSparagus! My favorite fast food!")

During the growth period when they need it most, teenagers are likely not getting adequate dietary folic acid. Female teenagers reaching menarche (the beginning of menstruation) are therefore malnourished. Folate undernutrition is probably a factor in endometriosis.

Other nutrients recommended to help combat endometriosis include vitamin C in quantity, the vitamin B complex, essential fatty acids (found in lecithin or primrose oil), iron, iodine, calcium, and magnesium. Dietary supplementation makes sense to try.

124

Raspberry leaves are rich in magnesium and have a long tradition of uterine usefulness. I have seen raspberry-leaf tea reduce pregnancy problems and delivery times in humans. We fed piles of raspberry leaves to our rabbit, who rewarded us with ten young practically while our backs were turned. That is a large litter even for a rabbit.

THE BENEFITS OF MAGNESIUM

Magnesium relieves muscle and menstrual cramps and spasms. It also eases childbirth. In addition to oral supplements and raspberry leaf tea, magnesium can be taken transdermally. That is duded-up lingo for an Epsom-salts bath. It is cheap and easy, not to mention just plain wonderful on one of "those" days.

Reference

Sircus M. Magnesium Baths for Safer Pregnancy and Birth, 17 June 2010. Accessed October 2011, http://blog.imva.info/ medicine/magnesium-baths-for-safer-pregnancy-and-birth.

Pregnancy and endometriosis are not in a cart-and-horse relationship: it is not known for certain which one influences the other. But I think the less sure we are, the more we should look to nature for our examples. What is good for heifers is good for humans. I vote for a bovine diet, plus supplements.

Recommended Reading

Case HS. *The Vitamin Cure for Women's Health Problems.* Basic Health Publications., 2012.

Dean C. *The Magnesium Miracle.* Ballantine Books, Updated edition, 2006.

125

> *"What is important is the weight of evidence*
> *that impelled me to take the steps I did.*
> *My personal actions may not have justified the evidence,*
> *but I think the evidence justified my actions."*
>
> —ROGER J. WILLIAMS, PH.D., *NUTRITION AGAINST DISEASE*

Sarah and her fiancé Richard wanted to have children as soon as they were married. Sarah had just been diagnosed with epilepsy, however, and was taking phenobarbital as therapy. She and Richard read up on the drug, and now knew, as did their doctor, that a pregnancy on barbiturates was not ideal.

"So we want to look into other options," Sarah said to me in the office. "Could vitamins replace the drug?"

"I'm not sure," I said. "My mother has been medicated for grand mal epilepsy for fifty years now and it's a real long shot to think that a nutrient could be enough. Still, Sarah, you have the advantage of being young. There is evidence that epilepsy in teenagers can be connected with magnesium deficiency. You've had blood tests done?"

"Oh, yes," she said. "Tons of them, and here's the latest." She handed me a copy. No one had even looked for serum magnesium. I told Sarah to ask her doctor to check next time. So they did. Sarah's serum magnesium levels were so low as to be actually unmeasurable.

"The doctor was a bit surprised at that," Sarah said the next time we talked. "So now what?"

"Let's try a large quantity of magnesium, starting with a supplement of 800 mg per day. That's just over twice the RDA, so it is not completely unreasonable. Then you can gradually work up from there if need be. You'll know if you are taking too much: the biggest side effect of too much magnesium is diarrhea. You've heard of milk of magnesia?"

"The laxative, sure."

"That is a magnesium preparation. Your supplement will be better absorbed, though. Especially if you take the right form, take it often, and really need it. Then your body will soak it up like a sponge. Try magnesium citrate, or magnesium gluconate. Divide your daily intake over four or more doses, at least. Then let's see what we get."

A few weeks later, we met again. Sarah had new bloodwork results in hand. Her magnesium level was just barely measurable, and she was taking 1,200 mg a day.

"Wow! Where's it all going?" Sarah asked. "I've had no loose bowels at all."

"Your body is evidently using it. This suggests a long-standing deficiency on your part. Most young men and nearly all young women do not eat even the RDA of magnesium. But this is beyond that. You have a special need for this mineral. The tests confirm that."

"But shouldn't the blood levels be going up more?" Sarah said.

"You'd think so, but not necessarily. You are more than your blood, important though blood certainly is. Serum tests fail to indicate how much of this or that is actually inside your body's cells. There are, after all, some 40 trillion of them. Magnesium is involved in hundreds of chemical reactions throughout your body. It is needed everywhere and always. Oddly enough, the cells can be critically low in magnesium and some of the mineral will often still show up in the serum. In your case, it's more the other way around. Now that you are supplementing with magnesium, your cells must be getting it, and there's not much left in the blood that transports it. There are a lot of tanker trucks on your highways, but they're empty. The cargo is delivered and now the fuel is in every home."

"So it looks like I need more magnesium than most people," said Sarah. "If I do take lots of it, will I need less of the drug?"

"That's the idea. Do you want to run it by your doctor? Ask him if he'd consider gradually decreasing your dose of phenobarbital down to the minimum that keeps you symptom-free."

She did, and he did. Sarah ended up on the lowest possible dose of the drug and a very high dose of magnesium. This was not a landslide victory for nutrition, but this book is about real solutions, not rhetoric: nutrition does not have to be an all-or-nothing proposition. Its greatest potential may be in maintaining optimally nourished bodies that then will thrive on vastly reduced medication. What are the long-term consequences of millions of Americans taking less of each of their many drugs? Healthier people, greater safety, and massive savings. Only the pharmaceutical companies could possibly object.

They do, of course. And, they heavily influence practicing physicians. When was the last time you saw a calendar, pen, ad, or prescription pad in your doctor's hand touting the benefits of magnesium?

Keep looking. It will be in some quack's office, no doubt.

Or not. L.B. Barnett, M.D., was onto this forty-five years ago. He published "Clinical Studies of Magnesium Deficiency in Epilepsy" in *Clinical Physiology* in 1959. Wonder why nobody listened?

Perhaps it is because no one cares about old papers. Our society prefers new lamps for old. New drugs invariably preempt old minerals. Too bad, when the old lamp or the old research may hold the genie.

"E" IS FOR EPILEPSY

Children using anti-epileptic medication have reduced plasma levels of vitamin E, a sign of vitamin E deficiency. So doctors at the University of Toronto gave epileptic children 400 IU of vitamin E per day for several months, along with their medication. This combined treatment reduced the frequency of seizures in most of the children by over 60 percent. Half of them "had a 90 to 100 percent reduction in seizures." This extraordinary result is also proof of the safety of 400 IU of vitamin E per day in children (equivalent to at least 800 to 1,200 IU/day for an adult). "There were no adverse side effects," said the researchers. It also provides a clear example of pharmaceutical use creating a vitamin deficiency, and an unassailable justification for supplementation. (Ogunmekan, AO and Hwang, PA. [1989]. A randomized, double-blind, placebo-controlled, clinical trial of D-alpha-tocopheryl acetate (vitamin E), as add-on therapy, for epilepsy in children. *Epilepsia* 30(1):84–89.

A CASE HISTORY FROM A READER

"In early 2005, I read an article written by you about magnesium and seizures, in which magnesium was used to reduce drugs but still control the seizures. Honestly, I did not credit it as possible to stop my seizures. I was diagnosed with epilepsy as a child. I was having petit mal seizures (also called absence or psychomotor seizures). When I was sixteen years old I had my first temporal lobe convulsion. So then I was taking two drugs for two types of seizures. Then I started having grand mal seizures . . . and now three drugs. When I was nineteen years old, I decided to train as an EEG (electroencephalograph) technician. My motivation was that I wanted to see if there were any treatments for epilepsy besides drugs. My parents and I had been told by neurologists in Canada, England, and the States that I would have to take drugs for the rest of my life.

"I trained at two teaching hospitals affiliated to universities in Canada. There was nothing in allopathic medicine for epilepsy except drugs. I took drugs for forty-nine years, and this is well documented as I had EEGs every year or two.

"Because of what I learned from your article, I started using transdermal magnesium chloride every day on my feet in whole-tub baths, plus occasionally in footbaths also. I had something called peripheral neuropathy in my feet. At that stage I had lost most of the feeling in my feet, plus I was also getting very sharp pains in my feet at night. I was very concerned that I would end up in a wheelchair.

"I no longer have peripheral neuropathy—it took almost two years to get all the feeling back in my feet. I noticed during this time that I was not having as many seizures. My temporal lobe and grand mal seizures had been controlled for the most part, but not my petite mal seizures unless I took such a high dose of the drugs that I was literally drugged out of my mind. I started taking oral magnesium everyday with B_6. At the same time, I decreased the drugs I was on. It worked. I have not taken any drugs at all since October 3, 2007, and I have not had any seizures of any kind.

"One of the symptoms of magnesium deficiency is seizures, and according to studies I have read, most epileptics are magnesium deficient. I wish I had found this out forty years ago. Now I can even drive a car and ride a bike. It is so wonderful not to have seizures anymore, not have to depend on drugs all the time, and of course, be free of drug side effects.

"I am so thrilled that I am over the moon about this—it is more wonderful then I can express. It is possible to not have seizures anymore if you get your magnesium levels up. Since some drugs deplete magnesium, it is no wonder that for many epileptics their seizures get worse with time

"When I trained as an EEG technician, we were told that when a nerve cell (neuron) became irritated, it gave off an extra large burst of electricity and this is what caused a seizure. The kind of seizures depended on what part of the brain the burst of electricity originated from as well as how far down the brain stem the burst of electricity went. Magnesium appears to calm the irritated neurons and prevents extra large bursts of electrical activity. There is a "catch" to this, however: it is hard to get magnesium levels up and oral magnesium alone may not be enough. When I suggest to anyone that they get their magnesium levels up whether it is because of seizures, heart issues, migraine headaches, high blood pressure, and so on, I also suggest that the easiest and surest way to get magnesium levels up is with magnesium chloride IVs, or injection, or transdermal magnesium chloride."

"Life in all its fullness is Mother Nature obeyed."

—WESTON A. PRICE, D.D.S.

If I assert that you can probably accomplish more with bean sprouts than with laser surgery, you'll call me some kind of a nut, which, to some people, I am.

Terri certainly thought I was. Terri was going blind, and she was miserable. She had a somewhat rare condition where her eyesight was tunneling. That is, Terri's peripheral vision was fading fast. She was still in her thirties. "This has just gotten worse and worse," she told me. "My sight is limited to what is right in front of me, and that's not very clear either. I can't drive. I can hardly even read any more."

"What has your ophthalmologist told you?" I asked.

"That there is nothing he can do, except monitor how much vision I've lost," she said. "A lot of good that does me."

"Surgery? Medications?"

"He said none are any help with what I've got," she said, her mouth firmly set. "I don't suppose you have any great ideas?"

I did have an idea or two, but she wasn't going to like them. "Naturopaths have accumulated decades of evidence about the food enzymes in uncooked foods, especially sprouted beans and sprouted grains. Cooking temperatures as low as 130 degrees Fahrenheit destroy these enzymes, which are essential to keeping us youthful and healthy."

"That sounds pretty cutesy," said Ms. Congeniality.

"It does to me, too. But I cannot discount the possibility, since you have been offered nothing else, that this research might apply to you. You could try a 90 percent raw food, mostly sprouts, diet for a few months."

"A few months?"

"At least. What I have read emphasizes that while nature heals, it takes time. The nature-cure authorities generally agree that it took years for our body to develop an affliction, and it will take us months to get out of it."

"If it works at all," said Terri.

"Yes, if it works at all."

There was a long silence. Counseling training, plus years of teaching, had taught me when to shut up and wait for a student to elaborate on their initial answer. "I'll try it," she finally said, "but this had better be worth it. How much of this stuff do I have to eat?"

Familiar question to a health nut who raised two kids on sprouts. My children will readily tell you that I gave them sprouts for breakfast, carrot-zucchini juice for lunch, and borscht for supper. While that is true, it is not the complete story. My policy was "Eat this good-for-you item first, and then you can have what you want, within reason." My kids had plenty of ice cream, brownies, cookies, health-food store candies, and other goodies on a regular basis. I get a lot of heat from purists who think I was a sell-out. But I got far more heat from their mother and my in-laws about the weird health foods I fed those "poor children." Compromise is a fact of life. If you hold too firmly to your principles, you risk them being discarded lock, stock, and barrel.

But I felt that, in Terri's case, she would need to bite the nutritional bullet.

"You'll need to eat at least two jars full of sprouts a day," I told Terri. "By jars, I mean mayonnaise-sized or mason jars, about a quart and a half each. By sprouts, I mean a variety of alfalfa, wheat, lentil, radish, cabbage, clover, and mung bean. You can grow your sprouts yourself. That will save a lot of money, and they will be fresher and better for you."

"Ugh," replied Terri.

"Actually, sprouts taste better than you think. A lot of salad bars have alfalfa sprouts. Radish sprouts taste exactly like radishes. Mung bean sprouts are used in Chinese food. Try different varieties and mixtures. Any health food store or food co-op will have the seeds. Soak them overnight, and then rinse and drain them twice a day. Start two or three jars a day, and harvest and eat them in rotation as they mature. That's it."

"Eat them how?" asked the impatient patient.

"Raw, except perhaps for mung sprouts. Build your salads on a base of sprouts instead of lettuce. Eat sprouts in a sandwich instead of lettuce. Top sprout salads with tomatoes, cucumber, broccoli, cashew nuts, onion, salad dressing, anything."

"Dressing?" said Terri, with a glimmer of optimism. "I can have dressing on them? I thought dressing was full of salt and fat."

"Put anything you want on your sprouts to make them taste good. You want this to be as enjoyable as possible. I'll look the other way on whatever it takes to get you to consume as great a volume of sprouts a day as you can. The value of the sprouts far outweighs any drawback of the dressing. You can always make your own, if you really want to do it right. It really isn't that hard to eat a lot of sprouts. You can take nearly a jarful and press them down between two pieces of bread and make a sproutwich."

Silence.

"You'll also want to have fresh vegetable juices daily for all the carotenes, lots of vitamin B complex, vitamin C and vitamin E, a good multivitamin, extra zinc, and a little selenium." We went over the recommended dosages. I suggested 600 to 1,200 IU daily of vitamin E, 100 mg per day of zinc, vitamin C to bowel tolerance (see my vitamin C chapters), and 50 mg balanced vitamin B complex with each meal.

"Don't take too much selenium; 400 mcg a day is the maximum, and half that will probably be sufficient. The other nutrients have a safety record a mile long. The vegetable juice is better than beta-carotene supplements. Yes, it contains a great deal of beta-carotene—probably 40,000 IU or more per glass—but it also contains dozens of other carotenes, not just the beta form. Even a single carrot a day reduces a person's risk of macular degeneration by 40 percent."

"I'll be taking pills all day," Terri grumbled.

"All these nutrients have an especially vital role in the health of the eye. Carotenes, C, E, zinc, and selenium are all involved with the antioxidant cycle. Macular degeneration, cataracts, and diabetic retinopathy are distantly related conditions that have responded to these nutrients."

Off she went, certainly no more miserable than when she came in, but that isn't saying much. Terri fundamentally questioned what she was doing, but driven by a lack of options, with that bare desperation that can work wonders, she did it. Kicking and screaming, perhaps, but she did it.

One phone conversation five weeks later, I dared ask her if she was noticing anything good happening.

"No," she said. "I went to the eye doctor this week, and he said there was no change."

"But isn't that actually a good sign, Terri? Every other visit, didn't he say that your vision was diminishing?"

"Well, yeah, he did."

"Then 'no worse' is an early sign of real progress," I said.

"Maybe. I hate eating sprouts."

"Look, Terri, I give you permission to hate my guts if it will keep you on the wagon and help you see."

She asked if she could have some rye bread. She asked if the bread could be toasted. She wanted some yogurt. (I said yes to all three.) The other day she had a piece of chicken. It was a dietetic confessional each time she called. And she called often.

Another month later, she had been to the ophthalmologist again. "He looked and said things were a bit better. He tested my vision and confirmed it. He asked what I was doing, and I told him you'd call him and explain it."

So I did, hoping for the best. The ophthalmologist was actually very interested. He noted some of my references, expressed his pleasure that Terri was improving with a condition that never improved, and said whatever she was doing, she shouldn't change it a bit. End of conversation.

Months went by, and Terri's eyesight got better and better. In the end, two near miracles happened: Terri's eyesight was restored nearly 100 percent, and she thanked me for what I'd made her do.

Don't take this next section too far out of context; just give it a moment.

A fellow who was born blind was once treated by a man who was said to be some sort of healer. The treatment was a bit strange: the healer mixed dirt with his saliva and applied the resulting mud to the man's eyes. He told the blind man to go wash it off in a local pond.

The man did that, and came home, seeing.

Everybody, of course, asked him what had happened. He told them. This was all pretty unusual, so they brought the man to the authorities, who also asked him what happened. The man told them.

There was considerable, but inconclusive, debate at this point. The man was asked what kind of a person could have done this. He responded that it was perhaps some kind of holy man. Nobody bought that, either.

So they brought in the man's father and mother, to identify him and verify that he had truly been blind all his life. This they confirmed.

Then, the man was brought in for yet another round of questioning, which focused on the doubtful credentials of the supposed healer who did all this. The authorities said that the healer was a phony and a fraud.

The man replied, "Whether that is true or not, I don't know. But one thing I do know: I was blind, but now I see."

I will never forget what a wonderful feeling it was to have been the educational and motivational link that stopped Terri from going blind. It does not matter how a person gets their sight back. By divine healing from above, or by sprouted seeds of the earth; whatever works and restores something as precious as eyesight must be taken as genuine, and good.

131

DILUTE VITAMIN C EYEWASH

Vitamin C (as very dilute ascorbic acid) makes a good substitute for traditional boric acid eyewashes. Boric acid is commonly used to kill ants, by the way. (Setting traps with vitamin C as ant bait will just result in ants that don't get colds. That's humor, folks.) Yes, ascorbic acid is an acid. It is a weak acid, but it still *must be diluted* with quite a lot of water. I use maybe a 20th of a teaspoon of ascorbic acid crystals in about two ounces of water. If it stings more than a tiny bit, I rinse my eyes with water immediately and retry, this time adding more water to the vitamin C solution. I personally have found this mixture, dripped into the eyes, to relieve itching, inflammation, and redness. Commonsense caution: Consult your doctor before embarking on this. Better yet, ask your doctor to mix and administer it for you.

Recommended Reading

Smith RG. *The Vitamin Cure for Eye Diseases.* Laguna Beach, CA: Basic Health Publications, 2012.

*WARNING: This chapter should probably be rated "R,"
because the topic is (gasp!) . . . SEX.*

Let's be honest: it would not be a health-nut book without a chapter on sex, now, would it? Yes, this is the article that is sure to make me a millionaire and get me my own talk show. First, to put this discussion on a proper, high scientific plane: high-dose ascorbic acid increases intercourse frequency and improves mood according to the results of a randomized, controlled clinical trial published in *Biological Psychiatry:*

[In] a randomized, double-blind, placebo-controlled 14-day trial of 3,000 mg per day of vitamin C [a group of 42 healthy adults] reported greater frequency of sexual intercourse. The vitamin C group (but not the placebo group) also experienced a decrease in Beck Depression scores. This is probably due to the fact that vitamin C "modulates catecholaminergic activity, decreases stress reactivity, approach anxiety and prolactin release, improves vascular function, and increases oxytocin release. These processes are relevant to sexual behavior and mood" (Brody, S. [2002]. High-dose ascorbic acid increases intercourse frequency and improves mood: a randomized controlled clinical trial. *Biol Psychiatry* 52[4]:371–4).

Additionally, the amino acid arginine has its own special benefits in improving blood flow, benefiting persons with angina (*J Am Col Cardiol* 39:7, p 1199–1203, 2002) and even perhaps those with erectile dysfunction (*Int J Impot Res* 6: p 33–36, 1994).

Just wait until Howard Stern hears about this.

While giving a talk on vitamins at a local college, I mentioned British Captain James Cook, who was unusually dedicated in employing nutrition to wipe out scurvy on his ships. I mentioned that, on a long voyage, Captain Cook did experiments with his seamen. Boy, did that break the ice.

In the *Rig Veda,* one of the oldest religious writings on earth, one of the cosmic beings mentions that she and her lover had sex three times a day throughout their entire relationship. Aside from a honeymoon or a wild weekend, whose love life can possibly compare with that?

The answer is, maybe yours. Now some old saying states that if you put a penny in a jar each time you make love during the first year of a long relationship, such as marriage, and if you take a penny out each time you make love after the first year, that you will never empty the jar.

How depressing.

Of course, it does not have to be that way. A satisfying and frequent sex life can extend throughout middle age and old age, too. In the remote villages of the Hunza (north of India), men have been documented to father children at 90-plus. No one readily believes this, in a culture where you are assured that a man's virility peaks at 19 and a woman's somewhat later. But the truth is, that peak-at-19 stuff is a myth. Nope—not even close.

What do men and women do to keep doing? Here is an assortment of racy, R-rated advice that I have collected over the decades.

1. Make sex a priority, and find the time. Turn the TV off and turn each other on.

2. Exercise moderately, not excessively or never.

3. Have sex during the day. You are less tired then. And, when it is bedtime, you'll be a candidate for a second time.

4. Try setting your alarm half an hour earlier in the morning. Get up earlier and you'll get more. After a night's sleep, we are all more relaxed. This can translate into improved sexual responsiveness. Many men wake with an erection. And while it may merely be nature's way of clearing out the blood vessels in the penis, or prodding you to go to the bathroom, it is also nature's way of giving you an opportunity.

5. If you can't quite manage it first thing when you wake, during the day, or right as you go to bed, wait a while and you'll have the fun of trying again. In the morning, you may just not have your sex mind awake. During the day, you may be separated by work schedules or location. At night, you may be too tense. So wait a bit; if you fall asleep, there's the next morning again.

6. If you are always too tired, make a point to get more sleep. There are numerous other health- and relationship-building advantages to this.

7. If you have kids, arrange to have them properly supervised but out of the house. You can agree on this with your kids, in an age-appropriate manner. More couples with kids would be happier in bed if they got it straight that what unifies a couple also benefits the kids. Children cheerfully understand mutual parental affection at an early age. Without being graphic in the slightest, a Mommy and Daddy can reserve personal time.

Up until now, the advice proffered is not impossibly far from what a sex therapist, women's magazine, or supermarket tabloid would tell you. Grimaces or smiles may accompany what I just wrote, but rage from old-school dietitians is virtually guaranteed by what follows.

8. If you want to conceive, or just play as if you might, try having the man take megadoses of vitamin C for a few weeks prior. At least 6,000 milligrams a day, and as much as 20,000 mg a day guarantees very high sperm production. Divide the dose throughout the day for maximum effect. And that effect is what, exactly? More sperm, stronger sperm, and better swimming sperm all occurred, at even lower daily C doses, in a University of Texas study.

9. Listen to this, guys: zinc, and plenty of it, nourishes the prostate and increases seminal fluid production. There is scientific literature a mile long about zinc and male fertility. About five to ten times the RDA will do it. That is approximately 50 to 100 mg of zinc daily. For best absorption and best results, divide the dose into two, or better yet, four doses. Zinc gluconate is well absorbed, and zinc monomethionine better still. These are available at any health food store without a prescription.

For those eager to tell you that such levels of zinc are harmful, let them prove it with research. Truth is, most men don't even get the puny RDA of zinc, set laughingly at 11 milligrams. Zinc lozenges for the common cold are many times higher than this.

Continued very high doses of zinc can produce a copper deficiency, and sometimes a copper-deficiency anemia. This is very easy to compensate for. To begin with, most Americans have copper water pipes in their homes. Drink a glass or two of cold water first thing out of the tap every morning and you'll get copper. Secondly, eat more raisins and other copper-high foods. Third, take a multiple vitamin (as you should be doing anyway) with copper in it. Finally, do what those lovers in India have been doing for thousands of years. Buy a copper metal cup, fill it with cold water at bedtime, and drink it first thing the next morning. Make this Ayurvedic routine your routine.

10.   Assuming a monogamous relationship, find a birth control method that is easy, offers twenty-four-hour protection, and doesn't excessively interfere with the lifestyle or feeling for either the woman or the man. If you are not in a monogamous relationship, use every safe sex precaution you can. If you need encouragement to evolve toward monogamy, consider that married persons do in fact make love more times a month than unmarried persons do. I also wish to interject a moral thought and quote the Reverend Norman Vincent Peale: "The reason sex is so bad outside of marriage is because it is so good inside of marriage."

11.   Find a sex- or marriage-counselor who will tell you that each of you needs sexual fulfillment (which is true) and you should enthusiastically see to it.

12.   Use mouthwash. Get a tan. Do a few crunches (sit-ups). Bathe or shower. Trim your hair. Bring flowers. Keep the bathroom door closed when you use it. Meditate. Eat right and take your vitamins daily. Wear flattering underwear. But most of all, put on a smile: it is the best makeup on Earth.

13.   Attitude follows behavior, a very wise counselor told me. (Yes, same person as in number 11.) Make love a lot, and you'll want to make love even more. Afraid of this? You poor dear!

14.   If you are arguing, table it instantly by necking. Just go for it. You'll thank me in the morning.

So, all these yummy ideas, or even one of them for that matter, may be enough to whoop you up. To quote an old and unrelated commercial: Try 'em. You'll like 'em.

Then start knitting booties.

I have worked with supposedly "infertile" people who have tried "everything" to conceive a child. Clinical application of nutrition, especially zinc and vitamin C, is not even mentioned in any fertility textbook I've ever seen. I've received some nice postcards from couples who have taken an odd idea or two of mine and gotten pregnant within a month or two. It is a wonderful feeling, by the way, to have helped them bring a soul to the Earth.

The flipside of this is that 1) *bad nutrition is not a form of birth control,* and 2) if you are having sex, remember that *you are designed to get pregnant.* Be very sure to use safe, appropriate, and effective forms of contraception. Sex is more fun (and likely more frequent) if you are confident about the outcome.

References and Recommended Reading

Dawson EB, Harris WA, Rankin WE, Charpentier LA, McGanity WJ. Effect of ascorbic acid on male fertility. *Ann N Y Acad Sci.* 1987;498:312–23. PMID: 3476000.

Dawson EB, Harris WA, Teter MC, Powell LC. Effect of ascorbic acid supplementation on the sperm quality of smokers. *Fertil Steril.* 1992 Nov;58(5):1034–9.

Effect of ascorbic acid and vitamin E supplementation on semen quality and biochemical parameters of male rabbits. [*Anim Reprod Sci.* 2003] PMID:12559724.

Sperm quality and ascorbic acid concentration in rainbow trout semen are affected by dietary vitamin C: an across-season study. [*Biol Reprod.* 1995] PMID:7626724.

Birth Control

I get a lot of questions about natural birth control, usually about options to drug or barrier methods of contraception. Can a safe, natural alternative really cost nothing and be more than 99 percent effective? As a former school sex-education coordinator and author of a master's thesis on the subject, I will now offer a few very fertile thoughts.

Even if it is granted that birth control education should begin very early, and that fertility awareness is a desirable inclusion, some objections may remain. One such objection is that there is no reliable indicator of fertility. This erroneous belief is widely held. A woman's cervical mucus secretion is a most reliable indicator of fertility. Using this fact to prevent conception is the basis for the Billings Method of birth control.

The Billings Method is named after Drs. John and Evelyn Billings of Melbourne, Australia, who first developed, tested, and promoted this natural birth control method in the 1950s. It is also known as the Ovulation Method or the Mucus Method. It is not the Rhythm Method. In fact, the reason the Billingses began their investigation of natural birth control in the first place is because the Rhythm Method is not reliable.

Natural birth control often conjures up images of ineffectiveness and Catholicism. This is unfortunate. Even the Rhythm Method, when carefully employed, may be 80 percent effective in preventing pregnancy. But since that failure rate is still far too high, there have been attempts to improve on it. The Temperature Method is one of the best-known refinements on rhythm. It is based on an observed temperature rise at the time of a woman's ovulation each month. Three days after this temperature rise, she is infertile until at least the next menstrual period. While temperature indicates ovulation, it fails to predict it. Intercourse before the thermal shift, then, again becomes a matter of rhythm-style calendar estimation. Another drawback is identifying the temperature rise. A significant temperature rise may be as low as 0.1 degree centigrade, making this otherwise reliable method difficult to use.

The Billings Method simplifies natural birth control greatly. Its refinements are that it requires no equipment (no thermometer, no calendar), no guesswork, and that it will predict ovulation. It is simple enough that, according to the Billingses, "Experience has shown that an overwhelming majority of women, probably nine out of ten, can immediately interpret their own mucus system. . . . The remainder can also be taught to do so."

The Billings Method is a one-step reading of a woman's cervical mucus, performed by the woman herself in a moment and without internal examination. Every day, she gently wipes her labia with clean, dry, white toilet paper. She looks at the paper to see if there is any mucus on it. If there is, she is likely to be fertile. If the mucus is wet and slippery, and can be easily stretched, then she is very fertile. If the paper stays dry, she is likely to be infertile that day. On the day of the most wet, slippery, clear mucus, she is most fertile of all. This day is called the peak day, and is the very day she ovulates. She will also feel wettest on this day. She remains fertile for three days after the peak.

It does not matter how old the woman is, nor does it matter how long her menstrual cycles are. Unlike the Rhythm Method, there is no need for regular menstrual cycles. There is no need to fit into a normal, clockwork 28-day model. If a woman has short menstrual cycles, she will ovulate early. If they are long, she will ovulate late. The mucus is there at ovulation, regardless. If she misses a period, there will simply have been no ovulation, and therefore no fertile, wet mucus that cycle. A woman does not even have to know how to read and write to use the Billings Method effectively. Trials in the South Pacific nation of Tonga between 1970 and 1972 showed high levels of acceptance and success with the Billings Method.

Abnormal temperature, such as a low fever, will interfere with the temperature method of birth control. It will not obstruct accurate readings with the Billings Method, however. Abnormal vaginal discharges, also, do not prevent a woman from recognizing her state of fertility. Given the knowledge, any woman can use the Billings Method for her entire reproductive lifetime without financial cost. And, obviously, unlike medical methods of birth control, there are no harmful side effects with the Billings Method.

Few physicians and nurses know of the ovulation method's effectiveness, and fewer still teach it. Pity, since, according to John Billings, "The combined biological failure rate and user failure rate of the ovulation method in Tonga was 0.69 percent." This is very low indeed, since some experts place the birth control pill failure rate at 1.2 percent. Planned Parenthood says that excellent use of natural birth control can be up to 99 percent effective.

A nurse-midwife taught my wife and I the Billings Method in half an hour. It took another few hours to read their book, *The Ovulation Method.* We subsequently used the Billings Method for fifteen years and the method, properly used, never resulted in an unplanned pregnancy.

Caution: As with any birth control method, the Billings Method should be learned from an experienced instructor. Even more important, it obviously provides no protection whatsoever from sexually transmitted diseases. This is one of the most important reasons why it is appropriate only for strictly monogamous, long-term relationships.

By the way, you can use the method backward to assist conception, since the days on which a woman is ovulating are when she is most fertile.

Recommended Reading

Billings J. Cervical mucus: the biological marker of fertility and infertility. *International Journal of Fertility* 26 (1981):182–195.

Billings J. Ovulation method of family planning. *The Lancet* 2 (1972):1193–94.

Billings J. *The Ovulation Method.* Collegeville, MN: Liturgical Press, 1978.

Billings J. In *Sex and Pregnancy in Adolescence,* Zelnik M, Kantner J, and Ford K, ed. Beverly Hills, CA: Sage, 1973, 164–70.

Billings J and Billings E. Teaching the safe period based on the mucus symptom. *Linacre Quarterly* 41 (1974): 41–51.

Clift AF. Observations on certain rheological properties of human cervical secretion . *Proceedings of the Royal Society of Medicine* 39 (1945):1–9.

Doring GK. "Detection of Ovulation by the Basal Body Temperature Method" in *Sex and Pregnancy in Adolescence* by Zelnik M, Kantner J, and Ford K, ed. Beverly Hills, CA: Sage, 1973.

Klaus H. Valuing the precreative capacity: a new approach to teens. *International Review of Natural Family Planning* 8 (1984): 206–13.

Klaus H, et al. Fertility awareness—natural family planning for adolescents and their families: Report of multisite pilot project. *International Journal of Adolescent Medicine and Health* 3 (1987):101–19.

Klaus H, Labbok M, and Barker D. Characteristics of ovulation method acceptors: a cross-cultural assessment. *Studies in Family Planning* 19 (1988): 299–304.

National Directory of Billings Ovulation Method Teachers. Washington, D.C.: Natural Family Planning Center of Washington, D.C.,1988.

"Teen STAR program." [pamphlet] Bethesda, MD: Natural Family Planning Center of Washington, D.C., 1986.

Weissman MC, et al. A trial of the ovulation method of family planning in Tonga. *The Lancet* 2 (1972): 813–16.

"What's the best method of birth control for me?" Rochester, NY: Planned Parenthood of Rochester and the Genesee Valley, 1986.

"A smart mother makes often a better diagnosis
than a poor doctor."
—AUGUST BIER

Is a strict raw foods diet the most promising natural approach to uterine fibroids? Here is a comment from a woman physician who ought to know:

I have suffered from fibroids for 16 years. Because I am so slender, the fibroid is easily palpated from the abdomen. Mine has shrunk from the size of a lemon to the size of a $1/4$" thick pancake about 1 inch in diameter. I tried many diets and supplements over the years and gave up dairy and meats. It finally responded to coffee enemas daily and a raw foods diet. It took 5 weeks. This is much simpler than many other things that I triedt. (Jennifer Daniels, M.D.).

Dr. Daniels is describing a diet very much like the Gerson therapy. A quick Internet search for "Gerson" will bring up a great deal of information on this type of treatment. It is well worth a therapeutic trial.

Max Gerson, M.D., was once asked, "Can fibroid tumors be dissolved?" (See www.doctoryourself.com/gersonspeech.html for more of the conversation.) Dr. Gerson answered: "Fibroid tumors are mostly benign. Benign tumors take 10 to 20 times as much time to absorb as malignant tumors. This goes for adhesions and scars. Fibroid and benign tumors are dissolved only very slowly because they are not abnormal. It is difficult for the parenteral system to bring its digestive powers to bear on these benign tumors. But when they turn malignant, then they are quickly dissolved." (Editor's note: a fibroid turns malignant only very rarely.)

Menopause

Fibroids often shrink or go away on their own, especially after menopause. Menopause is a big hormonal change for a woman. Hormonal therapy may help. Doing nothing and waiting for menopause may also work, too.

A reader says:

"I had a partial thyroidectomy at age twenty-two and then was never "allowed" to have thyroid meds, based on "normal" TSH. I depended on tons of vitamins to get by but developed fibroids in my forties. When I finally got Armour thyroid and realized I had been hypothyroid all my life, I also needed other hormones like progesterone and DHEA because my adrenals were exhausted. Fibroids disappeared with hormonal support, but also I am fifty-five and postmenopausal now."

Vitamin E

Fibroids are very possibly caused by vitamin E deficiency according to Evan Shute, M.D., writing in *The Vitamin E Story* (1946). Dr. Shute was an obstetrician. Vitamin E is very intimately involved with the body's hormonal balance.

Weight Management

Even though fibroids themselves are mostly muscle tissue, they are related to fat. Generally speaking, the more overweight you are, the more fat you carry. The more fat, the more estrogen in your body. Fibroids thrive on extra estrogen. Exercise helps reduce fat, and is therefore likely to reduce estrogen, too.

Meat-Eating or Vegetarian?

Meats are dietary sources of estrogen. A very-low-meat diet is a good idea . . . for so many reasons.

Iodine

Iodine is important for proper estrogen balance in the body. Fibrocystic breast disease in animals can be produced by iodine deficiency.[1] And, human fibrocystic breast disease has been found to respond to iodine supplementation.[2] One study reported that, "In 1,365 patients, using an aqueous saturated solution of iodine in daily amount based on body weight, estimated at 3–6 mg iodine/day, 74% of the patients had clinical improvements both subjectively from breast pain and objectively, form breast induration and nodularity." Results have been seen in less than two months.[3] Iodine may also be effective against uterine fibroids.[4] Effective doses are considerably larger than RDA quantities. The RDA for iodine is 150 *micrograms (mcg) per day; therapeutic doses are 2 to 50* milligrams/day. That is 2,000 to 50,000 micrograms/day. In other words, 13 to over 300 times the RDA. Kelp and other sea vegetables are excellent dietary sources of iodine. Kelp tablets are the cheapest supplemental source. They are also very safe. Iodine solution or tincture is very concentrated and poisonous if swallowed in quantity. However, iodine solutions can be applied to, and safely absorbed through, the skin. Common sense caution: consult with your health care provider before using very high intakes of iodine.

References

1. Krouse TB, Eskin BA, Mobini J. Age-related changes resembling fibrocystic disease in iodine-blocked rat breasts. *Arch Pathol Lab Med.* 1979 Nov;103(12):631–4.

2. Ghent WR, Eskin BA, Low DA, Hill LP. Iodine replacement in fibrocystic disease of the breast. *Can J Surg.* 1993 Oct; 36(5):453–60.

3. www.vitamincfoundation.org/iodine.htm.

4. Lekhtman MN, Lekhtman SM. [Medical procedures in uterine fibromyomas]. Zdravookhr Kirg. 1979 Sep-Oct;(5):48–55. [Article in Russian]. See also: Sol's'kii IP, Chizhova PS, Ivaniuta PI. [Function of thyroid gland in uterine fibromyoma]. *Pediatr Akus Ginekol.* 1968 Sep-Oct;5:55–8. [Article in Ukrainian]

For Further Reading

Fibroid Tumors & Endometriosis Self Help Book, by Susan M. Lark Lark, M.D., Celestial Arts, 1995.

Case HS. *The Vitamin Cure for Women's Health Problems.* Basic Health Publications, 2012.

THE "OTHER" WORLD-FAMOUS BACH

Dr. Edward Bach, a graduate of London's University College Hospital, was a bacteriologist with a successful practice on Harley Street. That is the English equivalent to having a Fifth Avenue professional address in New York City. In 1930, he left medicine irretrievably far behind when he ran off to the country to study, and heal with, flower blossoms of all things. He floated them in spring water (but never in "dead" tap or distilled water) in glass containers, placed in the sun. The energy from the flowers was thus collected, then diluted hundreds of times to make it stronger, and dropped onto patients' tongues and wrists. Somewhere—anywhere—in here you can find enough nuttiness to begin snickering.

The eccentric Dr. Bach believed that disease was, at its root, a matter of diseased temperament. He researched a dozen common flowers known as the Twelve Healers (also the title of his first book). Over two dozen more were to follow, bringing the total to thirty-eight. Impatiens seemed to cure impatience. mustard ended black depression "like a dark cloud has overshadowed life, blotting out all enjoyment." A combination of remedies, known as Rescue Remedy, was a first aid preparation for shock and trauma to the mind. Clematis relieved suicidal tendencies, and holly dissipated hatred. Honeysuckle dispelled excess nostalgia, and there were several remedies for fear, classified as to whether fear was from known or unknown causes, worldly or unfounded, or otherwise.

Dr. Bach is especially easy to dismiss. First, he was British; so to many an arrogant Yankee, he was not a real scientist, like, say, Faraday, or Newton, or Kelvin, or Boyle, or Turing, or Darwin . . . (That's a joke, son.) Second, flowers, especially common blossoms like impatiens and holly that served as their very names would suggest, offer no satisfaction to the scientific-spectacle-seeking patient.

Third, the idea that dilution increases potency is a homeopathic one, utterly in opposition to orthodox medical thought. The works of historian Harris Coulter, especially the three-volume masterwork *Divided Legacy*, will provide readers with very ample, very rational support for homeopathy and there is no need to try to justify it here. Homeopathy, itself regarded as quackery by many, is practiced by a large minority of licensed medical doctors worldwide. It is at least close enough to reason that over-the-counter homeopathic remedies are sold in discount stores, and the federal government both codifies and approves the manufacture of such remedies in the Homeopathic Pharmacopoeia of the United States. Double-blind, tightly controlled studies of homeopathic remedies have indeed verified their statistical significance to a very high degree, and their record of safety is unassailable even by the Food and Drug Administration. A single Google search for "homeopathy" (over 20 million listings) will keep you busy for a spell.

Back to Bach: his flower remedies seemed to work. Medical doctors would follow him, leaving a broad trail of case notes, published articles, and textbooks in their wake. It is a bold move to dismiss all these physicians as quacks without at least trying the remedies first. I have seen firsthand how they help people.

My favorite book on the subject is *The Bach Flower Remedies* by Edward Bach and F. J. Wheeler. (New Canaan, CT: Keats, 1979). This volume is a compilation of three short books in one: *Heal Thyself* and *The Twelve Healers* by Bach, and *The Bach Remedies Repertory* by Wheeler. Both were medical doctors. Wheeler's repertory (an index of symptoms and appropriate remedies for each) is simplicity itself to use. This is the best introductory volume available. Ask your librarian to help you get a copy.

Fibroids and Homeopathy

You may wish to investigate the following homeopathic remedies for treating fibroids:

- Caulophyllum thalictroides
- Cimicifuga racemosa
- Vinca major
- Galium aparine

Homeopathic remedies are produced under the auspices of the United States Homeopathic Pharmacopoeia, and are generally recognized as very safe. To learn more read William Boericke's *Homeopathic Materia Medica* (There are many available, updated editions of this century-old book . . . which was already in its ninth edition in 1927!

It is a comprehensive, one-volume listing of homeopathically active substances provides the framework on which to build an intermediate knowledge of the "like treats like" science of homeopathy. Several hundred remedy resumes are provided with over 350 pages of cross-indexing, symptom by symptom. This standard work is unusually inexpensive (because of the publication date) but is in clear need of revision, especially in the Therapeutic Index, which does not always agree with the much more comprehensive and superior Repertory immediately preceding it. Other more recent and more expensive Materia Medicas await the detailed needs of the more experienced homeopath, but Boericke's eighty-five-year-old text is hard to beat for everyday reference and home use. (1,042 pages, cloth)

John H. Clarke's *The Prescriber* (Ninth Edition, Essex, England: C. W. Daniel Co., Ltd., 1972) is just what the title indicates: a homeopathic prescription guide that is the next best thing to having a personal homeopathic doctor. Clarke's work has stood the test of time. In this one volume, the reader will first find the best sixty-page introduction ever written on just how to use homeopathic remedies, plus a list of abbreviations, and then over 300 pages of foolproof cross-indexing (repertory). With *The Prescriber,* a Materia Medica, and study, one can become a competent homeopath. Simple to use and to the point, *The Prescriber* is an essential reference for a healthy home.

No one is a better historian of homeopathic and allopathic (drug) medicine than Harris L. Coulter, M.D. (*Homeopathic Science and Modern Medicine,* Richmond, CA: North Atlantic Books, 1981). Dr. Coulter is also a fine spokesman for homeopathy, and here in just over 100 pages makes a strong, logical, and well-researched case for "the physics of healing with microdoses." If you've always wanted to know how and why "like cures like" and to read a fine review of the literature on infinitesimal dosage, here's the book. Although merely a pamphlet compared to Coulter's multivolume homeopathic treatise *Divided Legacy,* this little book still provides over 250 citations from medical journals, a handy table of remedy dilutions, and an annotated bibliography. A 31-page article by J. T. Kent, M.D., on case-taking and prescription is also included. (157 pages, paper)

*"So join the thousands of happy, peppy people
and get a great big bottle of . . . this stuff."*
—LUCILLE BALL, FROM THE "VITAMEATAVEGAMIN" ROUTINE

What natural approaches might help fibromyalgia?

Radical decapitation, perhaps?

After all, how many times have folks been told that their nagging pain and intense soreness are all in their heads? As late as 1982, "fibromyalgia" was not even an entry in the doctor's standard clinical reference book, the *Merck Manual.* You can find "myalgia," though, which is described as simple muscular pain. An utterly predictable medical recommendation promptly follows: take an aspirin!

The most effective therapy I know for fibromyalgia is saturation of vitamin C along with the use of calcium/magnesium supplements. This seems too easy for a problem that so many have really suffered from, I know. And this chapter looks all to brief to have merit. But just ask anyone with fibromyalgia this question: *Have you tried it yet?* If they still have the condition, I'll bet they haven't tried it. Large doses of vitamin C seem to have exceptional anti-inflammatory properties. Saturation of vitamin C is easily reached through frequent oral doses, and is fully described in the chapter "Vitamin C Megadose Therapy."

Media scare-stories to the contrary, the safety and the effectiveness of large amounts of vitamin C are well established. Vitamin C is *far* safer than aspirin. Do not be put off the very thing that can help the most until you have looked into it for yourself.

Calcium and magnesium supplementation, even at rather low RDA levels (about 1,000 mg calcium and 400 mg magnesium daily, in divided doses), can make a big difference in muscle health and happiness. A deficiency of either mineral can cause muscle pain and muscle problems. Dietary deficiency is the rule, rather than the exception, with both of these important minerals.

Gentle to moderate exercise can often help, too. Start light and gradually work up. Yoga stretches and walking are two good choices. Heavy weight-bearing workouts may set you back, so take it easy.

Want one more secret weapon? Vegetable juicing! I never feel so good, so energetic, so un-sore (is that a word?) as when I juice bigtime. Again, if you have not tried this utterly non-toxic approach to better health, why not? See "Juicing Hints" in part two.

Or you can just get some nice hydrocortisone injections to go along with the aspirin.

Fistulas and Boils

*"(You are not) obliged to give me a hearing,
since this may be read or not as anyone pleases."*
—BENJAMIN FRANKLIN, *AUTOBIOGRAPHY*

Todd was two, nearly. His mother brought him in to discuss options, if any, to scheduled surgery for his anal fistula. Todd had had a boil right next to his anus, and it had been lanced by a doctor. As is often the case, the drainage of pus left a pocket, which opened into a crevice. Nice, huh?

I first learned about this standard course of events from a surgical resident as he lanced the ugliest boil I could ever imagine. It was an inch long, half an inch wide, and immediately above the anus of a man, lying face down on an examining table, whose legs and butt were the only things protruding from under a white gown. At the time, I was a student observing at the emergency and outpatient surgical section of a local hospital. I rotated among several house staff, who showed me the ropes, among other things. The resident put a beige plastic cup between the guy's legs as he lay there, spread-eagled. A few jabs of lidocaine, and then a single stab with the knife. A fountain of white pus gushed from the incision. It was several teaspoons, easily. Gross. The resident matter-of-factly said that the man would probably develop a fistula there, which would need to be dealt with when it happened.

My mind came back to the present, where Todd was wandering around my office, hauling a few toys out of the box I kept handy for bored kids. He looked over at his mother, smiling. Had Todd known what was in store for him, he wouldn't have smiled at all. He was to travel to Boston for surgery at a specially selected hospital that allowed parents to stay overnight with their children. In the meantime, however, his mother asked if there were any alternatives to the surgical repair itself.

"I doubt it," I said. "It's asking a lot of a vitamin to close up a fistula without suturing it."

"What about the pus that keeps oozing out?" the mother asked. "This has been going on almost daily since the boil was drained."

"Perhaps there is something that might help that," I said. "You could try a homeopathic remedy called silicea. It's a harmless, over-the-counter preparation that has been used for pus-producing conditions for over a century. It's actually a microdilution of the main mineral in common sand, silica."

"A mineral? That sounds safe enough. Where would I buy it?" she asked.

"Any health food store. I usually used the 6X potency with my kids. The "X" is like the Roman numeral; it stands for ten. The "6" means it has been diluted six successive times. That's less than one part per million."

"Your kids had fistulas, too?" asked Todd's mom.

"No, but they've had a boil once or twice elsewhere, and so have I," I added. "The silicea cleared it up in a day or two. Never had any medicine or needed lancing. As long as you're waiting for the surgery anyway, it's worth trying it in the meantime."

Because of the number of time I'd seen silicea work, I was actually pretty confident that it would stop the pus problem. And, because of what I'd seen of fistulas, that's all I expected.

A joyful woman was on the phone a week later. "The fistula is gone!" said Todd's mother. "Not only did it stop the pus, the fistula closed up! Could the silicea have done all that?"

"Can't argue with success," I said. "Take Todd into his pediatrician and have her take a look."

"Already did that!" said the mom. "We canceled the surgery!"

Calls like that make my day. Calls like that make surgeons mad.

*"The fellow who has not had any experience is so dumb
he doesn't know a thing can't be done,
and he goes ahead and does it."*
—CHARLES F. KETTERING

The oldest records we have establish gout as a disease of overfeeding of protein foods. The simplest preventive solution is vegetarianism. The simplest therapeutic solution is raw-food vegetarianism and fasting. Those who are not whooped up about fasting might be able to do a "pseudo-fast" by simply not eating meat and drinking lots and lots of water.

A reader says:

"Until about a year ago I was suffering from increasingly frequent attacks of gout mainly in my big toe joints. The relief came from prescriptions of indomethacin. As I avoid drugs wherever possible, I decided that something different should be found. For reasons which now escape me, I decided to drink large quantities of water, i.e., about 2 liters per day. I have now been free of gout for over a year. This may be coincidence and this is why I have called the evidence inconclusive. However, my doctor observed that this has the effect of stimulating the kidneys. A very recent item on UK radio by a nutritionist and doctor came to the conclusion that we do drink too little water and that many can be suffering dehydration.

"My brother rang me and mentioned he had gout. This was last Saturday. I recommended he try drinking as much water as he could handle. It may be his gout was already going into remission, but anyway by Sunday the pain was receding and gone by Tuesday. Could be coincidence, but . . . he took no drugs.

"My advice is, go for that water."

More antigout hints: Increased vitamin C consumption improves urinary excretion of uric acid (Cheraskin, Ringsdorf Jr., and Sisley: *The Vitamin C Connection,* New York: Harper and Row, 1983). Use buffered ascorbate "C." But perhaps the tastiest solution is eating cherries. *Lots* of cherries, cherries by the bowlful. Sour cherries work best, but fresh sweet cherries will help a great deal as well. If you absolutely cannot obtain fresh cherries, canned unsweetened cherries will do. Frozen are better. Pie filling (and pie) are not acceptable. Do I really have to say that?

Water, vegetarian diet, and cherries. Such an odd-sounding but time-honored remedy package sounds too simple to work. And yet it does.

Out with gout!

"Of several remedies, the physician should choose the least sensational."

—HIPPOCRATES

Gum surgery is the last thing you want your dentist to tell you that you need. But that's exactly what Kate's dentist told her.

"I'd really like to avoid it," she said. "The very idea of getting my gums cut makes me queasy."

"You are on friendly turf here," I replied. "Dentistry in general makes me weak in the knees. Maybe that stems from my boyhood, when our dentist didn't believe in Novocain. Gum surgery sounds especially unpleasant."

"They've already scheduled it," Kate said. "They'll do the procedure next month. I'll do it if I have no choice, but I'd sure like to avoid it. Is there any way for me to improve my gums in the meantime?"

"Two things come to mind," I said. "The first is comfrey."

"Is that an herb?"

"Yes," I said, and spotting a chance to show off, added: "Comfrey has a four-hundred-year history of wound healing. It is favorably mentioned back in Turner's *Herball* of 1568, Gerard's *Herball* of 1597, Parkinson's 1640 *Theatrum Botanicum,* and Tournefort's 1719 *Compleat Herbal.* There have been monographs on comfrey throughout the centuries, and one of the active ingredients, allantoin, is found in salves and lotions today."

"Can I just buy some capsules at the store?" Kate asked.

"Yes and no," I answered. "You can buy comfrey capsules, all right, but they tend to contain dried comfrey leaf. The leaves are best used externally only, and fresh from the plant. Leaves taken internally, as with swallowed capsules, have little benefit, and negative side effects are much more likely. Comfrey, like medicinal herbs in general, is more a medicine than a food. It needs to be used appropriately. The root is what you want, and *the root is not to be taken raw.* Instead, you make a decoction. Basically, a boiled tea."

"And how do you make that?" said Kate.

"Take a bit of root, maybe a few inches, and wash it under water. Cut the root up, like you would a carrot, into thin slices or little chunks. Put the pieces into a Pyrex or stainless steel saucepan with a cup or two of water. Bring it to a boil, boil for five to ten minutes, and then let it sit and cool. The result is a dark-brown, not particularly unpleasant tea. A cup or two every other day will probably be enough. It can also be used as a mouthwash, and spit out afterward."

"Where do I get comfrey root?" Kate asked.

"Probably at a garden or herb store. I got mine fresh from a farmer who was trying to get rid of it. Comfrey grows like a big weed: very fast. If you mow it down or try to plow it under, it just comes back. Even a little bit of fresh root will grow a new plant. I'm here to tell you, there is nothing to growing your own comfrey. Cheaper that way, too."

"Is that it?"

"Not quite. The second approach you might consider is topical use of vitamin C—direct application of the vitamin to your gums."

"That sounds a bit weird," Kate said.

"It really does," I admitted. "However, vitamin C is so closely involved with wound healing in general and gum integrity in particular that it merits special attention. Vitamin C works as an anti-inflammatory agent. It also is essential for building collagen, the protein 'glue' that literally holds your cells together."

"I'm already taking 1,000 mg of vitamin C a day. Why hasn't that helped?"

"Either it's not enough, or it's not sufficiently concentrated where you need it most."

"But vitamin C is an acid—ascorbic acid, isn't it? I can't go putting that all over my gums and teeth."

"True enough. The trick is to use a nonacidic form of vitamin C called calcium ascorbate. Topical calcium ascorbate will not sting even sore gums, and it is safe to leave on the teeth. You can obtain it as a powder and spread about half a teaspoon on the gum surfaces. It has a bit of a metallic aftertaste, but it's quite bearable. Hold it for about ten minutes, then rinse."

For two weeks, Kate did exactly that, plus drinking the comfrey decoction. However, she did not cancel her gum surgery.

After a pre-op examination, her dentist canceled it.

"Always do right; this will gratify some people and astonish the rest."
—MARK TWAIN

From time to time I have told my students that, in all honesty, I am not particularly interested in nutrition as a subject. What I am interested in is people getting well, and nutrition is merely the best available means to that end.

Some even believe that. One undergraduate comes promptly to mind. He was twenty-one and suffered from a severe heart arrhythmia. Once every week or two his heart rate would violently soar, his pulse would get erratic, and he'd have to lie in bed for hours before it would return to normal. Sometimes he'd have to lie completely still, quite unable to get up without a recurrence. Occasionally he'd have to remain motionless for as many as six hours. He was an active fellow, and all this wasted time bothered him as much as the symptoms themselves.

Of course he'd seen a variety of doctors, including the obligatory specialists. Anxiety or panic attacks had been considered and ruled out. This problem was not in the lad's head. He'd had a lot of tests. The doctors had concluded by offering nothing except either some sort of pacemaker or a new drug packing the potential of serious side effects. Sitting in my office, he showed me the literature on the proposed drug, and I looked it up.

"This drug might indeed relieve your symptoms, Don," I said. "It can also cause myocardial infarction."

"That's, uh, that's a heart attack, isn't it? I'm way too young to risk a heart attack! And pace-makers are for old guys. There's got to be something else I can do."

"You could try nutrition and see how you do."

His mother had come along to the appointment, and spoke up now. "Nutrition? That couldn't hurt Don. His diet is terrible."

Don gave her one of those classic "Oh, Mom" looks, but that didn't stop her from telling me that he never ate breakfast and chose a lot of junk foods when he did eat. He was also under-weight, played a lot of sports, and had a busy work and social schedule. She was plain spoken and pulled no factual punches. She also sounded plenty worried about her boy.

"Let's look at it from the simplest vantage point," I said. If Don has not been eating well, he should start. If the heart is not well nourished, how could we reasonably expect it to work properly? The heart needs essential fatty acids for fuel. Especially linoleic and linolenic acid."

"I've read about them," said Don's mother. "Aren't they found in fish oil and flaxseed oil?"

"Right. Either source will do."

Don gave a sour look.

"In capsules, Don. Capsules."

He brightened up considerably.

"Vitamin E is next. At effectively large doses, vitamin E helps to strengthen and regulate the heartbeat. It works almost like one of the digitalis family of drugs. You'll need to take a lot, prob-ably over 1,000 IUs daily, perhaps as much as 2,000. You can work up this level gradually."

"What other vitamins?" asked his mother.

"The B complex and vitamin C would be wise, I think. A variety of cardiac and other muscle problems result from deficiencies in these vitamins. Don may need more of them than the average person. Or maybe his diet has just contained a lot less. I also would follow Dr. Hans Nieper's example and take gram-sized doses of both calcium orotate and magnesium orotate, in about a 2:1 ratio."

A reader says:

"Even as a kid I had arrhythmia, but at that time it was not considered serious. As I grew up, I occasionally had a little discomfort in the chest area. At the same time, as a kid I had hints of asthma and/or allergies, breathing issues, and so on. It all came home at age forty-four. I was working a high-stress job and eating only takeout. Got a small sore throat, but it just got worse and worse—rapidly. I went to an MD, and he just thought it was allergies. After six weeks, I couldn't speak, and was coughing and suddenly throwing up on myself. I was having asthmalike attacks to the point of repeatedly collapsing—totally unable to recover my breath, even coughing up blood. Three different MDs later: no help. Two of them didn't even explain to me what they thought I had. They just gave me drugs.

"The cough persisted with some attacks severe enough to literally put me on the floor. I had even tried "very large" doses of vitamin C, like one thousand mg/day. Then I found *your* website. I tried two, three, four thousand mg of C a day. By the end of *one* day I had no cough. When it would start to recur, I would take more C. I had also had angina symptoms, and my heart had been palpitating wildly as well. So I got vitamin E, and gradually worked up to over 2000 IUs per day. My problems were 90 percent better. I next added magnesium aspartate and—problem solved . . . for months now!

"The amazing thing is that I had read about vitamins, and believed in vitamins, but you specifically emphasize that if the dose is not large enough, it won't have a therapeutic effect. It will have nutritional benefit, but a certain dose is required if one has a disease condition. I eventually saw it as similar to taking just one mg of Tylenol when a standard dose is hundreds of mg. One mg will do nothing. The same is true for the vitamins."

And they did try it, cautiously, intelligently, and thoroughly. I had a follow-up session with them not long afterwards. Don was smiling. His mom was smiling. So I smiled too.

"How's it going?" I asked.

"Great!" said Don. "No sign of any heart problem at all."

Weeks later, we talked again. "I haven't had an attack since I started the vitamins," Don said.

We were all very pleased. I asked Don what he was taking daily, and he read it all off to me: "2,000 mg of vitamin C; 2,000 mg of flaxseed oil; 2,000 mg calcium orotate in four divided doses; 1,000 mg magnesium orotate in divided doses; two B-complex supplements; one multivitamin; and 1600 IU of natural mixed-tocopherols vitamin E."

Not a bad way to eliminate long-standing chronic tachycardia/arrhythmia events so promptly. No pacemaker surgery, no dangerous medicines. It's been a long time now and there has been only one recurrence. That was when Don skipped both breakfast and his supplements. He got back with the program and the symptoms were gone for good.

Another reader says:

A doctor had me on metoprolol for monthly arrhythmia episodes that sometimes lasted for up to two hours (I've had them since I was a teenager, but they were getting longer, more frequent, and worse). At the same time I started taking a common multivitamin. When I ran out of the vitamin, the arrhythmia returned although I was still taking the drug. After taking the vitamin, the arrhythmia went away in ten minutes. When I told my doctor this happened three times in a row, she laughed at me and said the vitamins don't do anything! I stopped taking the metoprolol six months ago, but continued with the vitamin and have not had the arrhythmia return yet. I am now convinced that good medicine starts with what we put in our bodies every day, and we have to research that for ourselves because the big drug companies don't make any profit when we effectively treat ourselves by simple vitamins and diet instead of paying them hundreds of dollars every month for specious drugs that only treat the symptoms.

"For duty and humanity!"

—DR. MOE HOWARD, DR. LARRY FINE, DR. CURLY HOWARD

The simple fact that you are actually reading this says something in itself. Perhaps you have nothing better to do, which I doubt. Or perhaps you have many better things to do, but you can't possibly get on with them until you relieve that itch. Whatever the case, here are my happy-heiney hints:

1. First, we can stop killing sharks (among our newest endangered species). Preparation H and its clones are made from shark liver oil. Use topical vitamin E instead. Medically speaking, "topical" means "applied directly to the surface." This really works, O hemorrhoid sufferers. Make sure the anus is clean and, even more important, dry. After a shower or bath, blot the area with a clean, white tissue and wait ten or fifteen minutes. Then, puncture a vitamin E capsule with a pushpin. (You might even like to keep a pushpin in the bottle, as long as it is out of reach of children and brightly colored so you can spot it, too.) Place the opened end of the vitamin E capsule right up against the anus, and squeeze the capsule. Spread the slightly oily vitamin E around and you will be pleased with the prompt results. Repeat twice daily.

2. Eat more fiber, as found in fruits, vegetables, whole grains, and legumes. This means softer, easier-to-pass stools. Just lovely, this chat we're having here, isn't it?

3. Drink more water. You need water for fiber to work. The bowel is your personal water recycling center, by the way. A human bowel movement usually contains only about 150 ml (that's about half a Dixie cup) of water. The rest, and we're talking quarts, is reclaimed by your body, which is itself two-thirds water. Dry stools are an adaptation for land animals, especially birds and reptiles, to conserve water. Although you are capable of forming a very solid stool, it is better for your butt if you don't.

4. Eat less meat. Meat contains no fiber, and fills you up before you get to the other fiber-rich foods.

5. Avoid surgery by doing the four steps above. Some almost personal experience: my dad had several hemorrhoid operations during his lifetime. (He actually watched them perform the surgery, thanks to the wonders of local anesthesia and cleverly placed mirrors. Now there's a lively answer for "What did you do today, Dear?") The simple fact that he had the same operation more than once tells us much about the value of such operations. Dad noted the proctologist's custom-made wallpaper, with its novel, abstract design. Turns out it was a pattern of assorted anal sphincters. This was in the man's professional office, and I am not making this up: my dad told me. Of course, there is a slim chance that he might have been making it up, and let's hope so.

The rest of this chapter has been pretty much on the level.

"A hospital bed is a parked taxi with the meter running."
—GROUCHO MARX

There must be *fifteen ways to love your liver.*

1. *Put the six-pack back, Jack.* Half of all the alcohol consumed in America is consumed by only 10 percent of the population. One in three adult Americans is a heavy drinker, with a liquor habit sufficient to be indistinguishable from an alcoholic. Such behavior wrecks livers. Cirrhosis of the liver is a rather rare disease—except among alcoholics, who make it the seventh leading cause of death in the United States! It usually takes half a quart of whiskey a day for ten years to abuse the liver to the point of cirrhosis.

The fibrous tissue that replaces normal liver in cirrhosis causes decreased liver function. This leads to fluid buildup, jaundice, and perhaps cancer of the liver. Cirrhosis is fairly easy to arrest by stopping alcohol consumption. But cure is difficult and generally considered impossible. Well, as they say in the Marines, the difficult we do immediately; the impossible takes a little longer. Reversing cirrhosis becomes merely very difficult if you employ the Gerson program (referenced below, and in cancer chapters) and very high doses of C and B-complex vitamins. The corticosteroids (prednisone) are commonly tried for this, but the side effects are undesirable, and in my opinion, the drug is generally ineffective.

Prevention is the way to go: stop drinking! Sure, as W. C. Fields said, "It's easy to give up drinking; I've done it a thousand times." But consider this: Fields, the highest-paid comic of his time, drank over a quart of hard liquor a day and was dead at age sixty-six.

That's not so funny.

2. *Avoid the virus, Iris.* The various forms of hepatitis are all diseases that attack the liver, causing symptoms ranging from jaundice, abdominal pain, and diarrhea to nausea, fever, and death. All viral forms of hepatitis respond remarkably well to extremely high doses of vitamin C, the B-complex vitamins, and the Gerson therapy (described below).

3. *Take a lot more C, Lee.* Vincent Zannoni at the University of Michigan Medical School has shown that vitamin C protects the liver. Even doses as low as 500 mg daily helps prevent fatty buildup and cirrhosis. 5,000 mg of vitamin C per day appears to actually flush fats from the liver. And vitamin C over 50,000 mg per day results in patients feeling better in just a few days, and actually eliminates jaundice in a matter of days. Frederick Klenner, M.D., found that such huge doses of vitamin C had his patients recovered and back to work in a week.

4. *Don't rely on the shot, Dot.* Even if you choose to vaccinate, it is immeasurably reassuring to remember this: Dr. Klenner showed that very large doses of vitamin C (500 to 900 mg per kilogram body weight per day) can cure hepatitis in as little as two to four days.

5. *Take vitamin B, Dee.* Especially vitamin B_{12}, which significantly reduces jaundice, anorexia, serum bilirubin, and recovery time. B_{12} is most effective if administered by injection, which your

doctor can easily arrange. If injection is not an option, there is an intranasal gel that improves absorption. Or, you can make your own B$_{12}$ paste by going to my vitamin B$_{12}$ supplementation chapter. This vitamin is nonprescription, utterly nontoxic, and has no contraindications or negative side effects.

6. *Eat veggies and greens, Gene.* The fiber and abundant nutrients in vegetables are a sure way to improve the health of practically any organ you can name, especially the liver. Vegetables are essentially fat-free. And greens are rich in the B vitamin folic acid. (*Folic,* as in *foliage.* Neat, huh?) Folate has been shown to help shorten the recovery time for viral hepatitis.

7. *Eat your food raw, Pa.* Or at least as much of it as you can. Max Gerson, M.D., believed that cancer in general is a disease of the liver, even if it occurs elsewhere in the body. Gerson's nutritional therapy is a raw-foods protocol that is often very effective against cancer, as well as other diseases. Cancer in the liver itself is often due to environmental toxins, such as dry-cleaning fluids. I have personally seen a terminal liver cancer case vastly improved with the Gerson program. Full dietary details are provided in his classic book *A Cancer Therapy: Results of 50 Cases* and in a more recent work, *Healing the Gerson Way,* by Charlotte Gerson and Beata Bishop.

8. *Get off the drugs, Doug.* Illegal drugs of all sorts (and more than a few prescription drugs as well) are rough on the liver. This includes anabolic steroids. The liver is the main chemical detoxification center for your entire body. Don't push it; quit now before your liver quits on you.

154

9. *Watch the fat, Matt.* To help relieve indigestion, cut down on those fatty foods. Diseases of the liver can lead to reduced bile secretion. This results in a diminished ability to emulsify fats. ("Emulsify" means breaking down of fat into smaller pieces that can be more easily digested.) Your liver, an enormous four-pound gland, helps you digest fats by normally making up to a quart of bile every day. Most of your body's bile salts are reabsorbed by the intestinal tract after digestion and recycled by the liver. Often the same bile material will go through two or three recyclings during digestion of a single meal. That is how your body, with less than 4 grams of total bile salts in it, can secrete twice that amount (or more) in a single fatty meal. Gross, huh?

10. *Practice safe sex, Tex.* If you are not in a monogamous relationship, you are at increased risk for hepatitis.

11. *Wash your hands, Stan.* Good grief, is that so hard to do? Toilet paper is thinner than a politician's election promise. Do you really think the tissue keeps your hands squeaky clean? To put it another way, do you think it keeps someone else's hands clean enough for you? No? *Then wash your hands with soap and hot water!* I read once that over half of all physicians don't wash their mitts after using the toilet. I hope this is not true. I suspect that it is, however. When heads of state, billionaires, or doctors use the john, they are likely to do what you do. Think about that in your spare time today. And wash, Josh.

12. *Prevent that stone, Joan.* In addition to salts for emulsification, bile contains the pigment bilirubin, neutral fat, phospholipids, and high concentrations of cholesterol. About 33 ml of bile are stored in the average gallbladder. But the gallbladder is more than a storage receptacle. It concentrates bile by removing water from it. Sometimes the resulting cholesterol level becomes too high to remain in the bile solution, and cholesterol gallstones precipitate out. In addition to

hurting, gallstones obstruct the bile duct, thereby interfering with fat digestion. Low-fat meals help prevent future gallbladder problems by keeping your cholesterol levels low (the body uses fat to manufacture cholesterol). In addition, therapeutic vegetable juice fasting and large doses of vitamin C significantly reduce cholesterol production. And, as only animal foods contain cholesterol, try to go vegetarian.

NUTS REDUCE GALLSTONE RISK

A study at Harvard Medical School showed that men consuming five or more one-ounce servings of nuts per week had a 30 percent lower risk of gallstones than men that did not eat nuts. If you are concerned that nuts are fattening, it is worth noting that the study found that fat consumption had nothing to do with it. Furthermore, nuts are a "filling" food. As an eleven-year-old, I remember filling up on nuts while waiting, endlessly, for a wedding banquet to begin. When they served dinner, I was full. If you eat more nuts, you will eat less of other things. And have fewer gallstones. What a deal!

Reference

Tsai, CJ, Leitzmann, MF, Hu, FB, Willett, WC, and Giovannucci, EL. (2004). A prospective cohort study of nut consumption and the risk of gallstone disease in men. *Am J Epidemiol.* 160(10):961–8.

13.   *Eat lecithin, Lynn.* Phospholipids in bile help emulsify cholesterol. Lecithin is loaded with phospholipids (also known as phosphatides), to the tune of about 1,700 mg of phosphatidyl choline and 1,000 mg of phosphatidyl inositol per tablespoon. Lecithin therapy is therefore almost certainly worth trying for threatened gallstones. Three to five tablespoons daily is more likely to be effective than a just few capsules. Even a really large 1,200 mg capsule contains only about $1/8$ tablespoon lecithin because of size limits and added carrier oils. Lecithin is harmless and without side effects. Bulk granules run $8–15 per pound. Lecithin is available over-the-counter at any health-food store.

14.   *See your Doc, Rock.* Take the doubt out of it all. Get tested. Be monitored. Listen to your doctor. I said *listen,* not "obey." Go and hear what the doctor has to say, and then decide for yourself what you want to do. Negotiation skills and how to shape your doctor into a natural healing practitioner are discussed in other chapters of this book.

15.   *Be well-read, Fred.* You can start with the references cited below, and then move on to this book's bibliography.

Recommended Reading

Campbell RE and Pruitt FW. The effect of vitamin B-12 and folic acid in the treatment of viral hepatitis. *American Journal of Medical Science* 229 (1955): 8.

Campbell RE and Pruitt FW. Vitamin B-12 in the treatment of viral hepatitis. *American Journal of Medical Science* 224 (1952): 252. [Cited in Werbach, M. *Nutritional Influences on Illness.* New Canaan, CT: Keats Publishing, 1988.]

Cathcart RF. The method of determining proper doses of vitamin C for the treatment of disease by titrating to bowel tolerance. *Journal of Orthomolecular Psychiatry* 10 (1981):125–32.

Gerson C and Bishop B. *Healing the Gerson Way: Defeating Cancer and Other Chronic Diseases.* Carmel, California: Gerson Health Media, 2nd Edition, 2009.

155

Gerson M. *A Cancer Therapy: Results of Fifty Cases and the Cure of Advanced Cancer.* San Diego, CA: The Gerson Institute, 2000.

Jain ASC and Mukerji DP. Observations on the therapeutic value of intravenous B-12 in infective hepatitis. *Journal of the Indian Medical Association* 35 (1960): 502–05.

Klenner FR. Observations on the dose of administration of ascorbic acid when employed beyond the range of a vitamin in human pathology. *Journal of Applied Nutrition* 23 (Winter 1971): 61–68.

Ray O and Ksir C. *Drugs, Society and Human Behavior,* chapter 9. St. Louis, MO: Mosby, 1990.

Ritter M. "Study Says Vitamin C Could Cut Liver Damage," Associated Press (11 October 1986).

Smith LH, ed. *Clinical Guide to the Use of Vitamin C: The Clinical Experiences of Frederick R. Klenner, M.D.* Portland, OR: Life Sciences Press, 1988. Originally titled: *Vitamin C as a Fundamental Medicine: Abstracts of Dr. Frederick R. Klenner, M.D.'s Published and Unpublished Work.* Reprinted 1991. The full text of this book is posted at www.seanet.com/~alexs/ascorbate/198x/smith-lh-clinical_guide_1988.htm.

"One grandmother is worth two M.D.s."

—ROBERT MENDELSSOHN, M.D.

You may or may not believe this, but even at the risk of bending the Medical Practice Act, I just had to include it. I got this hiccup cure from my outlaws, er, in-laws, and it is as effective in practice as it is ridiculous in description.

To cure ordinary hiccups, do the following: *Drink out of the far-side rim of a glass.* It may also be described as "drink out of a glass upside down," although you aren't really upside down. Even so, it looks weird enough when you try it, because you have to bend yourself forward to do it.

My experience has been that it takes a full cup of water and about thirty seconds of this type of sipping for the hiccup reflex to cease. It has never failed me. Since I wanted you to gain all possible practical benefit from this book, I couldn't resist mentioning it. (Mag. Phos. 6X, a Schuessler cell salt in homeopathic potency, is also effective against hiccups.)

A probable explanation for the success of the drinking-out-of-the-other-side-of-the-glass technique is that your bending-over posture and your concentration on performing such an unusual feat serves to restrict the spasmodic inhalation characteristic of hiccups. The act of drinking itself might create new nerve messages to displace the hiccup reflex, calming the glottis and diaphragm. Whatever; it works.

"If you care to go to school, go to the honey bees, fowl, cats, dogs, goats, mink, calves, dairy cows, bulls and horses and allow them to teach you their ways."

—D. C. JARVIS, M.D.

Honey and cider vinegar as a remedy became well known and somewhat well respected by Deforrest Clinton Jarvis (1881–1966), who received his M.D. from the University of Vermont Medical College and was a member of the American Academy of Ophthalmology and Otolaryngology. Practicing in Vermont, Dr. Jarvis's decades of observation and experience seem to have given him good reason for his major dietary recommendation: acidify your diet. He states that one may do so by drinking a teaspoon or two of cider vinegar, dissolved in water with a little honey, every day.

Dr. Jarvis's book, *Folk Medicine* (1958), fully discusses why and how to prepare and use this obviously harmless self-treatment. Essentially, a tablespoon or two each of honey and cider vinegar is dissolved in a glass of water and taken several times daily as needed. White (distilled) vinegar is not recommended, by the way. Dr. Jarvis states that numerous common ailments, including colds, infections, rheumatism, arthritis, and many other everyday illnesses may be relieved and even cured with this simple treatment.

But Why Vinegar?

One rationale for the vinegar-honey regimen is that a person's internal environment tends toward becoming alkaline through a modern diet of fats, starches, and de-vitalized processed foods (here we go again, right?). Dr. Jarvis found that the acidity of cider vinegar, although weak, is enough to correct this excess alkalinity, and that a slightly acidic body prevents and fights infection. Since vinegar solution in a teakettle dissolves mineral buildup, Dr. Jarvis also suspected that calcium deposits in the joints might also be dissolved by a slight acidification. He experimentally proved both of these theories with patients of his, after first studying cows.

"Milk fever" in cows is usually treated with calcium injections by the veterinarian. A critically ill cow generally then makes an immediate recovery and is often on her feet again in minutes. Dr. Jarvis reasoned that vinegar must be dissolving calcium into the bloodstream, for when he gave cows with milk fever some vinegar, they too recovered immediately. This lent support to his premise that calcium deposits could be dissolved from the joints of the body in arthritic persons.

By observing cows out at pasture, Dr. Jarvis saw that they preferred eating the most acidic of the plants and grasses. He also noted that the modern diet of a high-producing dairy cow under intensive milking lacks these acidic greens and is high in alkaline-producing grains. At the same time, these heavy milkers are prone to mastitis, an infection of the udder. Dr. Jarvis felt that their alkaline diet facilitated infection, so he gave cows a few ounces of cider vinegar daily in their feed. The cows so treated failed to develop mastitis. This lends support to the belief that vinegar is anti-infective.

And Honey?

Honey added to the vinegar naturally makes the mixture more drinkable for people. Honey also contains subtle amounts of beneficial food factors suspected for ages but just beginning to be fully understood. Curative powers of honey were known about in the most ancient civilizations, and naturally minded doctors recommend it still. It is what is not known about honey that is probably of greatest medicinal value.

As a sweetener, honey is more than just the sum of its sugars. Traditional nutritional authorities say that sugar is sugar, and that the source or state of it doesn't matter nutritionally. You may choose to believe that or not. I think that there is quite a significant difference in life-supporting qualities between processed white sugar and dark, raw honey. The darker, cloudier, and less filtered the honey, the better. Light, crystal clear, pasteurized honey lacks the trace factors that nature had the bees put into the comb.

Honey is by nature pure; why on earth anyone would pasteurize it is beyond me. Heat does in fact destroy valuable enzymes in the raw honey. In addition, bacteria can grow on the surface moisture left under the cap of *processed* honey as a result of heating and condensation. Raw honey actually contains natural antibiotics. So eat the honey the way the bees made it; the very best way is comb and all. (It's delicious and makes a great sandwich spread. Honey in the comb doesn't leak through your bread as much.)

Honey has a self-limiting effect on the appetite. A person who could eat a one-pound chocolate bar with ease might have great difficulty eating a quarter-cup of honey all at once. Try it on your kids next time they are pestering for candy: give them a teaspoon or two of honey. Dates and raisins work the same way. Who do you know that can eat a couple of handfuls of dates right down? Nature has put more into many foods than we fully realize.

Acidify or Alkalize?

There have long been divergent opinions on acid/alkaline foods and how they affect body pH. Occasionally, there have been attempts to co-opt Dr. Jarvis's work in order to support consuming an alkaline diet. This misrepresents his work. Some sources will tell you that distilled or "white" vinegar acidifies, but apple cider vinegar is actually an alkalizing food. That is incorrect. Both acidify. As found in stores, apple cider vinegar and distilled vinegar have about the same acidity. The acetic acid in either type of vinegar is still acetic acid. Acetic acid is not alkaline. Vinegar has a pH of about 3. Neutral is 7. This stuff is definitely an acid.

Distilled vinegar is made from ethyl alcohol, which is commonly made from corn or another carbohydrate source. Indeed, if you take no-preservative apple cider and let it sit for a week or so, you get hard cider, as the sugar converts to ethanol (beverage alcohol). If you let the hard cider sit for a week or two more, it will turn into vinegar. Same with grapes, which ferment into wine, and then further to vinegar. I have done both. It's easy.

But neither are very strong vinegars. Distillation makes them stronger. Then, for sale in grocery stores, they are reduced (diluted) to about 5 percent acidity.

One might speculate that the potassium in cider vinegar is what supposedly could alkalize the cider vinegar in the body. Yes, potassium on the periodic table of the elements is an "alkali metal." But you do not consume potassium metal. You consume potassium ions, taken in as dissolved potassium salts.

Cider vinegar is made from apples. Dr. Jarvis advocated potassium, and apples are high in it. But apple cider vinegar, in the one- or two-teaspoonful dose Dr. Jarvis recommended, would

159

only provide around 10 mg of potassium. Even if potassium ions were wonderfully alkali forming, that would not matter a whit in the large amount of potassium that you eat every day. The U.S. RDA for potassium is 4,700 mg/day for an adult. Even if you did not meet that, you'd still be taking in several thousand milligrams of potassium daily. Plant foods (fruits, vegetables, nuts, beans) are all good sources of potassium. To increase your dietary potassium, you can eat more fruits and vegetables and their juices. And even if you didn't, meat and dairy products contain potassium.

So there is a whole lot more acetic acid in cider vinegar than there is potassium. Consuming an acid does not alkalize. Indeed, Dr. Jarvis specifically wanted to acidify the urine, and in *Folk Medicine* he discusses this in some detail. Urine is what your kidneys filter out of your blood for excretion. If it is in your urine, it was in your blood. Your blood, however, is constantly buffered by an amazing chemical mechanism that keeps your blood pH very close to 7.4. That is slightly alkaline. It is also automatic and not dependent on your diet, fortunately for us all.

But you can, and Dr. Jarvis did, measure urine pH and see that urine can be acidified. Vitamin C as ascorbic acid does that, too. This slight acidification helps prevent urinary tract infections (UTIs). Dr. Jarvis believed that it also prevented colds, sinusitis, neuralgia, digestive ailments, headaches, and quite a few other illnesses.

Whether you go along with that or not is up to you. However, to know what Dr. Jarvis thought, we need to go directly to what he wrote. You might want to start with Chapter 6 and also page 75 of *Folk Medicine*. I urge all interested to read his books and make up their minds for themselves. As my father always said, "Go to the organ grinder, not the monkey."

References

Jarvis D. C. *Folk Medicine.* New York: Holt, 1958.

Jarvis D. C. *Arthritis and Folk Medicine.* New York: Holt, 1960.

Yes, these texts were written a long time ago. But nothing has changed about the way honey and vinegar work.

"Without health there is no happiness. An attention to health, then, should take the place of every other object."

—THOMAS JEFFERSON, 1787

Here's a very common question about a very common problem: "My doctor has recently declared that I have blood pressure that has to be treated and wants to put me on blood pressure pills (the reading was 150/100). Is there a way I can reduce my blood pressure without medication?"

You bet. Switching to a good, near-vegetarian natural diet would certainly be a good place to start; there is no downside to eating right. More fiber, less sugar and fat, and more fruits, vegetables, and grains are all great for the ticker. So are Dr. Jacobus Rinse's supplement suggestions, which we will come to shortly.

Garlic may help reduce moderate hypertension. A number of clinical studies have shown significant benefit.[1–4] The effect is not dramatic, but an effect does not have to be dramatic to still be valuable and useful. High regular intake of garlic requires working with your doctor, because garlic may interfere with some medications. I eat a lot of fresh garlic, and I grow even more. Dracula will not be raiding my vegetable garden anytime soon.

Your BP is significantly higher when you are anxious, and a false reading may result in unnecessary medication. Take your own blood pressure at home, or have a friend do it. You may find that you already have a partial cure for hypertension: avoid doctors' offices! This is more than just rhetorical hyperbole. A daily program of stress reduction repeatedly has been proven to reduce high blood pressure without drugs. (See my chapter "Stress Reduction" for specifics.) Exercise works, and so does weight loss. Please look at my chapters on these uncomfortable but important subjects.

Certainly stress raises blood pressure. Want to really make it soar? Arguing is one of the best ways; repressing anger is another. Sometimes high bold pressure is due to straining against lifestyle conflicts that you cannot fully resolve: kids, job, where you live, family, traffic, or whatever turns you off. Take a look at your life and reduce the stresses that you can reduce, accept the ones you can't, and as the old saying goes, have the wisdom to know the difference. If your "stresses you can't reduce" box is too full, prescription anti-anxiety or sleeping medication might be a reasonable medical compromise.

Commonsense caution: If these measures do not work, and your blood pressure remains consistently high, medication is no longer optional: it is necessary.

Back to cardiovascular health in general. Let me tell you about Dr. Jacobus Rinse. When he was only in his early fifties, Jacobus Rinse's doctors told him he had but a few years to live. Cardiovascular disease had ravaged his body. Medicine had little to offer him but hope, and not much of that. So Dr. Rinse, a chemist, decided to look into matters for himself. He hit the books and collected an enormous pile of nutritional research. Some studies suggested that he might be able to delay death with vitamins and other food supplements. He had little to lose, so he tried it. His payoff? Rinse lived for another third of a century.

I drink a modified version of Dr. Rinse's breakfast supplement drink nearly every morning in winter and spring (and juice fresh veggies instead during summer and fall). You can find the recipe for this in my chapter "Breakfast Blast."

My last suggestion, many will note with great joy and considerable relief, has nothing to do with nutrition. Transcendental Meditation is just as effective as prescription drugs for the treatment of high blood pressure. According to a study published in the November 1995 issue of *Hypertension,* TM is twice as effective at lowering blood pressure as is progressive muscle relaxation. Even more important, the results with meditation proved to be just as good as those obtained with pharmaceutical medication. Exactly how good? "Over a three-month interval, systolic and diastolic blood pressure dropped by 10.6 mm Hg." This cannot be written of as a fluke, because a similar study at Harvard yielded the same data: TM for three months reduced systolic blood pressure by 11 mm Hg.

The American Heart Association has said, "People with high blood pressure may want to medicate and meditate." Perhaps they should say it a good bit louder.

For more information on hypertension and nutrition, you may wish to look at Hickey S and Roberts H. *The Vitamin Cure for Heart Disease* (Basic Health Publications, 2010)

References

1. Ried K, Frank OR, Stocks NP. Aged garlic extract lowers blood pressure in patients with treated but uncontrolled hypertension: a randomised controlled trial. *Maturitas.* 2010 Oct;67(2):144–50.

2. Sobenin IA, Andrianova IV, Fomchenkov IV, Gorchakova TV, Orekhov AN. Time-released garlic powder tablets lower systolic and diastolic blood pressure in men with mild and moderate arterial hypertension. *Hypertens Res.* 2009 Jun;32(6):433–37.

3. Reinhart KM, Coleman CI, Teevan C, Vachhani P, White CM. Effects of garlic on blood pressure in patients with and without systolic hypertension: a meta-analysis. *Ann Pharmacother.* 2008 Dec;42(12):1766–771.

4. Ried K, Frank OR, Stocks NP, Fakler P, Sullivan T. Effect of garlic on blood pressure: a systematic review and meta-analysis. *BMC Cardiovasc Disord.* 2008 Jun 16;8:13.

Recommended Reading

"In Search of an Optimal Behavioral Treatment for Hypertension: A Review and Focus on Transcendental Meditation" in *Personality, Elevated Blood Pressure, and Essential Hypertension.* Washington, DC: Hemisphere Publishing, 1992.

Prousky J. *Anxiety: Orthomolecular Diagnosis and Treatment.* CCNM Press, 2007.

Rinse J. Atherosclerosis: prevention and cure (parts 1 and 2). *Prevention* (November and December 1975).

Rinse J. Cholesterol and phospholipids in relation to atherosclerosis. *American Laboratory Magazine* (April 1978).

Roberts H, Hickey S. (Saul AW, series editor). *The Vitamin Cure for Heart Disease.* Laguna Beach, CA: Basic Health Publications, 2011.

TM combats heart disease. *Vegetarian Times* 221 (February 1996).

Transcendental Meditation, mindfulness, and longevity: an experimental study with the elderly. *Journal of Personality and Social Psychology* 57 (1989): 950–64.

Immune Dysfunction

"The germ is nothing; the terrain is everything."

—LOUIS PASTEUR

Like a country veterinarian, I drove my red '78 Ford pickup along a vacant road to a client's rural home out near Pavilion, New York. Driving along in the middle of nowhere (and even in New York State there are still such places) to a house call was not my usual routine, but on a sunny spring day like this, it was a taste of the life of James Herriot.

I pulled up the long driveway to the cedar-shingled house where my appointment was scheduled. Going to the side door, I met the father and mother, who showed me into the dining area, where I met a perfectly normal-looking nine-year-old boy. He was blond, fair-skinned, and a bit skinny. His name was Charles.

Charles had no immune system to speak of. His mother told the tale. "He's been in and out of Children's Hospital, again and again. He's home, he gets a sniffle, then he clogs up and can't breathe, then it's pneumonia, then he's back to the hospital. This happens every few weeks, over and over again, and has been going on for years. The doctors said there is nothing they can do except give him antibiotics. They said his immune system isn't working. They do not know why. They are out of ideas, and we are at our wits end over this." She really did look wrung out.

"What can you do?" asked the father. He looked like his nerves were frayed, too. "Nothing has done him any good. All the doctors do is tell us to stick him in a steamy shower when he can't breathe, and we have to keep him there all night sometimes. Then he gets bronchitis. Last time, it went to meningitis."

"Does he take vitamins?" I asked.

"A multivitamin, nearly every day," the mother answered. "Sometimes I give him some vitamin C, but it hasn't helped."

"Maybe his body needs more of it," I said, taking the plunge. "There are fifty years of scientific literature on successful vitamin C megadose therapy. Much of it comes from the two dozen or so published papers of Frederick Robert Klenner, M.D., of Reidsville, North Carolina."

"How much did he use?" the father asked.

"A whole lot; more than you'd ever imagine giving to a nine-year-old."

"We've given Charlie 500 mg sometimes," said his mother.

"Dr. Klenner gave that amount or more per kilogram of body weight per day," I explained. "A kilogram is 2.2 pounds. What do you weigh, Charlie?"

"Seventy-five pounds, I think," Charlie said. "Maybe a little less."

"All right, that's about thirty-three kilograms or so. Dr. Klenner would have given you somewhere between 11,000 and 30,000 mg."

"A day?" said his mother.

"Yes."

"That seems like an awful lot of vitamin C," said his father. "How safe is it?"

"Klenner was a very competent doctor, who practiced for some thirty-five years. He wrote that vitamin C is the safest and most effective substance available to the physician. You could start raising Charlie's daily vitamin C intake, and really take it up high if he starts to get sick."

"How high?" asked the father.

"If he gets sick? At least 11,000 mg a day, maybe twice that. Enough so his symptoms stop."

If John Dillinger had told J. Edgar Hoover that he'd never even been in a bank, you could not have gotten a more skeptical look than the one I got then.

"All right, thank you," said the father.

I left without much confidence in this one. It was only days later that I got a call in the morning from Charlie's mother, and she was not happy.

"It's started again," she said. "Charlie is sneezing and coughing and gasping, and we've just put him in the shower. What am I supposed to do again?"

I went over the protocol once more: give Charlie as much vitamin C as he could hold, at least 11,000 mg before the day was over.

"OK," she said. "This had better work."

That's what I was thinking, too. That night I got another call.

"I can't believe it," came the voice of Charlie's mother. "I cannot believe it. He's actually getting better. He's getting better!" She told me that Charlie's symptoms had gone away during the afternoon. He'd had around 12,000 to 14,000 mg of vitamin C that day. No medicines. No more showers. No hospital visit.

"No kidding!" I said. "That's really great."

"Now what?" said the mother.

"As a preventive, continue to keep his vitamin C level high each day, maybe 4,000 mg or so. Dr. Klenner said that children can take their age in grams (thousands of mg) of C each day, as a maintenance dose. My own kids seemed to do fine with around half that. The exact amount will be the amount that keeps Charlie well. Remember that we don't take the amount of C that we think we should take; we take the amount of C that does the job. My corny little jingle is, 'Take enough C to be symptom free, whatever that amount might be.'"

A reader says:

"I had pneumonia a couple of years ago. The minute a cold starts, I know I am in trouble. Pneumonia likes me. I took control of my health and body. Vitamin C works. I am now off all medicines, except my high blood pressure meds. Coworkers tell me I have more energy and can tell when I walk with a bounce. They ask me questions and want my advice and I say, 'Vitamin C, and lots of it.' They look at me funny and my comment is, 'Hey, you're the one that is sick, not me.' With health insurance becoming out of control, I decided changes had to be made. At age sixty, I finally got smart. Best thing I ever did."

"So when he's sick, give him enough to get him well, and when he's well, give him enough to keep him that way?"

"Right," I replied.

"That seems too simple to be the answer," said his mother.

"The hospital tried everything else, true?" I reminded her.

"Yes."

"And what worked?"

"The vitamin C is the only thing that's worked," she said. "Normally he'd be in the hospital by now. There must be something to this."

There is. And for such a good idea, the spread of this knowledge has been exceptionally slow. Furthermore, for such a useful therapy, medical-political hindrance has been unbelievably high. Nowhere is this more apparent than in the case of Dr. Linus Pauling.

Linus Pauling, Ph.D., is one of history's great chemists, and his textbooks and huge output of scientific papers continue to influence generations of research. Pauling is the only person, ever, to win two unshared Nobel prizes. The first, normally enough, was for pioneering work into the detailed nature of chemical bonds. The second was for peace, after it was eventually appreciated that Pauling's position against atmospheric nuclear weapons testing was the correct one. Neither of these awards prepared the world for what was to follow: Pauling suggested that vitamin C might be effective against the common cold. It would be difficult to imagine that the practical medical applications of ascorbic acid would cause more of a ruckus than Pauling's complete overhaul of our knowledge of chemistry, or the vicious blacklisting Pauling got from the U.S. government when he opposed nuclear testing. But it is true nonetheless.

> *"Linus Pauling never lost a horse race."*
> —ABRAM HOFFER, MD, PHD

Pauling reviewed several dozen supposedly open-and-shut papers concluding that vitamin C was apparently unsuccessful at slowing, stopping, or preventing the common cold. He found that the researchers had failed to interpret their own work fairly, or even accurately. In virtually every instance, Pauling found that the effect of vitamin C was, at the very least, statistically significant. Again and again, the authors of the studies had written biased opinions and passed them off as valid summaries of their work.

These authors were simply wrong: science repeatedly demonstrates vitamin C is indeed an effective antiviral. There are other widely known, but completely false, "facts" about vitamin C. Here are two:

VITAMIN C MYTH #1: *"Your body doesn't absorb extra vitamin C. All you get from taking vitamin supplements is expensive urine."*

Urine is what is left over after your kidneys purify your blood. If your urine contains extra vitamin C, that vitamin C was in your blood. If the vitamin was in your blood, you absorbed it just fine. Think about that.

You can swallow a marble (but please don't) and find it in the toilet bowl a couple of days later. That is because your food tube, or alimentary canal, is essentially just a twenty-five-foot hose connecting your mouth to your anus. That swallowed marble is "in" your body geographically, but it is not in your body the way your blood is. If you stick your finger through the hole of a donut, you might say your finger is "inside" the donut, but it is not in the donut the way the flour and sugar are. We can turn you upside down and shake you, and you'll probably barf up your most recent meal, maybe even that marble. Your blood won't come out, though. If something is in your blood, it is really in you, fully and utterly absorbed.

If water is coming out of the overflow spillway on a dam, then the reservoir is full and is dumping the excess water. If there is not enough water in the reservoir, nothing comes out. Wasting indicates fullness, just as a cup overflowing is truly a full cup. Urine spillage of vitamin C indicates that you have some to waste, then and there. But such does not indicate bodily sat-

165

uration; bowel tolerance (loose stool) indicates saturation. Therapeutically, one takes enough C to stay just below that level.

It is the absence of water-soluble vitamins such as vitamin C in urine that indicates vitamin deficiency. If your body excretes vitamins in your urine, that is a sign that you are well nourished and have nutrients to spare. It is easier to put a twenty in the Salvation Army pot at Christmas if you have a few grand to spend shopping. So many Americans are credit-card shoppers and deficit spenders. We are also deficit eaters, trying to obtain a ridiculously low RDA of vitamins from a selection of nutritionally wimpy foods that cannot really meet any of our vitamin or mineral needs abundantly. Vitamin supplements are a solution, not a problem.

A reader says:

"I now swear by, and will tell anyone who will listen, about vitamin C crystals. I just sent my son at college a bottle of them. They knocked out my cold in days. I take 7,500 mg a day as maintenance and can probably increase that now. That was my saturation point in the beginning. A side benefit has been that it's helped an achy joint in a finger and my lower back. I'm a happy woman."

VITAMIN C MYTH #2: *"Vitamin C causes kidney stones."*

I have never seen any scientific evidence to back up that statement. I've had literally hundreds of students and health practitioners looking for years for any controlled study demonstrating a vitamin C–caused kidney stone and so far I have received . . . nearly one submission. In other words, none. The vitamin C kidney stone myth is one of the better-known nonfacts in existence. Every medical doctor has heard of one, yet none of them has ever seen one. Vitamin C does not cause kidney problems; it prevents them (see the chapter on Kidney Disease for more information).

It's hard to believe that a vitamin can start a scientific civil war, but Pauling speaks from much experience as he discusses this in his exceptionally interesting book *How to Live Longer and Feel Better*. I urge you to read this book, along with Lendon Smith's *Clinical Guide to the Use of Vitamin C;* Hickey and Saul's *Vitamin C: The Real Story;* and Thomas Levy's *Vitamin C, Infectious Diseases, and Toxins: Curing the Incurable*.

I read them all, and then I was glad I did because I needed them myself, badly. Because I seem to have this little problem with pneumonia.

The first time I had viral pneumonia, I was sick as a dog. My wife had bronchitis at the same time. We looked so awful that my father took us both to the doctor. The doctor saw my wife first and prescribed erythromycin, an antibiotic. Then it was my turn. He gave me erythromycin, too.

"But isn't that useless against a virus?" I asked him.

"Yes. It's for the secondary bacterial infection that often follows the viral infection," he told me. "There's not much we can do about the virus except have you rest in bed."

So I did, knocked silly by codeine cough medicine. For two, perhaps three days, I was in la-la land, not knowing or caring if I ate or not, or if it was day or night. I could barely tell if I was asleep or awake. Nice vacation though it was, neither the codeine nor the erythromycin really cured the pneumonia. The body did, and it took something less than two weeks for me to recover.

The next time I got pneumonia, I did it my way (well, their way) and followed the Klenner/Pauling protocol: take enough vitamin C to get well, no matter how much it may be. This initially makes a lot more sense if you are really, really sick. Pneumonia sets that part up effectively enough.

TODAY'S GORILLA BEHAVIOR HINT

When you use weights (bar or dumbbells), tap your chest lightly with them with each repetition. This stimulates your thymus gland, located just above your heart. The thymus is part of your immune system. Is that why gorillas pound their chests? Or maybe all of this is just to impress the "gorilla my dreams." (If you didn't catch that right away, say it slowly, out loud.)

So there I was, coughing without pause with a fever of nearly 104, playing Scrabble. I literally emptied a bottle of 1,000 mg tablets onto the table, lined them up two by two, and took 2,000 mg of vitamin C every six minutes. In three hours, that amounts to 60,000 mg. And three hours is what it took to lower my fever three degrees and stop my cough completely.

Here's another true confession from my sordid past. I lived off campus as a college senior. Boy, that was fun. Four friends and I closely inhabited one third of a rented house, near the university but well out of reach of the local board of health. We demonstrated our pragmatism, our existentialism, and our sloth on a daily basis. We reduced housekeeping to its most rudimentary form. Plan A: if the dishes in the sink had more than an inch of black mold on them, it was time to clean up. Plan B: forget that, throw them out instead. Plan C: go out for pizza.

Plan C got a lot of use.

We were never sick. Sure, we were young and our immune systems were at their peak. But we were surrounded with germs, as all people are who live outside of a bubble. *This is the whole point:* we live in a world filled with pathogens, but only some of us are sick. There are survivors to every massacre. As a former teacher, I can attest that when the flu comes through school, your absence rate can instantly soar to over one-third of all students. But the other two-thirds, exposed to the same viruses, coughs, and flying phlegm of the school lunchroom, are quite well.

The classic contagious disease would be bubonic plague. The Black Death killed better than one in four Europeans during the fourteenth century. We are talking 30 million people now, plus 45 million more dead in Asia. Pretty awful. Keep in mind, though, that nearly three in four *lived through it.* How? How did the great majority of people *not* die?

It comes down to this: If your immune system is strong (and a strong vitamin-nutritional component therein is indisputable) you will be among the ones who don't get the plague. Or a cold. And if your resistance is down, there is something you can immediately do about it: promptly take vitamin C to saturation, just as those vitamin C "quacks" recommend.

Vitamin therapy is about curing the real diseases. It is not limited to prevention, and it is certainly not reducible to a few cute platitudes about better food choices. One bold example is a study released in December 1993.[1] At Johns Hopkins, 281 HIV-positive men were studied for six years. Half received vitamin supplements. The other half didn't. There were only *one-half* as many full-blown AIDS cases in the vitamin group as in the no-vitamin group. If this were a new *drug* that reduced new AIDS cases by half, it would have been front-page news.

A 2004 Harvard study[2] *also* found that vitamins slow the progression to AIDS by 50 percent. In addition, vitamin supplementation **cut AIDS deaths by an astounding 27 percent**. The authors wrote that vitamins "resulted in significantly higher CD4+ and CD8+ cell counts and significantly lower viral loads."

I'll bet that you have not seen one TV, newspaper, journal, or classroom mention of this. And for those who have died, we grieve. How much would they have liked to have known about vitamin antivirals?

References

1. Tang, AM, Graham, NM, Kirby, AJ, McCall, LD, Willett, WC, and Saah, AJ. (1993). Dietary micronutrient intake and risk of progression to acquired immunodeficiency syndrome (AIDS) in human immunodeficiency virus type 1 (HIV-1)-infected homosexual men. *Am J Epidemiol.* 138(11):937–51.

2. Fawzi, WW, Msamanga, GI, Spiegelman, D, Wei, R, Kapiga, S, Villamor E, Mwakagile, D, Mugusi F, Hertzmark, E, Essex, M, and Hunter, DJ. (2004). A randomized trial of multivitamin supplements and HIV disease progression and mortality. N Engl J Med. 351(1):23–32.

Recommended Reading

Hickey S and Saul AW. *Vitamin C: The Real Story.* Basic Health Publications, 2008.

Levy T. *Vitamin C, Infectious Diseases, and Toxins: Curing the Incurable.* Philadelphia: XLibris, 2002.

Pauling L. (1986; revised ed. 2006). *How to Live Longer and Feel Better.* Corvallis, OR: Oregon State University Press.

Smith L. *Clinical Guide to the Use of Vitamin C.* Tacoma, WA: Life Sciences Press, 1988.

"As the warden said, 'I wouldn't want them all to break out at once.'"

—CONCERNING A POSSIBLE CASE OF RASHES IN *THE BRADY BUNCH.*

"**B**ugs" get their nickname for a reason: they just bug you, and especially bug me. I have always had considerable sensitivity to mosquito bites, but the worst of all for me are fleabites. When I was about eight, we had cats with the run of the neighborhood, and consequently, fleas. My parents wisely (and considering their budget, generously) replaced our living room couch when it became infested with fleas. Flea powder didn't help. I have seen fleas tunnel right through a pile of the stuff.

And then there is poison ivy and its noxious cousins. Behind my parents house was a wild, tree-and-bushes area, and further behind that, the four tracks of the Baltimore and Ohio Railroad. It is a forgone conclusion that this became our playground of choice. It was blissfully almost free of poison ivy, but not totally. My father happened into some, somewhere, and he swelled up, itched, and I do declare, swore about it for some time.

As one of my education professors said: "All children learn every day: the question is, learn what?" I learned how to scratch, how to apply calamine lotion, and how to leave three-leaves alone. As I grew in woodsman's wisdom, running free with my friends in "our" woods, I also learned to avoid belladonna plants. The lovely, glistening, petite red berries are very toxic. The vine is no prize pig, either: a rash from contact with belladonna vines (often growing on garden fences or in shrubbery) will give you a near-poison-ivy experience. And then there is poison sumac: same problem, same itchy rash.

The good news is that they all have the same solution:

Topical Vitamin C

It's true: direct skin application of vitamin C stops the itch, swelling, and even the rash of poison ivy, belladonna, poison sumac, and other poisonous plants. Rashes from plants with alkaloid toxins are also greatly relieved with plain vinegar. When I come in from the garden or the bush, I wash off any ungloved or otherwise uncovered skin with vinegar. Cider or white or wine; doesn't matter. The acetic acid is what you want, and vinegar has it. Vinegar is more acidic than ascorbic acid vitamin C. The acidity alone therefore helps. (There is more on the internal value of vinegar in the "Honey and Cider Vinegar" chapter.)

However, independent of its acidity, vitamin C is an actual, bona-fide antitoxin. Dr. Frederick Robert Klenner, discussed earlier, and Dr. Thomas E. Levy have discussed this at length in their writings.[1–5] You can demonstrate the truth of this by applying calcium ascorbate powder (a non-acidic vitamin C) and it will also work. In fact, if the rash is especially raw, or if there is a cut or other break in the skin, calcium ascorbate is much preferred because it will not smart when applied.

References

1. Smith, LH. *Clinical guide to the use of vitamin C: The clinical experiences of Frederick R. Klenner, M.D.* Portland, OR: Life Sciences Press, 1988. Originally titled: *Vitamin C as a fundamental medicine: Abstracts of Dr. Frederick R. Klenner, M.D.'s published and unpublished work.* Reprinted 1991. The full text of this book is posted at www.seanet.com/~alexs/ascorbate/198x/smith-lh-clinical_guide_1988.htm.

2. Klenner FR. Observations on the dose of administration of ascorbic acid when employed beyond the range of a vitamin in human pathology. *J Applied Nutrition,* 1971, Winter. Vol 23, No 3 and 4, p 61–68. www.orthomed.com/klenner.htm and www.doctoryourself.com/klennerpaper.html

3. Klenner FR. Case history: The black widow spider. *Tri-State Med J,* 1957, December.

4. Klenner FR. Case history: Cure of a 4-year old child bitten by a mature Highland Moccasin with vitamin C. *Tri-State Med J,* 1954, July. The Highland Moccasin, a viper, is also known as the copperhead.

5. Levy, T. (2004). *Curing the Incurable. Vitamin C, Infectious Diseases, and Toxins.* Henderson, NV: MedFox Publishing. Earlier edition: Levy, TE. *Vitamin C, Infectious Diseases, and Toxins: Curing the Incurable.* West Greenwich, RI: Livon Books/MedFox Publishing, 2002.

Phil writes:

"Our six-year-old, Tommy, unknowingly played in a poison ivy patch, along with a friend of his. Once I knew what I was dealing with, I mixed a paste of calcium ascorbate, then gently rubbed it onto the rash and made him rest for fifteen minutes with the paste in full contact. I then slowly dissolved the paste onto his skin by misting him with distilled water. After that, I misted his skin with a solution of calcium ascorbate several times a day, while making him eat 2,000 mg an hour, to bowel tolerance.

"He was free of any evidence of poison ivy in less than three days. His buddy Sam was a mess for almost two weeks and has the scars to prove it. Sam also took some kind of steroid which didn't help him too much. Sam's mom would not heed my advice, because I'm the "vitamin quack" in our circle of friends. Needless to say, Tommy now has a poster with eighteen pictures of poison ivy so that he knows what to look for, and a dad who knows just what to do if he grabs the wrong vegetation in the woods.

"I would never have believed it if I hadn't tried it myself."

"Health is the fastest growing failing business in western civilization."
—EMANUEL CHERASKIN, M.D., D.M.D.

Kidney diseases kill 60,000 Americans a year and afflict at least 26 million more. When I wrote the first edition of this book 9 years ago, that number was 8 million. Things are not looking up. Worldwide, the annual death toll from kidney diseases is about 800,000. Dialysis and transplants are expensive, costing billions of dollars annually just in the US. To that, add the emotional and physical costs in pain.

How do your kidneys work? The answer is: constantly! Twenty-four hours a day, your two kidneys filter your blood somewhat like an aquarium filter filters the water in a fish tank. The functional unit of the kidney is the *nephron,* a tissue unit that not only filters, but also recycles and excretes. The nephron cleans the blood, maintains the body's acid-base ion balance, recycles needed substances (water, minerals), and excretes wastes in a concentrated urine. In a manner of speaking, urine is filtered blood, or more exactly, blood is filtered urine. Following are the common diseases with a kidney connection.

Diabetes and Hypertension

Diabetes and hypertension (high blood pressure) are major causes of long-term kidney problems. Each topic is discussed in a separate chapter of this book.

Inflammation and Infection

The role of massive doses of vitamin C is profound in the case of kidney infections, providing prevention and treatment at saturation levels. Since vitamin C is filtered and "wasted" through the kidneys, it is a virtually custom-made targeted therapy.

Degeneration

A chronic excess of dietary protein almost certainly taxes the kidneys and leads to gradual degeneration. Reducing protein intake helps prevent the protein-breakdown-induced nitrogenous overload that is responsible. Vegetarianism is the rational solution to this nationwide pattern of protein abuse. Increasing carbohydrates is also recommended to reduce the catabolism of proteins and prevent ketosis. Again, a regular vegetarian diet, which is high in complex carbohydrates, will assure this.

Nephrotic Syndrome (protein in the urine)

This condition results from tissue damage and impaired nephron function. Its association with collagen diseases (such as rheumatoid arthritis and lupus) is hardly accidental, for chronic deficiencies of vitamin C (and vitamin C's helpers, the bioflavonoids) cause degeneration of the walls of the kidney's blood vessels, enabling protein to escape into the urine. Capillaries, those tiniest and most numerous of all blood vessels, get leaky in the absence of ample vitamin C. Easily bleeding gums are an example of this. Easily bleeding kidneys need C.

171

Acute Renal (Kidney) Failure

Early successful management of infectious disease greatly reduces the likelihood of renal failure. Saturation with vitamin C is a very effective, broad-spectrum treatment for infectious diseases. Vitamin C stops the formation of oxalate stones, and actually dissolves phosphate and struvite kidney stones (see below). If kidney failure is suspected, don't be a martyr: see your doctor early in the game. (Remember: I favor always listening to your doctor, but not always obeying your doctor.) Even conventional nutrition texts mention (correctly) the need for supplemental vitamin C and the B complex for kidney tissue healing. Just up the doses if you want the best results.

In early renal failure, no protein should be given. Vegetable-juice fasting may work well here. If liquids are restricted, put the vegetables through a blender and eat as a salad puree. It tastes better than it sounds.

BLENDER SALAD

1 SMALL TOMATO	JUICE OF $1/2$ LEMON OR LIME
1 RED OR GREEN PEPPER	6 LEAVES ROMAINE LETTUCE
$1/2$ SMALL CUCUMBER	4 STALKS FRESH FENNEL OR CELERY

Cut up tomato, pepper, and cucumber and place in blender. Add lemon juice, and blend until smooth. Add romaine leaves one at a time, to avoid clogging the blender. Add celery or fennel; blend a minute or two longer. The consistency depends upon personal taste; some like it smooth and watery, others thick and crunchy. Eat your blender salad immediately. Crushed raw food does not keep at all.

Chronic Renal Failure

Continued deterioration means loss of vital kidney participation in the activation of vitamin D_1. The result can be osteodystrophy: calcium deficiency in the bones or poor bone formation during childhood. Supplementation with vitamin D and calcium are therefore required.

Amino acid supplements have shown promise in treating chronic renal failure, when coupled with a greatly curtailed amount of dietary protein of only 20–25 grams per day. As an advocate of vegetable juice fasting, I personally think the protein restriction may have done as much as the amino acid supplementation. Why? Because typical hospital "protein-restricted diets" provide 40 g per day of protein!

Consider this: the typical American eats over 100 g of protein per day, and frequently exceeds 120 g, which is *way* too much. So a so-called "restriction" to 40 g per day is simply a correction. Most of the world's peoples would be pleased as punch to be able to eat 40g per day of protein. But we happily chow down three times that, call it normal . . . and then line up for dialysis. The hidden cost of eating meat may ultimately be over $75,000 per year for dialysis. During dialysis, the water-soluble vitamins (B complex and C) are lost from the blood. Supplementation is *essential* and must be both high-potency and frequent.

Kidney Stones

There are five types of kidney stones:

1. *Calcium phosphate stones* are common and easily dissolve in urine acidified by vitamin C.

2. *Calcium oxalate stones* are also common but they do not dissolve in acid urine.

3. *Magnesium ammonium phosphate (struvite) stones* are much less common, often appearing after an infection. They dissolve in vitamin C-acidified urine.

4. *Uric acid stones* result from a problem metabolizing purines (the chemical base of adenine, xanthine, theobromine [in chocolate] and uric acid). They may form in a condition such as gout.

5. *Cystine stones* result from a hereditary inability to reabsorb cystine. Most children's stones are this type, and these are rare.

The very common calcium phosphate stone can only exist in a urinary tract that is not acidic. Ascorbic acid (vitamin C's most common form) acidifies the urine, thereby dissolving phosphate stones and preventing their formation.

Acidic urine will also dissolve magnesium ammonium phosphate stones, which otherwise require surgical removal. These are the same struvite stones associated with urinary tract infections. Both the infection and the stone are easily cured with vitamin C in large doses. Both are preventable with daily consumption of much-greater-than-RDA amounts of ascorbic acid. Think grams, not milligrams! A gorilla gets about 4,000 mg of vitamin C a day in its natural diet. The RDA for humans is only 60 mg. Someone is wrong, and I don't think it's the gorillas.

The common calcium oxalate stone can form in acidic urine whether one takes vitamin C or not. However, if a person gets adequate quantities of B-complex vitamins and magnesium, this type of stone does not form. Any common B-complex supplement twice daily, plus about 400 mg of magnesium, is usually adequate.

Ascorbate (the active ion in vitamin C) does increase the body's production of oxalate. Yet, in practice, vitamin C does not increase oxalate stone formation. Drs. Emanuel Cheraskin, Marshall Ringsdorf, Jr. and Emily Sisley explain in *The Vitamin C Connection* that acidic urine reduces the union of calcium and oxalate, reducing the possibility of stones. "Vitamin C in the urine tends to bind calcium and decrease its free form. This means less chance of calcium's separating out as calcium oxalate." Also, the slight diuretic effect of vitamin C reduces the static conditions necessary for stone formation in general. Fast moving rivers deposit little silt.

Furthermore, you can avoid excessive oxalates by not eating much rhubarb, spinach, or chocolate. If a person is especially prone to forming oxalate stones, they may take their vitamin C in a buffered form. Instead of ascorbic acid, they might use vitamin C as nonacidic "ascorbate." Magnesium, calcium, sodium, and potassium ascorbates are all nonacidic. Other "buffered" vitamin C preparations are usually made from ascorbic acid mixed with powdered limestone (dolomite). Linus Pauling says you can take a little sodium bicarbonate with ascorbic acid to neutralize it.

Ways for *anyone* to reduce the risk of kidney stones:

1. Maximize fluid intake, especially water. Also drink fruit and vegetable juices. Orange, grape, and carrot juices are high in citrates, which inhibit both a buildup of uric acid and also stop calcium salts from forming.

173

2. Control urine pH. Acidic urine helps prevent urinary tract infections, dissolves both phosphate and struvite stones, and will not cause oxalate stones.

3. Eat your veggies. Studies have shown that dietary oxalate is generally not a significant factor in stone formation. I would go easy on rhubarb and spinach, however.

4. Skip the soda. Stone-formers are often advised to reduce their calcium intake because most kidney stones are compounds of calcium. Sounds sensible until you think about it. Kidney stones are found in calcium-deficient people. Most Americans are already calcium-deficient (we average only about 500–600 mg of dietary calcium per day, and the RDA is 800–1,200 mg per day). Worse, excess dietary phosphorous causes calcium washout, which we can ill afford. So instead of lowering calcium intake, reduce excess dietary phosphorous by avoiding carbonated soft drinks, especially colas. Soft drinks contain excessive quantities of phosphorous in the form of phosphoric acid. This is the same acid used by dentists to etch tooth enamel before applying sealant.

5. Take a magnesium supplement of at least the RDA of about 400 mg per day. (More may be desirable in order to maintain a 1:2 balance of magnesium to calcium. Some sources even recommend a 1:1 ratio.)

6. Be certain to take a good B-complex vitamin supplement daily that contains pyridoxine (vitamin B_6). B_6-deficiency produces kidney stones in experimental animals, and deficiency is very common in humans. B_1 (thiamin) deficiency also is associated with stones.

7. Additionally, low calcium may itself *cause* calcium stones.

8. For uric acid/purine stones (gout), *stop eating meat!* Nutrition tables and textbooks indicate meats as the major dietary purine source. Naturopathic treatment adds juice fasts and eating lots of sour cherries. Increased vitamin C consumption also helps by improving the urinary excretion of uric acid. Use buffered ascorbate C.

9. Persons with cystine stones (only 1 percent of all kidney stones) should follow a low-methionine diet and use buffered C.

10. Kidney stones are associated with high sugar intake, so eat less (or no) added sugar.

11. Infections can cause conditions that favor stone formation, such as overly concentrated urine (from fever sweating, vomiting, or diarrhea). Drink plenty of water. Practice good preventive health care and it will pay you back with interest.

Recommended Reading

Carper J. Orange juice may prevent kidney stones. [syndicated column] (5 January 1994).

Cheraskin E, Ringsdorf M, and Sisley E. *The Vitamin C Connection.* New York: Harper and Row, 1983.

Hagler L and Herman R. Oxalate metabolism II. *American Journal of Clinical Nutrition* 26 (August 1973): 882–89.

Pauling L. Are kidney stones associated with vitamin C intake? *Today's Living* (September 1981).

Pauling L. Crystals in the kidney. Linus Pauling Institute *Newsletter* 1 (Spring 1981).

Pauling L. (1986; revised ed. 2006). *How to Live Longer and Feel Better.* Corvallis, OR: Oregon State University Press.

Smith LH, et al. Medical evaluation of urolithiasis. *Urological Clinics of North America* 1 (June 1974): 241–60.

Thom JA, et al. The influence of refined carbohydrate on urinary calcium excretion. *British Journal of Urology* 50 (December 1978): 459–64.

Williams SR. *Nutrition and Diet Therapy,* 6th edition, chapter 28. St. Louis, MO: Mosby, 1989.

"Never go to a doctor whose office plants have died.

—ERMA BOMBECK

Without showing any slides, photographs or home movies, I'd now like to address a very common question asked of me: "What did you do to keep your family healthy?" Over the years, people looked at my two children, raised as near-vegetarians, and wondered why they look so good. To a great extent, it is because they were raised as near-vegetarians! From what I've seen, I'm convinced that eating virtually no meat at all is a tremendous health advantage for children. Our kids were certainly the only ones in the neighborhood that had never tasted meat in any form.

When my wife and I started out with our first baby we didn't know what to do. We'd never been parents before, and we, like you, wanted only the best for our kids. For this reason we decided to raise our children from day one on as natural a diet as possible. We soon realized that this meant breast milk and vitamin supplements for the first six months or so, with the gradual addition of whole-grain cereals, mashed vegetables, fruits, and juices. We couldn't quite bring ourselves to feed dead animal muscle to an infant. Now we didn't know beyond a shadow of a doubt that this would be the best baby diet, but we'd read about it, and we had friends with exceptionally healthy, active, bright-eyed babies who were totally vegetarian. We reasoned that we could always add meat to the children's diet if they really wanted or needed it. So, we decided simply to wait until they asked. They were each about eight years old before they did so.

It is fun to be the parent of little vegetarians. I regularly took my three-year-old son with me when shopping at the local supermarket. Inevitably, we had to pass through the meat department. My son pointed to the blood-red packages and loudly asked me, "What's that Daddy?" I replied, much more quietly, "That is meat." He then said, just as loudly as before, "We don't eat meat, do we, Daddy!" He was correct, of course, and I told him so. He smiled, and in a voice that could easily be heard in the produce department on the other side of the store, declared for all to hear: "We don't eat meat! We're not Italian!"

I think he meant to say, "We're vegetarian," but I kinda like it better his way.

But another fun aspect of vegetarian children is to see how happy and healthy the little beezers are. Our children have been much healthier than most children. They missed only a day or two of school a year. We kept a close eye on their health, though, believe me. But aside from the usual colds and such, they were simply healthy. This was largely due to their natural, vitamin-supplemented, virtually meatless diet, in our opinion. What we thought would be best for them has proven in our experience to be best for them. What better evidence is there than success?

The children's good health is owed to the continued grace of God and nature. My wife also gets a lot of credit for having taken the time to feed them right, and also for taking exceptionally good care of herself during both pregnancies. She ate a small amount of meat during the first pregnancy, and less during the second as we both learned more about the benefits of vegetarianism. She also ate a lot of peanut butter, all dairy products, and fish, becoming a near-vegetarian over time. And, of course, she took her vitamins.

You know, neither of us was raised a vegetarian. As a youngster, I'd attack a hot dog or hamburger just as any other kid would. My wife and I eventually settled on what I call a "near-vegetarian" diet, meaning we avoided meat and poultry in favor of eggs and some fish, and especially cheese, yogurt, and milk. The point that I'd like to make here is that children do not specifically require meat to get their protein. I'm sure that little children should not be started on meat, and it should not be offered to older kids until they ask for it. And if your home meals are complete without meat, they're not likely to ask.

Perhaps you'd like more details on just how the children ate. Each child got a simple but balanced vegetarian diet consisting of at least two servings each, each day, of corn, beans, and squash. You will remember these as the "three sisters" of the Iroquois. Corn, beans, and squash together make up a complete protein, just like meat, only without the toxins resulting from meat metabolism. However, fear not: my kids didn't live entirely on corn, beans, and squash! They also got dairy products in many forms, especially a wide variety of easy-to-digest cultured cheeses. This was no hardship at all, for they really loved cheese.

For years, their mother baked all of our bread, which was partly but not entirely whole grain, and made with organically grown flours. The children ate peanut butter, walnuts, almonds, and other nuts (under parental supervision when they were younger), ice cream, lots of fruits, all kinds of vegetables, salads, home-baked desserts, casseroles, juices, pasta (including whole-grain macaroni and spaghetti), and really quite an array of foods. They were not finicky eaters, either, for these real foods appeal to children's appetites. Try them on your kids and see for yourself. Start early, preferably in infancy, and you too will have the distinct pleasure of seeing your daughter eat borscht, your son drink lettuce juice, *and your visits to the doctor vanish.*

Each of our children always received a quality multivitamin (liquid, chewable, or tablet, depending on age) twice each day plus extra vitamin C at each meal. As babies, they had liquid vitamin C, then chewable C's (which they loved) when they got a bit older. Before they could swallow capsules, every other day they got a few drops of vitamin E (about 50–90 IU) squeezed from a capsule onto their tongue. Believe it or not, they liked the taste of it. It's simple to do, and you can easily control the number of drops you give them. Vitamins A and D, plus the B vitamins, are all in the multivitamin. For kids, choose a multiple preparation containing a natural, chelated form of iron. You can powder a tablet between two spoons and mix it with an infant's pureed fruit. This trick works for vitamin C as well.

MULTIVITAMINS DANGEROUS?

The following purports to be a transcript of a recent meeting at the World Headquarters of Pharmaceutical Politicians, Educators, and Reporters [WHOPPER]:

"All right, all right! Please come to order, ladies and gentlemen. We know how excited you all are over the recent flood of antivitamin news coverage. But please have a seat! Thank you.

"First of all, congratulations on a job well done. We now have the public totally flummoxed about vitamins. We have persuaded the media that high doses of supplements are dangerous, and that low doses are also dangerous. We have scared the people away from taking any nutrients at all. Why, we have even sold the idea to the press that a once-daily multivitamin is dangerous. Nice work, everyone!

"Funny thing about multivitamin supplements: if you look at each individual nutrient in a multi-

176

vitamin, it is of course good for you. Thousands upon thousands of research studies confirm the body's absolute need for each and every vitamin. So, we urge people to eat a "balanced diet" to get all their various vitamins from food . . . while simultaneously convincing them that a balanced multivitamin supplement is bad! Essential vitamins from foods are good; essential vitamins from pills are not. Then, truly a stroke of marketing genius, we push processed foods devoid of vitamins, advertising day and night.

"We hardly have to spell it out, now do we? The fewer nutrients people consume, the more sick they will become. The more illness, the more drugs the public will have to take. After all, if vitamin therapy is "dangerous," what's left? Us, that's who. Our pharmaceutical plants running 24/7 can produce millions of pills a day, for pennies apiece, to retail at ten dollars per tablet. Cha-ching!

"Even better, the government will pay for it all. "National health care," as you already know, is really "national pharmaceutical insurance." The Feds will pay all right. After all, we sold them on the flu vaccine, didn't we? Even when it was shown that the vaccine was worthless at best?[1] "You can see other ways that the Feds listen to us. We have set it up so that food stamps cannot be used to buy vitamins.[2] A bag of cookies or a box of donuts, yes. But not vitamins. The ban includes supplemental vitamin D, which is widely known to prevent bone diseases in children and the elderly, and to prevent lung cancer, colon cancer, prostate cancer, breast cancer, and a dozen other cancers.[3] "Is it just me, or have you noticed how hot it is in here? Well, at any rate, you have all done one Hell of a nice job. Our Boss is proud of you."

References

1. http://orthomolecular.org/resources/omns/v04n17.shtml.

2. www.fns.usda.gov/SNAP/faqs.htm#10 section 10.

3. http://orthomolecular.org/resources/omns/v04n11.shtml and http://orthomolecular.org/resources/omns/v06n10.shtml.

177

We never used fluoridated vitamins, nor did our community have fluoridated water. Our kids have had only a very minimal number of cavities. To this day, my son has only two fillings in his mouth. Always choose vitamins that contain no saccharin, no aspartame, and no other artificial sweeteners. Look for natural flavors, and look to avoid all unnatural additives. We used multiple preparations containing iodine, plus many additional trace minerals.

That's about it, aside from the fact that our children got no brightly colored (meaning artificially colored) "foods" like Jello, and no foods containing chemicals including, but not limited to, preservatives. Why feed children paint and poisons?

When our children showed symptoms of a cold or fever, which was seldom, we didn't use medicines, because we have seen that natural methods work better. Knowing that appetites should and do decrease during illness, we switched the kids to a pretty much all-fruit diet when illness came on. Think of it as a "kiddie fast." This light, tasty, cleansing diet is very effective for reducing the severity of any illness, naturopaths believe. I would have to agree, and I follow this same plan for myself when I'm not feeling well. The all-fruit diet continues for a few meals or a few days, as long as there's a fever, or sore throat, cough, or runny nose. Remember that these are symptoms of nature's decision to rest and clean the body. A fruit diet is accepted by the children quite easily, for it is just what nature wants them to have at this time. Fruit or especially vegetable juices, their usual vitamin supplements, and lots of extra vitamin C are given throughout the illness.

We monitored sickness in the usual ways, with temperature-taking, common sense, and bed rest. *Be sure to consult your doctor for your own situation.* During a fever we didn't give milk or other dairy products. Milk and dairy products can be mucus-provoking. When kids expel a lot of mucus, fewer dairy items in the diet may be helpful. High temperature, of course, needs due attention: moderately cool baths (and immoderately high doses of vitamin C) will help lower it. As far as the baths go, Dr. Benjamin Spock in his *Baby and Child Care* standby tells exactly how to do this without aspirin or Tylenol. We ignore the drug parts of the book, and use the rest when needed. *How to Raise a Healthy Child In Spite of Your Doctor,* by Robert Mendelsohn, M.D., is radical but recommended reading for parents with a sick child. For best results, read it in advance.

When your child is sick, you will feel a lot more confident if you keep in personal touch with a knowledgeable, naturopathically oriented physician or teacher, especially at first.

Believe me, this is what I did! It's one thing to write a how-to book for other parents; it's another to have that real inner assurance that you're right when it's your own child. The confidence and experience come as you learn by doing. Make it easy on yourself and keep in contact with someone who has been through this before. Someone both supportive and knowledgeable of nature's ways of healing is best. With time you will see your own self-sufficiency, and ability to help healing, grow and grow.

Remember the Four Vs:

1. **V**egetarian diet, or as close to it as you reasonably can.

2. **V**egetable juices.

3. **V**itamin supplements.

4. **V**ery liberal quantities of knowledgeable support.

Very effective!

How effective? Aside from routine school physicals, my son had two visits to a pediatrician in his life, and both were for checkups in infancy. My daughter never even met her pediatrician. Yes, we had pediatricians. *The secret is that we never needed them.*

For Further Reading

Campbell, R, Saul, AW. *The Vitamin Cure for Children's Health Problems.* Laguna Beach, CA: Basic Health Publications, 2011.

Mendelsohn RS. *How to Raise a Healthy Child in Spite of Your Doctor.* NY: Ballantine Books, 1987.

Lactose Intolerance

"The best doctors in the world are Dr. Diet, Dr. Quiet, and Dr. Merryman."

—JONATHAN SWIFT

First of all, you probably aren't lactose intolerant, even if you've been told you are. The majority of supposedly lactose intolerant people are not, and can and do eat ice cream and small amounts of milk. A definitive medical test for lactose intolerance is the breath hydrogen assay, which you can have your doctor arrange for you. Only about one in three people initially diagnosed lactose intolerant will turn out to be truly so. I personally speculate that lactose intolerance may be mostly the result of a poor colon bacteria environment, from eating too much of the wrong foods, or even too much of the right foods.

There are several ways to proceed here. First, just avoid milk products completely. Many people simply fare better without any dairy at all. Try for a couple of months and see if you are one of them. Dr. Benjamin Spock (yes, *the* Doctor Spock) recommended against milk, even in growing children. Milks contains lactose, which is digested by the enzyme lactase. Lactase production in humans decreases after age five, and in other mammals not long after birth. A good argument for vegans, perhaps. Be sure you get enough calcium and other bone minerals from moo-less sources such as lots of fresh vegetables. Greens are a great nondairy source of calcium, and whole potatoes are surprisingly good as well. The fruit with the highest calcium content I know of is, believe it or not, the fig! Molasses and almonds are two other ways to bone up without abusing Bossy.

If you are really hooked on the white of the cow (and I confess that this includes me), try limiting yourself to yogurt, kefir, and aged cheeses. These and other cultured milk products are very digestible. Speaking as a former dairyman (I milked over one hundred head twice a day), I will say that fluid milk is perhaps the least desirable dairy product of all, and is also the most likely form to provoke a reaction.

Recommended Reading

Ramig VB. Make your own yogurt. *Mother Earth News Health, Nutrition and Fitness* 11 (1984): 26–28.

Rowell D. What acidophilus does. *Let's Live* (July 1983).

Sandine WE. Roles of bifidobacteria and lactobacilli in human health. *Contemporary Nutrition* 15 (1990).

Savaiano DA and Levitt MD. Nutritional and therapeutic aspects of fermented dairy products. *Contemporary Nutrition* 9 (June 1984).

Sehnert KW. *The Garden Within: Acidophillus-Candida Connection.* Burlingame, CA: Health World, 1989.

"Live your life so that whenever you lose, you're ahead."
—WILL ROGERS

My dad used to say that I learned to talk early and haven't shut up since. Not exactly: I've had laryngitis several times. Once, rather famously, was when I had to give a public presentation in a small Vermont town. I put the highlights of my speech on enormous cue cards, held them up to the audience, and was a hit. Perhaps success was due to the fact that old Vermonters often let you know that they didn't talk much but they thought a lot. The experience also pressed me to look into and find some simple and reliable ways to find a lost voice. Here they are:

1. Saturation, or bowel tolerance, of vitamin C will stop laryngitis in a matter of hours. If you take as much C as you can hold, as often as humanly possible, your voice will be back before your friends get to appreciate the silence. People who take megadoses of vitamin C every day preventively are unlikely to ever lose their voice in the first place. When I do weekend seminars, I am speaking for six consecutive hours on two consecutive days. I take about 3,000 mg every hour, and never lose my voice.

2. The homeopathic remedy Ferrum Phos 6X works for loss of voice due either to overstraining or simple inflammation. This remedy works best taken promptly, preferably as soon as you notice the slightest huskiness or hoarseness. A homeopathic remedy is taken until the symptoms begin to improve. Then Mother Nature takes over and your body heals itself.

3. An ounce or two of cider vinegar, straight up, will do wonders for a simple sore throat and laryngitis. When I do this, I get the impression that the vinegar is absorbed into the throat on the way down and never even reaches the stomach. If you immediately, and I mean immediately, follow the vinegar with a "chaser" of an especially sweet fruit juice, you will barely taste the vinegar at all. Be sure to rinse your mouth with water afterward, to remove any lingering acidity. If your stomach is delicate, taking a calcium supplement along with the vinegar will buffer it in the tummy.

4. Avoid dairy products. Dad liked to sing barbershop harmony. Years ago, the men's chorus director (who was also one of my favorite music teachers in elementary school, by the way) told him not to drink milk or eat ice cream before a choral concert. This cannot be just an old wives' tale, because men know of it! Try and see: leave out the dairy if you are going to give us a speech or break into song.

"Keep to moderation;
keep the end in view;
follow Nature."

—LUCAN (MARCUS ANNAEUS LUCANUS)

What a beautiful animal the angelfish is. I killed a whole tankful of them with lead, and never knew it.

As a teenager, I was really into tropical fish, successfully breeding Siamese fighting fish at age fourteen. That was a rather strange experience. The babies started to fight at a surprisingly tender age, so of course I had to isolate each one. Until I sold them, I had forty baby-food jars of fighting fish in my bedroom. But they were far from alone; I also kept a large bluegill sunfish (by himself) and an assortment of other species in several more aquariums, utterly filling up my rather small part of the house. Walking into my room was like a visit to Jacques Cousteau's rumpus room.

I always wanted to breed angelfish. I had a number of really fine angels which I moved to a private tank furnished with some beautiful plants. The plants were held down with some metal "plant weights" that I bought at the local pet shop. Aquatic plants, you see, often get uprooted and float to the surface. So when I saw the package of nice, easily bendable, made-to-order soft metal strips, I bought it.

The weights held the plants down admirably.

All the angelfish died.

It was pretty awful. It is sad to see sparkling silver angelfish swimming on their sides, upside down, writhing in their death throes, and not be able to do anything about it.

It was not until I had taken chemistry at college that I had a guess at what had happened. Those plant weights were made of lead. The lead leached into the aquarium water, and the angelfish may have died of lead poisoning.

Over the years, we have all heard about the hazards of lead. These include lead-paint ingestion by children, lead dust inhalation by miners and metalworkers, lead in solder used in plumbing, and leaded gasoline contaminating cattle pastures. We know that lead poisoning can cause severe mental retardation. Lead has been clearly linked with Alzheimer's disease.

We have been told to avoid lead in the home and to stop lead pollution of our environment. But we have not been told how to remove it from our bodies at home. No drugs are needed; vitamin C megadoses will do the job efficiently. Saturation, or bowel tolerance, doses of vitamin C will chelate lead right out of a person. (http://orthomolecular.org/resources/ omns/v03n07. shtml)

That is good news for everybody.

HAIR ANALYSIS

I am sometimes critical of hair analysis, as it is too often employed unscientifically (and for profit) by vitamin salespeople to prescribe supplements. As a rule, hair analysis is not a reliable method to determine your body's levels of nutrients. It is, however, a very good way to determine your body's levels of heavy metals. Forensic pathologists use hair analysis to measure lead, cadmium, mercury, and other toxins. A "before" and a few "after" readings can be most useful for diagnosis and also be most encouraging as they indicate improvement with vitamin C treatment.

Lead-Avoidance Checklist

Avoiding and removing lead remain the best ways to steer clear of problems with it. The good news is that environmental lead pollution is way, way down, making it one of the great hippie eco-freak contributions to world health. I was there, and saw it happen. The EPA and our much tighter environmental laws are largely 1970s products of 1960s activists.

There is still more to do, though. Here's what is directly in your power:

1. Do not use lead solder for plumbing projects. Make sure your plumber doesn't either.

2. Have lead paint and lead products taken away by your community's Hazardous Waste Disposal Unit. And you do have one; check the phone book's Government Listings, or call the EPA, toll-free, or hit their website, for help.

3. When a lead-painted room, house, or barn is repainted, have the contractor use all precautions, including collection and removal of all paint scrapings.

I grew up in a house with a lead-paint exterior. When I was a kid, my dad used barn paint on our house because it was a buck cheaper per gallon and, he believed, longer lasting than regular house paints. We had the only barn-red house in the neighborhood, and maybe even the city. Pop also made a large wood and metal star to display on our white front door at Christmas time. He painted it with the red barn paint, too. Imagine, if you will, the overall patriotic effect of a bright-red house, with a bright-red star on the door . . . during the McCarthy era. Dad (who was fortunately well known as a very American WWII veteran) finally realized the humor of the whole thing and painted a one-inch green border around the star. The house stayed red for years until Pa was making more money and finally caved in and painted it brown . . . with lead-free latex paint. So like many houses, the lead is still there, entombed under a twenty-year durable new coating. It is only a problem if disturbed by something like paint-scaping. Hence the suggestion that began this section.

4. This next idea is pretty cool: plant sunflowers. Yes, sunflowers, those giant yellow smiley-faces of the farm, will suck up lead from contaminated soil. Their roots silently clean the dirt as their huge blossoms follow the sun across the sky. I make it a policy to border house, garden, garage, and barn with sunflowers. This is all the more vital if that barn is an old one, and most wood barns are. Each autumn, after the sunflowers dry and die, be sure to throw them out in the trash, along with the lead they have soaked up. Do not burn them or compost them.

The ancient Romans used rot-proof, rustproof, cheap-to-make, easy-to-use lead pipe for their plumbing. In fact, "plumber" comes from the Latin word for lead, *plumbum,* and the chemical symbol for lead remains "Pb" to this day. When I recently visted Bath, England, I saw original Roman lead plumbing still in its original place. There is some speculation that the decline of the Roman Empire, complete with its mad emperors, violence, and general dissolution, was the result of chronic lead poisoning of drinking water and food.

Fanciful revisionism? Maybe not. Geologic cores in the arctic and elsewhere have shown that the ancient Romans polluted as much as half the world with lead many centuries ago. Smelting metal ores often drives off lead fumes, and they travel with the weather. Autopsies of the corpses of ancient Romans have revealed unusually high quantities of lead in their bodies. They, like my angelfish, never knew what made them sick. Now we know, and we know what to do to get the lead out.

Recommended Reading

Dawson EB, et al. The effect of ascorbic acid supplementation on the blood lead levels of smokers. *J Am Coll Nutr* 2 (18 April 1999):166–70.

"One-quarter of what you eat keeps you alive.
The other three-quarters keeps your doctor alive."
—ATTRIBUTED TO ANCIENT EGYPTIANS

It is just amazing how tough the human body can be sometimes. Beggars in India were found to have fewer—yes, fewer—dental cavities than well-fed persons in wealthy Western countries. Years ago, one study of 160 beggars found cavities in only two of them. The overall health of the beggars was remarkably similar to that of a comparison group of eighty medical students.

Please do not hurry to catch the next boat to Calcutta, however, just to try to stop Mother Theresa's workers from helping the destitute. The truly poor and the sick need all the help they can get. Still, there is a puzzle here. Is it what the beggars ate, or what they didn't eat, that enabled them to survive in impossible nutrition conditions?

The above study indicated that beggars ate less and were always underfed. And there we may have the answer. The medical students were perhaps overfed, but undernourished, eating more sugar and processed foods. The study also proposed that the beggars had better intestinal flora, or friendly digestive-tract bacteria, to synthesize more of certain B vitamins for them. That would figure, for beggars would receive far fewer courses of antibiotics than "properly" cared for students. At the very least, I think we are left with the suggestion that we should eat less in general, eat less sugar in particular, and eat some more yogurt.

We've tried a few impromptu nutritional experiments in our house. My son had a gerbil that ate fresh seeds, grains, nuts, and garden vegetables. We also fed the gerbil raw bean sprouts. There definitely were times when my son forgot to feed the animal at all. The sleek, shiny, and slim gerbil's name was Mister Chubb, and don't ask why from a boy who invented a dish called "dogstocket." Mister Chubb lived six and one half years. That is very, very old for an animal whose heart beats hundreds of times per minute. Oh, I do wish I'd contacted the *Guiness Book of World Records* on this one, but who would have thought to have certified the birth date of a rodent?

We've also had some rather long-lived cats, and even a catfish that is surely eligible for a pension. The cats get raw egg yolk; what the catfish eats is indescribable. Our dog gets carrot pulp left over from the juicer mixed into her dog food, and has never needed to go to the vet, except to be spayed. My wife raised an amazingly ancient parakeet. It would eat sprouts, too. (Hey, everybody in this family eats sprouts!)

There is, believe it or not, a point to all of this show-and-tell, and here it is: the common thread connecting all these domestic Methuselahs is that we systematically underfed them. I do not mean that they have been starved, but they are seldom allowed to eat their fill. All our pets are a little hungry. In nature, this seems to be the rule by necessity. With pets, and their keepers, it is a healthy rule by design: planned undereating promotes longevity. The best exercise is still to push yourself away from the table. Or the dog dish.

Scientific support for undereating for increased longevity will be found in UCLA Medical

School professor Roy Walford's book *Maximum Life Span*. Walford, a medical doctor and distinguished gerontologist, insists that we can live much longer than we'd expect, perhaps to over 120 years of age. This prediction is based on his laboratory experiments that have greatly extended the lifespan of mice, rats, and fish.

And here is the plan: you keep the animals hungry, just like we've been doing at home. Dr. Walford's research found that systematic underfeeding leads to longer lives for animals. And, he submits, it will do the same for people. He calls it "intermittent fasting." You eat every other day, or eat less every day. It's all about "undernutrition without malnutrition." Choosing nutritious foods and taking vitamin supplements are therefore essential. Dr. Walford daily supplements his diet with 1,600 mg of vitamin C and a very substantial 600 IU of vitamin E.

I am pleased that Dr. Walford has openly proclaimed that he takes megadoses of supplemental nutrients. Every medical doctor making such an admission helps patients the world over. Nobel prize winners Linus Pauling and Roger Williams both publicly advocated vitamin supplementation for decades, and both, perhaps not so coincidentally, lived into their mid-nineties.

But the real key to Dr. Walford's plan is what you don't do: eat. This whole topic becomes ever more vital as our years click by. If normal life expectancies are to be believed, my life is already more than half over. Most of us are generally going in the wrong direction: we regularly overeat. Obesity is an epidemic in the United States. And no wonder: in his book, Dr. Walford provides a map of downtown Washington, D.C., showing the locations of no fewer than sixty-four food lobbyists' offices—all within a few blocks of the White House.

The idea that the long-sought Fountain of Youth may consist simply of undereating is pretty wild. But then, think of the money you'd save. Think of the years you'd gain.

Those beggars in the India study would almost surely have been healthier with a better balanced diet and vitamin supplements. I think we all would be. But with many vitamins, the B-complex in particular, deficiencies can actually rise with unhealthy food intake. If you avoid unnecessary calories, your vitamin need can decline. This also means that if you overeat, your vitamin need is going to be higher. Unfortunately, just eating more of the standard American diet of empty calories from foodless foods does not provide healthy quantities of vitamins. Eating more of the wrong thing is no solution.

The Best Health and Longevity Bargains Ever

1. The don't-stuff-yourself vegetarian diet, or as close as you can get to it.

2. The high-potency, natural multivitamin-multimineral supplement, twice daily.

3. The use of extra vitamin C and extra vitamin E daily.

4. Eating lots of raw foods (like salads and sprouts) and fresh raw vegetable juices.

Medical and nutritional research supports this plan. So do the experiences of millions of vegetarian or near-vegetarian Americans who take vitamin supplements each day. So does our family's pet menagerie. And, I am happy to say, our kids prove it, too. Whenever I give a nutrition lecture, people listen to me but want to see my kids. So sometimes I tote them along as exhibits. I suppose I could take some pets instead, but the kids answer questions better.

MAXIMUM LIFE SPAN AND DR. ROY WALFORD

"In my own laboratory at UCLA Medical Center, we have extended the maximum life span of fish by 300 percent." This is the voice of Roy Walford, M.D., who insists that we can live longer than we expect, much longer, but it can only be done by slowing down our actual rate of biological aging. And he has a very specific prescription to do it: eat less food.

So who is this guy? Hang on; he's a real scientist, and the author of five books, one of which is *The Immunologic Theory of Aging*. Dr. Walford has been on the medical faculty of UCLA for over thirty years, and is a member of the National Academy of Sciences' Committee on Aging. He has received shelves full of awards, including the American Aging Association Research Award, the Kleemeir Award of the Geriontological Society, and the Henderson Award of the American Geriatrics Society. The doctor is an acknowledged heavyweight in the field of aging research.

Dr. Walford, while calling death the ultimate crime against consciousness, also tells us that "Sponges do not age. Nor do sea anemones." Not a lot of consciousness there, admittedly. He has tripled the life span of fish (who cares?) and greatly extended the life span of mice, rats, and some assorted microscopic critters (again, who cares?). Well, I do, for one. I at least want to know how he did it. I do have an aquarium full of moderately valuable fish.

So here is the plan: you keep the animals hungry. Dr. Walford's research found that systematic underfeeding leads to longer lives in pets.

But on the other hand, hasn't modern medical science extended our lives? Well, yes and no. Our average life expectancy has increased, but maximum life span has not. There have always been a small number of people living to 110 or so, and it is largely unchanged today. Honest documentation of old age has been historically hard to come by. The confirmed leader in modern times appears to be Fanny Thomas (no relation to Danny, a short-lived smoker). Fanny is certified to have lived to be 113, attributing her longevity to the fact that she ate applesauce three times a day and never married.

Interestingly, Walford torpedoes a common myth: It's probably not true that women age more slowly than men, because there's no difference in maximum life span between the sexes. Where lifestyles are equal, men live as long as women. So you can do what Fanny did. And maybe even if you are a man and married, perhaps, and have only a moderate passion for applesauce.

Dr. Walford provides dozens of references to back up his statements in his book, *Maximum Life Span*. I also like the map of downtown Washington, D.C., showing the locations of no fewer than sixty-four food lobbyists offices all within a few blocks of the White House.

But mostly I like Dr. Walford's utterly unapologetic attitude that death is to be beaten back for a good solid 120 years (thats about forty years longer than most people expect to live, Dr. Jack Kevorkian notwithstanding). I also like Dr. Walford's expressed appreciation for Nobel prize winners Linus Pauling and Roger J. Williams, both of whom publicly advocated vitamin supplementation for decades, and both of whom, perhaps not so coincidentally, lived into their middle nineties.

I am pleased that Dr. Walford openly proclaims that he takes megadoses of supplemental nutrients. Every medical doctor making such an admission helps patients the world over. But the real key to Dr. Walford's plan is what you don't do: eat. Aye, there's the rub, for how many people would just as soon eat now and die young than sacrifice the joys of pigging out for a mere forty extra years of existence?

Dr. Walford died in 2004 at age seventy-nine. He was two-thirds the way there. Longevity remains a work in progress. However, I know a few very elderly folks that, to me, seem to have instinctively been in line with Dr. Walford's ideas. One is ninety-three and you can hardly keep up with her. I called a friend in Vermont on her ninety-ninth birthday. She wasn't home.

Recommended Reading

Pathak CL. Nutritional adaptation to low dietary intakes of calories, proteins, vitamins and minerals in the tropics. *American Journal of Clinical Nutrition,* March–April 1958, 6:151–58.

Walford RL. *Maximum Life Span.* New York: W.W. Norton, 1983.

"Always do whatever's next."

—GEORGE CARLIN

Lizards, Bananas, Frogs . . . and Gin

My partial alma mater is the University of Ghana at Legon, a suburb of Ghana's capital, Accra. I attended graduate school there in 1974. The entrance building to the campus will always be memorable to me because the university's rather inadequate supply of toilet paper was all stored here. Hey, I tell it like it is.

Once on campus, on the grand steps there was one little tan lizard per square meter of stonework, whether vertical or horizontal. The lizards were everywhere, always sunning themselves, but hard to catch. I tried. I failed. As we walked this main thoroughfare, local children would appear seemingly out of nowhere in order to sell us fresh fruit. Until you have had tree-ripened African bananas, you do not know what "sweet" really means.

During the rainy season, nearby garden areas had rectangular pools that, in a matter of hours, filled with water. This phenomenon was promptly followed by another: thousands of enormous frogs. The frogs were not quite as big as small chickens, but close to it. At night, their incredibly loud collective croaking was ubiquitous and mind-numbing. If you wanted to have a conversation with a friend, even inside a building, you literally had to shout to be heard at arm's length.

One night in Ghana, a bunch of us just could not take the heat and humidity any more. Someone bought a bottle of really cheap gin; someone else produced some limes and enough quinine water (tonic) to fill every glass we could find. We sat in the dark, trying to hide from the mosquitoes, and had a great old time.

The particular mosquitoes we were attempting to evade carry a single-celled parasite, called a plasmodium, which causes malaria. As far as I know, my paternal grandfather, who worked on the similar-ecosystem Panama Canal, did not get it (or yellow fever either, thank heaven). Incidentally, I have his pickaxe, and I've personally been through the entire Canal. Grandpa did good work, and he lived a good long life.

However, malaria has been, and remains, one of the major killers on our planet, perhaps taking as many as 2,500,000 lives a year. A high percentage of those fatalities are children.

Does anyone know exactly how many bites from malaria-carrying mosquitoes it takes to give a person malaria? If the number varies, then why does it vary? How come many people get this severe parasitic disease, and yet most people do not, including people that live right beside them?

The World Health Organization (WHO) says, "Science still has no magic bullet for malaria and many doubt that such a single solution will ever exist." WHO recommends mosquito netting for prevention. (See www.who.int/inf-fs/en/InformationSheet01.pdf.)

While there now are a number of costly drugs used to fight malaria, drug-resistant strains of the disease have rendered them increasingly untrustworthy. I think it is significant that the conventional medical treatment of malaria still relies on the use of quinine, even after some 300 years. While heavy dosage of quinine has its side effects, in moderation it appears to have worked for me, and presumably for my grandfather. Modern antimalarial drugs also have significant, often serious, side effects. (See www.rph.wa.gov.au/labs/haem/malaria/ treatment. html.)

WHO says that "40 percent of the world's population—mostly those living in the poorest countries—is at risk for malaria," and that over 300 million people a year get the disease.

Let us explore the numbers, and therein the risk.

Our planet currently contains over 7 billion people. Forty percent of that is over two and a half billion, the number WHO says are "at risk for malaria." Of that number, over 300 million actually get the disease. If we estimate 350 million, that is an infection rate of 14 percent of people, mostly poor, who live 24/7 with lots of mosquitoes and far too little insect repellant.

If 350 million have malaria, and we accept the high estimate of two and a half million who die from it, that is a death rate of 0.7 percent of those infected. The world's people have far more to fear from war, poverty, malnutrition, poor sanitation, and cigarette smoking.

While there is no joy to be found in any mortality statistics, these suggest to me that malaria is effectively a symptom of poor living conditions and low resistance to illness in general. These are the real angles to explore in order to eliminate malaria, and for that matter, most other diseases.

Can Malaria Be Prevented with Vitamin C?

What most physicians will tell you about malaria prevention, including medication side effects, can be found at www.rph.wa.gov.au/labs/haem/malaria/prophylaxis.html.

The antibiotic doxycycline is one of the drugs used for malaria prophylaxis (www.trav doc. com/ptrav4.html). Since vitamin C has a history of successful use as an antibiotic, I speculate that daily high dosages of vitamin C may work to prevent malaria, and do so with fewer side effects. I only took 500 mg vitamin C daily when I was in the tropics nearly forty years ago. Knowing what I know now, I would take a vastly higher daily dose should I return.

"Ascorbic acid. . . when given in massive repeated doses. . . in acute infectious processes is favorably comparable to that of the sulfonamide or the mycelial antibiotics, but with the great advantage of freedom from toxic or allergic reactions" (Klenner 1953).

Yes, Vitamin C Stops Malaria

But even that 500 mg/day I took might have done the trick. Recent research has validated this hypothesis.

Researchers "measured the serum concentration of the antioxidant, ascorbic acid, in 129 patients presenting with acute falciparum malaria infection and in 65 healthy individuals (and found that) ascorbic acid plays a significant role in the pathogenesis of acute falciparum malaria in adults. Infected children also need to be given supplemental doses of ascorbate in view of the weakness of their immune system." (Hassan GI, Gregory U, and Maryam H. Serum ascorbic acid concentration in patients with acute Falciparum malaria infection: possible significance. Braz J Infect Dis., 2004 8(5):378–381.)

Note the words *"supplemental doses* of ascorbate."

What practically no physician will tell you about malaria treatment:

Garlic

No, it's not just "the smell would keep the mosquitoes away." It's biochemistry:

"In cell culture studies, sulphide compounds such as those found in garlic were active against malaria-infected human cells and against cultured melanoma cells. The compounds ajoene and dysoxysulphone may act by affecting an enzyme that allows malarial parasites to infect cells, and which is also present in malignant cells. Despite the garlic's pungent nature, these compounds deserve further study" (Crandall I, et al.[2001]. Paper at American Society of Tropical Medicine and Hygiene Meeting, Toronto. Abstract cited at www.everybody.co.nz/ nutrition/ nnoct22_01maleria.html).

Arginine

A study of African children showed those with the lowest levels of the amino acid arginine suffered most from malaria. Arginine can be given orally, which is easy and relatively inexpensive, especially for developing nations. Arginine promotes relaxation of smooth muscle and blood vessels, and promotes circulation by keeping arteries flexible. Malaria parasites secrete arginase, an enzyme that breaks down arginine (www.dgp-nvp-2002.de/abstract/ d13.htm).

The study authors wrote that "hypoargininaemia was significantly associated with cerebral malaria case-fatality" (Lopansri BK, et al. [2003]. Low plasma arginine concentrations in children with cerebral malaria and decreased nitric oxide production. *Lancet* 361[9358]:676–8).

ABC reported this news, showing a beautiful picture of a smiling, bright-eyed African child, with this caption: "One of the children in the study; although infected with malaria, high levels of arginine appear to have protected him." ABC added: "Associate Professor Nick Anstey of the Menzies School of Health Research in Darwin, Australia, one of the authors of the study, said, "We found that (low) arginine was a strong predictor of death even when other factors were taken into account" (Anna Salleh, ABC Science Online, MSNBC, Feb 21, 2003, www.abc.net.au/science/news/health/HealthRepublish_789706.htm).

There is no need to make urgent donations to relief agencies in order to buy arginine supplements for poor African children. Grains, seeds, and especially nuts are loaded with arginine. And developing countries can and do grow lots of nuts. If local, small-scale, self-sustaining agriculture is encouraged, the problem will solve itself. That is a political problem that money will not solve. People need their own land. They need to raise crops, not cattle. They need to raise peanuts, not more corn. George Washington Carver was right: eat peanuts.

Peanuts

When I was in Africa, the best dish on the table was "groundnut soup." Groundnut is another name for peanut. Having previously heard musical satirist Tom Lerher's distressing description of "peanut butter stew," I was skeptical, to say the least, about that wide, steaming bowl of brown liquid placed in front of me at the dining hall of the University of Ghana. It really was peanut soup. It sounds dreadful.

It was delicious. Try it with lots of pepper. What's that? You want the recipe? Hit the Internet and you will find many to choose from. Some use fresh peanuts, and believe it or not, some recipes actually use peanut butter.

When you buy peanut butter, select the "natural" (all peanuts, no added sugar, no added fat) variety. How do you know if nuts or nut butters are fresh? The nose knows: fresh nuts smell good; stale or rancid nuts smell "off," harsh or bitter. Only buy fresh. Smell nuts and nut products before you buy. This certainly will make you immensely popular at your local market. When you get them home, I recommend that you keep nuts and nut butters refrigerated.

As George Washington Carver demonstrated to nineteenth-century America, peanuts are versatile, tasty, vegetarian, a cheap source of protein, and they can grow in lousy soil. In third grade music class, after learning that peanuts were formerly known as "goober peas," we all delighted in belting out the chorus to the folk song of the nearly-starved Confederate Civil War soldier:

> "Peas, peas, peas, peas
> Eating goober peas;
> Goodness how delicious
> eating goober peas!"

This may all be coincidence, but when I went to West Africa, I did not get malaria prophylaxis. I did eat a ton of peanut soup. I took 500 mg of vitamin C daily. I did not get malaria. Maybe it was coincidence. Maybe it was the placebo effect. Maybe it was luck. Maybe it was all that arginine and ascorbate.

References

Klenner, FR. (1953). The use of vitamin C as an antibiotic. *Journal of Applied Nutrition* 6:274–278, and posted at www.seanet.com/~-alexs/ascorbate/195x/klenner-fr-j_appl_nutr-1953-v6-p274.htm.

McCormick, WJ. (1951). Vitamin C in the prophylaxis and therapy of infectious diseases. *Archives of Pediatrics* 68(1):1–9,and posted at www.seanet.com/~alexs/ascorbate/195x/mccormick-wj-arch_pediatrics-1951-v68-n1-p1.htm).

McCormick, WJ. (1952). Ascorbic acid as a chemotherapeutic agent. *Archives of Pediatrics* 69(4):151–155, and posted at www.sea-net.com/~alexs/ascorbate/195x/mccormick-wj-arch_pediatrics-1952-v69-n4-p151.htm.

"A smart man learns from his own mistakes.
A wise man learns from the mistakes of others."

—PROVERB

Genitalia and related peripherals aside, there are few health issues that are not men's—or women's—health issues.

Cardiovascular disease is not only the number-one killer of men; it is the number-one killer of women, too. Lung cancer is the greatest cancer killer of women, just as it is of men. Smoking is the number-one preventable health danger for women, as with men. Bad diet and vitamin malnutrition is every bit as common with women as with men. From a holistic or naturopathic point of view, the prevention and systemic treatment of breast or ovarian cancer is essentially the same as for any other cancer.

"OK, then where's the Woman's Health chapter?"

Parity check: Ladies, you are right: there is no Woman's Health Issues chapter in this book. Many health issues of special interest to women warrant their own chapters, and these topics are listed in the table of contents accordingly: endometriosis, fibroids, menopause, miscarriage, PMS, pregnancy, and lactation.

Some additional woman's health topics (UTIs, yeast infections, menstrual irregularities, postpartum depression, and osteoporosis) are discussed in my other book, *Fire Your Doctor.* Guys, that is also where you will find a chapter on prostate health. Both genders: herpes and HIV/AIDS are discussed there, too.

Additionally (and here comes the commercial) my daughter Helen Saul Case has written a book called *The Vitamin Cure for Women's Health Problems.* It is practical, fun to read, full of attitude, and full of facts. That's it: my nepotism outburst is over now. (Case, H.S. *The Vitamin Cure for Women's Health Problems.* Laguna Beach, CA: Basic Health Publications, 2012.)

But this chapter here is for males. And for the women who care for them.

The health disadvantages of being male start at conception and continue throughout the man's nearly six-year-shorter life expectancy. While women have a backup (XX) sex chromosome pair, men have an XY pair. This means there is no genetic safety net, no duplicate backup for gene defects such as hemophilia and colorblindness, and that is why it is almost always men who have these infirmities.

But this is just the beginning. Males are far more likely to be diagnosed with ADHD; far more likely to go to prison; far more likely to be victims of violent crime; far more likely to accept, and die from, a dangerous occupation; infinitely more likely to be drafted and consequently far more likely to die in service to their country. Males are more likely to be separated from their children by their job's demands if they are married, and separated from their children by the courts if they divorce. No wonder men die sooner from heart attacks, and are much more likely (at all ages) to die from suicide.

In fact, **men are more likely than women to die of the fifteen leading causes of death,** whether it be accident or disease.

Pretty grim stuff, and these and more facts fill the books of Warren Farrell, PhD. Guys, if you have not yet read *Why Men Are the Way They Are*[1] and *The Myth of Male Power*[2], you want to do so without delay. In spite of, or perhaps because of, all the statistics that Farrell presents (hundreds of references back up his statements), his books are not downers but are in fact very uplifting. He offers many insights and much practical advice, which I have personally found to be genuinely helpful. Here is reading that will make a guy feel better right away, and be a better man and a better person. This has to have real benefits for the ladies in our lives, too.

Farrell's 1999 book, *Women Can't Hear What Men Don't Say*[3] contains some notable thoughts:

• We "care more about saving whales than saving males."

• It hurts either sex less to be rejected by an object than by a person.

• "More hate for men will hurt women." Why? Men will stay away from committing to women even more. Children raised without fathers are more likely to end up in prison. Companies will fear, not respect, women, says Dr. Farrell, and, he thinks, will outsource, downsize, and avoid hiring them to avoid legal issues such as harassment.

• Men feel that they are "obligated to earn money that someone else spends while he dies sooner." This is not power. This is powerlessness. The author's father was reduced to selling Fuller brushes to support his family.

I am especially impressed with this one. In dialogue (read "arguing"), "try to criticize so the other will still be willing to listen." That is tricky, but Farrell tells you how, very specifically and step-by-step. I greatly value his advice for couples to "identify your loved one's best intent, the best spirit of her or his strongest argument, without distortion." This is masterfully effective, and you have got to try it. When we feel heard, Farrell tells us, we feel loved, understood, and secure. We can then stand valid criticism far better.

Farrell also notes that "recent studies show that even when income was the same, both the boy and the girl child did better brought up by a single dad than by a single mom" (p. 63). Statements like that cannot be taken lightly, or made lightly. Fortunately, Dr. Farrell provides hundreds of research references to support such statements. That "hundreds" figure is a number not to be taken lightly, either. Like it or not, and we shouldn't like it at all, we currently live in a male-despising society. Farrell calls for men to speak up when they are discriminated against.

Myths abound. Farrell challenges them all, taking each one down like metal ducks in a shooting gallery. Here is a really bold example: The average man, Farrell says, works five hours per week more than the average woman . . . job, commuting, and housework included. And Farrell itemizes a list of fifty-four household tasks generally done only by men (pp 100–106).

Farrell openly debunks man-bashing myths with study after study, citing feminist researchers' own statistics to show that headlines and legends alike are simply false. Talk about a second opinion!

This book makes good reading. Others of his do, too.

References

1. Farrell, W. (1986). *Why Men Are the Way They Are.* New York: McGraw-Hill.

2. Farrell, W. (1993). *The Myth of Male Power.* New York: Simon and Schuster.

3. Farrell, W. (1999). *Women Can't Hear What Men Don't Say.* New York: Tarcher/Putnam.

QUICKLY NOW: WHAT ANIMAL HAS THE WORLD'S LONGEST SPERM?

The Blue whale? The elephant? You're going to love the answer:

The fruit fly.

Yes, the fruit fly: *Drosophila bifurca,* to be specific. And each sperm is about 2.3 INCHES long, 20 times as long as the fly itself. The fly is found in Central America, Mexico, and Arizona. There's something to think about before you swat again. (Source: Fruit fly dwarfed by its sperm. *The Associated Press.* May 11, 1995, citing an article in *NATURE* of the same date by Scott Pitnick et al.)

Ménière's Syndrome and Tinnitus

"Doc, I have a ringing in my ears." "Don't answer!"

—HENNY YOUNGMAN

It shook me deeply to see my father have to crawl to the bathroom to vomit. Dad was only in his mid-fifties and was already using a cane to stand up, when he could stand at all. He had a really bad case of Ménière's syndrome, a miserable collection of symptoms including recurrent ringing in the ears, dizziness, and nausea. Perhaps it was a defining moment for me. Seeing your father reduced to helplessness is enough to make anyone want to know more about getting well. When you look this one up, the treatments you come across, whether pharmaceutical or surgical, are primarily aimed at the symptoms, because the cause of the illness is pretty much unknown.

Enter natural healing. By trial and error, I have found some drugless, scalpel-less options for Ménière's. While the solutions may shed some light on the cause, I, like you, am interested in results.

Chiropractic or osteopathic adjustment of the upper cervical (neck) vertebrae is worth trying.

Some twenty years ago, I met a young man so dizzy that he could not read or even watch TV without having to lie down. Ménière's, aptly described in the *Merck Manual* as "prostrating," certainly is capable of flooring a person. Such was the case with Lowell, a college dropout. He had a gentle but persistent series of chiropractic manipulations that restored his life. He was able to read again, to return to school, and to live again. How so? The practitioner discovered that his two top neck vertebrae, the atlas and the axis, were practically at right angles to each other, and to the skull as well. This seemingly impossible state of affairs turned out to be due to a summer job Lowell had a few years before: he was a sparring partner for boxers in training. He had almost literally had his block knocked off.

Pa refused to go to a chiropractor until his Ménière's was so bad he could not take it any more. He'd been on various ineffective medications from various ineffective physicians, none of whom gave chiropractic the time of day. But I managed to get him to a D.C. for a visit or two. Pa said it did not help one bit.

He then began taking vitamins, notably the B complex in fairly high doses. Pa had no praise for that, either. But over a period of months, his specialist-diagnosed Ménière's went away.

I had persistent suspicions that the natural approach helped him.

Since then, I have come across references showing that niacin has been used for Ménière's syndrome since the 1940s. In long-term therapy, improvement has been obtained with only 150–250 mg daily. This may explain why Pa's improvement was so gradual, yet in the end, profound.

I think that Ménière's syndrome, and perhaps a number of other difficult-to-tag neurological problems, could be a manifestation of untreated, long-term **B_{12} deficiency**. I discuss this, and what to do about it, in the chapter "Nasal Administration of Vitamin B_{12}."

The late Lendon Smith's newsletter *The Facts* mentions that **aspartame** ("Nutrasweet") may "trigger or mimic" a Ménière's attack. Dr. Smith specifically lists nausea, vertigo, hearing loss, and tinnitus as symptoms that say, "Stop using aspartame."

A **low-fat, low-sodium, no alcohol, and especially** *no sugar* **diet** may help a wide variety of illnesses. Ménière's seems to be closely connected with chronic low blood sugar, sometimes diagnosed as hypoglycemia or type 2 diabetes. Caffeine may aggravate the condition, as might manganese deficiency.

Zinc supplementation and moderate additional amounts of B_6 (pyridoxine) are also worth a several-month therapeutic trial.

For uncomplicated simple ringing in the ears, dizziness, or nausea, a 6X potency of **Kali Phos** (a homeopathic remedy) may be surprisingly helpful. I have personally used this remedy for thirty years, as I have a motion-sickness problem that my flight instructor insists he's never seen topped. If it were not for Kali Phos, not only would I not have passed my flight test, I think I would have thrown up right in the FAA examiner's lap over the Batavia, NY, airport.

My Dad, fully recovered from Ménière's, walked four miles a day for the rest of his life. His dizziness and nausea were gone for good. His sense of humor was not, however. If you ever asked my father how his hearing was, he'd invariably shout back at you, "WHAT?" But he did it smiling, and standing up straight.

"There's nothing wrong with you that an expensive operation can't prolong."

—MONTY PYTHON

Menopause has been medicalized into a disease. It is not. Just as menarche (the start of menstruation) is a natural process, so is its cessation also a natural process. The symptoms we associate with menopause still need to be addressed, of course, but perhaps from a slightly different angle.

It is interesting that the medical profession, which is set against treating vitamin deficiency with vitamin supplements, has no difficulty treating hormonal deficiency with hormonal supplements, even though estrogen supplementation carries a known cancer risk.

I do not think estrogen/progesterone supplements or creams are a good idea. The body's hormonal system is a beautifully (if delicately) balanced one, and not to be messed with. If you gave me a new Porsche, and I went under the hood with a wrench, I could only do harm. The same with your endocrine system.

On the other hand, frequent oil changes, good gas, safe driving, and lots of preventive maintenance can really prolong the life and beauty of a car—or a woman. Such a systemic approach is best done through nutrition. Here are some helpful suggestions collected by a guy who has, at least so far, only experienced menopause secondhand.

Hot Flashes: vitamin E, 800 IU daily, may help, as may a supplement of primrose oil.

Constipation: vegetable juicing is the world's best cure for this.

Dizziness, Headache: chiropractic or Kali Phos 6X (see chapter on Ménière's syndrome)

Heart Palpitation: magnesium (400–600 mg) and calcium (800 mg), especially as orotate or aspartate. The citrate form is okay.

Difficult Breathing: all of the above, and perhaps some homeopathic Aconite 6X.

Depression: lecithin (several tablespoons), plus Niacin and Vitamin C (see "Dr. Saul's Super Remedy").

Vaginal Dryness: vitamin E topically. The natural form is best. Also drink more water.

Hypoglycemia: B-complex supplement, with each meal and between each meal. Be sure to increase your dietary fiber. Eat no sugar, little dairy, little meat, lots of raw veggies, cooked rice and beans, and whole grains.

Adrenal Support: vitamin C, and plenty of it (see "Saul's Super Remedy").

Stress Reduction: Meditation, yoga, and similar techniques (see my Stress Reduction chapter).

Recommended Reading

Case, HS. *The Vitamin Cure for Women's Health Problems*, Laguna Beach, CA: Basic Health Publications, 2012.

Multiple Chemical Sensitivity

"If man made it, don't eat it."

—JACK LALANNE

It was midsummer and Rhonda had gloves on. "I have to wear gloves whenever I read," she explained. "The problem is, I'm a librarian."

A librarian with multiple chemical sensitivity; talk about a handicap.

"Newsprint is especially bad. The ink on the paper gives me rashes. Even the smell of an open book sets me off gasping, in hives, with a sore throat. And I can't wear gloves for the odors," she added. "And then there's the air conditioning; the smell of the carpet and cleaners; the water from the water fountain that I can't drink; foods in the cafeteria that I can't eat; the unending weakness and fatigue; the depression about it all. What can I do? Aside from live in a bubble, I mean."

Rhonda, a prematurely gray woman in her forties, had been unhappily coping for years. She did indeed wear gloves at work. She'd probably have worn a respirator if they'd let her. She was a mess and, of the very few doctors willing to consider her plight, none had helped her.

Multiple chemical sensitivity (MCS) probably affects millions of Americans, but the medical profession is not doing any counting. MCS has been pretty much rejected as a legitimate illness. That's because "It may be the only ailment in existence in which the patient defines both the cause and the manifestations of his own condition." (Gots, RE. [1995]. Multiple chemical sensitivities: public policy [Editorial]. *J Toxicol Clin Toxicol* 33:111–113.)

Orthodox medicine generally regards people with MCS as sensitive, all right: sensitive in their heads. The stress, anxiety, and depression that doctors equate with MCS may all be results of MCS. Certainly Rhonda fit the description.

But this was not all in her head. It was in her whole body. You had only to look at her, or listen, to appreciate her misery. She was able to function, but only with the greatest of daily efforts.

It shouldn't have to be that hard. And, I do not think it has to be. But then, I am not a physician.

So let's ask some.

At their website, accessed June 2012, the American Academy of Family Physicians (AAFP) offers polite, lukewarm compassion, but essentially still regards MCS as a nonentity. (Multiple chemical sensitivity syndrome. Magill, MK and Suruda, A. [1998] American Family Physician, Sept 1, 1998. http://www.aafp.org/afp/1998/0901/p721.html)

As evidence, the AAFP refers to statements such as this one by the American Medical Association (AMA) in 1992:

"No evidence based on well-controlled clinical trials is available that supports a cause-and-effect relationship between exposure to very low levels of substances and the myriad symptoms reported by clinical ecologists to result from such exposure."

The American Academy of Allergy and Immunology made a similar statement in 1986, and the American College of Physicians likewise in 1989.

But the American College of Occupational and Environmental Medicine's 1993 statement must really irk MCS suffers: "The science is indeterminate about MCS as a specific entity and the cause and effect relationships have not been clearly established."

The U.S. Environmental Protection Agency (http://www.epa.gov/iaq/pubs/hpguide.html #faq1, accessed June 2012) states that "claimed or suspected MCS complaints should not be dismissed as psychogenic, and a thorough workup is essential."

Interestingly enough, according to a 1995 statement by Sheila Bastien, Ph.D., a neuropsychologist who has served on the environmental illness advisory panels for the State of California and the U.S. Agency for Toxic Substances and Disease Registry (ATSDR): "In 1988 workers of the EPA headquarters became ill when new carpets were installed and other remodeling took place. Some of the employees developed MCS. Some of these employees are still working at home, and many of them still have MCS or continuing illness. Some have not been able to go back to work." (www.california.com/~hawk/MCS-Ammunition.htm.)

You have to love the irony there, don't you?

Actually, the American Academy of Family Physicians' website is probably the most supportive "official" medical website an MCS sufferer will come across. For instance, it lists some thirty common chemical exposures from air fresheners and asphalt to tile cleaners and varnish, all of which may "precipitate" MCS symptoms. But then, AAFP goes so far as to advise alleged MCS sufferers to avoid "unproven therapies" including "rotating diets" and "extreme avoidance of chemicals." In my opinion, behind this one may sense unwritten industry-friendly assumptions that chemicals are our friends, whether in your food or in your environment.

Does AAFP share mottoes with Alfred E. Newman? Chemicals? What, we worry? "Don't worry; be happy" was a popular hit song. Adorable. But "Strength through joy" was the motto of the Nazis, the least environmentally conscious administration imaginable.

I do not think anxiety or depression causes MCS; MCS may certainly cause anxiety or depression. Either way, I am quite certain that "putting on a happy face" is not the cure.

Instead, I suggest that you look at ducks.

Ducks don't get wet. They don't, you know, even though they wade and swim and dive in water. Sure, the duck's feathers will feel wet to the touch. But that's not the real ducky part. The duck's skin and body stay nice and dry. When they preen themselves, ducks keep their feathers oiled, and the oily feathers trap a layer of insulating air between them and the duck's skin. This also serves to keep the duck warm, even during their extended swims in *Titanic*-temperature freezing waters that would kill humans from hypothermia in a matter of minutes. Winter after winter, I've watched pairs of mallards happily paddling around in the not-quite-completely-frozen waters of the Erie Canal that flow near my home in upstate New York.

The duck can't change its environment, so it fortifies itself against it. Whether it is fur on a polar bear or blubber on a walrus, animals are remarkably tolerant of their surroundings. I mean, what choice have they?

In my opinion, people with multiple chemical sensitivity have no practical choice, either. Certainly, reducing environmental pollution and one's exposure to known irritants has my complete support. But we live in a strikingly imperfect world, not in a bubble, and that is the way it is likely to stay until we make our governments change it. We, like ducks, do well when we strengthen our personal defenses against a hostile environment.

I am no friend of the toxic chemical industry, as those who have been following my involvement with the battle against the Diaz Chemical Corporation will instantly bear witness to. (See www.doctoryourself.com/diaz.html; scroll down the page for the background information on this issue. Incidentally, I was sued for libel by the chemical company; they dropped the case as soon as it got to a judge. Then the Feds went after them.)

But I digress.

My take on multiple chemical sensitivity is, in essence, not of chemical isolation but of nutritional insulation. Until we have cleaned up the world, you had better toughen up your body. Here's a fast-working approach that is worth a fair therapeutic trial: saturation of vitamin C.

At least that's what Rhonda did. She was in a real hurry to feel better, and got to bowel-tolerance saturation in a day. In fact, in a single morning. After taking nearly 50,000 mg of vitamin C in the hours before noon, she left the library and went out for a lunchtime walk. Saturation hit at that very moment. Into a nearby restroom . . .

Look, my job is to tell you what works. Why does mega-C dosing work? Several reasons come to mind.

One: Vitamin C is an antitoxin.

Two: Vitamin C is an antihistamine.

Three: Vitamin C is an antidepressant.

After this episode, Rhonda was a new woman.

"The very moment I reached bowel tolerance of vitamin C," Rhonda told me afterward, "I had a rush of energy and a huge upswing in my mood. It was as if I'd turned on a light in a dark room. It was amazing, truly like night and day."

You should have heard her "new Rhonda" voice. It was light and bubbly and filled with vitality. The woman was a changed person. She had drive. She had confidence. Most of all, she had bare hands.

"Nuts to the gloves," Rhonda said. "From now on, I'm taking my C, and plenty of it."

"The history of medicine is full of ideas and treatments which are acceptable today but which were rejected out of hand for 40 years and more."

—ABRAM HOFFER, M.D.

Americans generally do what their doctor tells them without many questions. I suggest they question their doctor extensively, listen attentively, and not necessarily do what the doctor says. Then hit the books for a really different second opinion. Here is an example why:

Miseries of Misdiagnosis

Jane was twenty-four and had always been in good overall health. She was lactose intolerant, or at least sensitive enough to dairy products that she didn't eat them. She had a two-year-old running around and had just had her second baby. And she was terrified.

"I was told I have MS," she said. Imagine hearing that, at her age, with two babies no less. "I've been having numbness in some of my fingers. My muscles will twitch and I get these weird feelings in my face. My GP told me that it might just be a calcium deficiency, since I don't eat dairy products and have carried and nursed two children. So he gave me a calcium supplement to take."

"And?" I asked.

"It didn't seem to help, so he sent me to a neurologist. The neurologist heard the symptoms and then and there said that I have multiple sclerosis."

I could see her eyes reddening and some tears forming.

"What am I going to do? What will happen to my kids? Can you do anything for me?" she said.

Now there's three good questions. I wasn't sure about any of them, but like a good one-trick pony, I began with what I always say.

"It can't hurt to take a look and see," I said. "Now what about that calcium supplement? How much are you taking?"

"About 1,000 milligrams a day," she answered. "I have the bottle with me."

That amount is close to the RDA, and actually exceeds it if you allow for some calcium in her foods. It was time to open my paisley bag, so to speak, and try to overturn Murphy's Law. I read the entire label.

"OK, how many of these tablets do you take each day?" I asked.

"Three," Jane said.

"Well, to begin with, the label says that it takes six tablets to make 1,200 milligrams. You are getting 600 milligrams."

"Mmm," she said.

"On top of that, you'd think that each tablet therefore supplies 200 milligrams of calcium but it doesn't. This is a calcium chelate, which is a good form to take all right, but in this instance they weighed the entire compound, not just the calcium it gives you. That's sort of like weighing the corn, the water, and the can. We want just the net weight. It is called the weight of elemental calcium in this case. That's only about a quarter of the label claim."

"Isn't that misleading people?" she wondered.

"Perhaps, but the consumer always has to read *all* the label, especially the side part with the smaller numbers. This section, right here," I said, pointing it out on the bottle. "You can't just go by the front label. It's the same with anything you buy: a car, a service contract, Twinkies; you have to read the fine print."

"So I need more," she said.

"Maybe, yes. And there is little harm, if any, in trying more. Nobody dies of calcium overdose."

"What about stones: gallstones, kidney stones, like that?" she asked. "Gallstones are cholesterol stones and have nothing to do with calcium. Kidney stones are caused by a deficiency of calcium, not an excess. Most nutrition texts still get that one wrong, but they'll come around eventually. Excess calcium is simply not absorbed. And you are certainly not getting an excess."

"How much was I getting?" she said.

"Let's see: each tablet provided about 50 milligrams of actual elemental calcium, and you were taking three. A hundred and fifty milligrams; not nearly enough to make a difference. You'd probably want to try a whole lot more, and this will sound kind of silly. With these tablets, we're talking around twenty."

"A day?" she exclaimed. "Twenty calcium tablets a day?

"Well, yes. That would give you about 1,000 milligrams, plus what you might pick up in your diet from green leafy vegetables, beans, tofu, sardine bones, whatever. That's not even a megadose. Several thousand milligrams of calcium have been given, and very safely too, in some studies. The biggest side effect of three thousand milligrams a day appears to be less colon cancer."

"Less colon cancer? That's not much of a problem," she said.

"You will also want to divide the dose. Your body absorbs calcium passively, and can't take in much at any one time. Take it all throughout the day, as often as humanly possible. It's a nuisance, I know, but you'll get more for your money."

So off she went, with equal parts hope and skepticism.

A little over two weeks later I heard from Jane again.

"They're gone!" she said. "My symptoms are gone!" What a happy voice on the phone that was, let me tell you. "The neurologist was wrong: it wasn't MS. at all!"

I tactfully kept my thoughts to myself: *What an ignoramus that "specialist" was, who had to be so fast with the big diagnosis.* Even if a patient clearly did have MS, you'd want to break the news a whole lot more gently than he did. But he never did any tests. The GP was smarter: he at least considered the less spectacular, less traumatic, and more likely possibility that her diet had something to do with it. His only mistake was not having sufficient nutrition experience to know how to tailor the dose to deliver the calcium Jane's body was really demanding.

No one is saying that multiple sclerosis is just a form of calcium deficiency, although the connection has been demonstrated.[11] This was an illustration of poor diagnosis, scaring the patient needlessly, and not using Dr. Roger J. Williams's precept "When in doubt, use nutrition first."

So what if someone, for sure, has multiple sclerosis? The answer, and it is a remarkably good answer, is to follow the MS protocol of Frederick Klenner, M.D., as described in *Clinical Guide to the Use of Vitamin C,* edited by Lendon Smith, M.D. Far from just considering vitamin C, this book urges and lists a comprehensive therapeutic program using a large variety of nutrients in significant quantity. Here are Dr. Klenner's most important nutrient recommendations for

MS (which also apply to myasthenia gravis, a disease involving the neuromuscular junction), all of which should be divided up throughout the day:

- Vitamin B_1 (thiamin): 1,500–4,000 mg per day, orally and by injection

- Vitamin B_2 (riboflavin): 250–1,000 mg per day

- Vitamin B_3 (niacin): 500 mg up to many thousands of milligrams daily, enough to deliberately cause repeated episodes of warm-feeling vasodilation ("flushing")

- Vitamin B_6 (pyridoxine): 300–800 mg per day

- Vitamin B_{12} (cobalamin): 1,000 mcg three times a week by injection

- Vitamin C (ascorbic acid): 10,000–20,000 mg per day

- Vitamin E (d-alpha-tocopherol): 800–1,600 IU per day

- Choline: 1,000–2,000 mg per day

- Magnesium: 300–1,200 mg per day

- Zinc: 60 mg per day

- Calcium, lecithin, folic acid, linoleic and linolenic acids, and a daily multivitamin-multimineral tablet supplement are also recommended.

A Claim Too Far?

"Arrest or reverse multiple sclerosis with nutrition? With megadoses of vitamins? That is just a bit too much!"

203

No, it is actually a time-honored and well-tested therapy. Vitamin therapy for MS goes back at least eighty years to when the *Archives of Pathology* published a paper indicating that MS was caused by an inadequate intake of B-vitamins.[1]

Then in 1940, niacin and thiamine were employed to treat MS.

Not long after that, Canadian physician H. T. Mount began treating multiple sclerosis patients with intravenous B_1 (thiamine) plus intramuscular liver extract, which provides other B-vitamins. He followed the progress of these patients for up to twenty-seven years. The results were excellent and were described in a paper published in the *Canadian Medical Association Journal* in 1973.[3]

Frederick Robert Klenner, M.D., of North Carolina, mentioned above, published "Treating Multiple Sclerosis Nutritionally" in *Cancer Control Journal* 2:3, pp. 16–20. His complete treatment program is now posted for all interested persons to read at www.tldp.com/issue/ 11_00/ klenner.htm and www.townsendletter.com/Klenner/KlennerProtocol_forMS.pdf.

Drs. Mount and Klenner were persuaded by their clinical observations that multiple sclerosis, myasthenia gravis, and many other neurological disorders were primarily due to nerve cells being starved of nutrients. Each physician tested this theory by giving his patients large, orthomolecular quantities of nutrients. Mount's and Klenner's successful cures over decades of medical practice proved their theory was correct. B-complex vitamins, including thiamine as well as niacinamide, are absolutely vital for nerve cell health. Where pathology already exists, unusually large quantities of vitamins are needed to repair damaged nerve cells.

"Let's See Some *Recent* Studies."

Okay. New research confirms that niacinamide, also known as vitamin B_3, is a key to the successful treatment of multiple sclerosis and other nerve diseases.[7] Niacinamide, say researchers at Harvard Medical School, "profoundly prevents the degeneration of demyelinated axons and improves the behavioral deficits." Other research indicates that NAD (nicotinamide adenine dinucleotide), produced by the body from the vitamin niacin, can arrest and reverse MS.[8–11]

Research indicating that vitamin D fights multiple sclerosis was first published over twenty-five years ago.[12] In recent years, the evidence is literally piling up.[13–17]

It is time to apply it.

References

1. Zimmerman HH, and Burack F. Lesions of the nervous system resulting from a deficiency of the vitamin B complex. *Arch Pathology,* 1932, 13:207.

2. Moore MT. Treatment of multiple sclerosis with nicotinic acid and vitamin B-1. *Archives Int Med,* 1940, 65:18.

3. Mount HT. Multiple sclerosis and other demyelinating diseases. *Can Med Assoc J.,* 1973, 108(11):1356–1358.

4. Klenner FR. Response of peripheral and central nerve pathology to mega-doses of the vitamin B-complex and other metabolites. Parts 1 and 2. *J Applied Nutrition,* 1973, 25:16–40. Free full-text download at www.townsendletter.com/Klenner/KlennerProtocol_forMS.pdf or www.tldp.com/issue/11_00/klenner.htm.

5. Klenner, FR. Treating multiple sclerosis nutritionally. *Cancer Control J,* undated(ca. 1970), 2(3):16–20. And, a similar, comprehensive MS/MG protocol is to be found in Smith's *Clinical Guide to the Use of Vitamin C: The Clinical Experiences of Frederick R. Klenner, M.D.* (reference below).

6. Smith, LH. *Clinical guide to the use of vitamin C: The clinical experiences of Frederick R. Klenner, M.D.* Portland, OR: Life Sciences Press, 1988. Originally titled: *Vitamin C as a fundamental medicine: Abstracts of Dr. Frederick R. Klenner, M.D.'s published and unpublished work.* Reprinted 1991. The full text of this book is posted at www.seanet.com/~alexs/ascorbate/198x/smith-lh-clinical_guide_1988.htm. It includes a multiple sclerosis protocol, which takes up about five pages. It discusses orthomolecular therapy with all vitamins, not just vitamin C. See also: www.doctoryourself.com/klennerpaper.html.

7. Kaneko S, Wang J, Kaneko M, Yiu G, Hurrell JM, Chitnis T, Khoury SJ, and He Z. Protecting axonal degeneration by increasing nicotinamide adenine dinucleotide levels in experimental autoimmune encephalomyelitis models. *J Neurosci.,* 2006 26(38):9794–804. www.ncbi.nlm.nih.gov/entrez/query.fcgi?CMD=search&DB=pubmed.

8. Penberthy WT. Nicotinic Acid-Mediated Activation of Both Membrane and Nuclear Receptors towards Therapeutic Glucocorticoid Mimetics for Treating Multiple Sclerosis.

PPAR Res., 2009, 2009:853707.

9. Penberthy WT, Tsunoda I. The importance of NAD in multiple sclerosis. *Curr Pharm Des.,* 2009, 15(1):64–99. Review.

10. Penberthy WT. Nicotinamide adenine dinucleotide biology and disease. *Curr Pharm Des.,* 2009, 15(1):1–2.

11. Penberthy WT. Pharmacological targeting of IDO-mediated tolerance for treating autoimmune disease. *Curr Drug Metab.,* 2007, 8(3):245–66. Review.

12. P. Goldberg, M.C. Fleming, E.H. Picard. Multiple sclerosis: Decreased relapse rate through dietary supplementation with calcium, magnesium and vitamin D. *Medical Hypotheses,* 1986, 21(2): 193–200. http://www.direct-ms.org/pdf/VitDMS/Goldberg%20Medical%20Hypoth%20Vit%20D.pdf

13. Hanwell HE, and Banwell B. Assessment of evidence for a protective role of vitamin D in multiple sclerosis. *Biochim Biophys Acta.,* 2011, 1812(2):202–12.

14. Solomon AJ. Multiple sclerosis and vitamin D. *Neurology,* 2011, 77(17):e99–e100.

15. Holick MF. Vitamin D deficiency. *N Engl J Med.,* 2007, 357(3):266–81.

16. Colleen E. Hayes, Margherita T. Cantorna and Hector F. DeLuca. Vitamin D and multiple sclerosis. *Exp Biol Med,* 1997, 216(1): 21–27.

17. Hayes CE. Vitamin D: a natural inhibitor of multiple sclerosis. Proceedings of the Nutrition Society (2000), 59: 531–535.

Why a large *variety* of nutrients? Because there is no such thing as monotherapy with nutrition. People often ask me, "What is this vitamin good for?" My answer is, "Everything." They give me the look, but it's true nevertheless. All vitamins are important. Which wheel on your car can you do without? Which wing on an airplane can you afford to leave behind?

Why large *quantities* of nutrients? Because that's what does the job. You don't take the amount that you think should work; you take the amount that gets results. The first rule of building a brick wall is that you have got to have enough bricks. A sick body has exaggeratedly high needs for many vitamins. You can either meet that need, or whine about why you didn't.

But why try to cure with nutrition? Well, why not? Must a cure be medical for it to be any good? There is no medical cure for MS; if there were, you would have heard about it. I say, if one doctor's black bag is empty it does not necessarily follow that all other doctors' black bags are. Go where you can get the outcome you need. The first rule of fishing is to put your hook in the water, for that is where the fish are.

Let's consider just one lone nutrient, thiamin, and one oddball disease, beriberi. Beriberi has been a problem for centuries in impoverished countries. It is a disease of the peripheral nervous system. Beriberi, the very description of nutritional exhaustion, literally means "I can't, I can't." It results in pain and paralysis, swelling and anemia, decreased liver function and wasting away. Note, please, the wide variety of symptoms.

No drug on earth, then or now, can cure it. For centuries, the question has been: what exactly causes it? In 1897, Dr. Christian Eijkman first cured beriberi. He had previously observed that many prisoners had the disease. They were fed a diet primarily of polished (white) rice, the stuff Americans eat to this day. Eijkman fed the prison diet to pigeons and watched the same beriberi symptoms emerge. He then fed the sick pigeons unmilled (brown) rice. The birds were cured. He tried whole brown rice on the prisoners, and they were cured. Completely. No drug had done that; it took brown rice, and something special in that unprocessed rice. Eijkman later received the Nobel prize for this work.

In 1911, Casmir Funk, a Polish chemist living in London, would discover that special something in the outer, usually wasted rice hulls. Because it was a nitrogen compound, he labeled it an amine. Because it was vital to health, it was a vital amine, or vitamine, or vitamin. The name stuck and became generic, like Kleenex. (Incidentally, "vitamine" is the English and Australian pronunciation to this day.)

Between 1909 and 1916, the Philippines-based American R. R. Williams began curing beriberi in young children with outstanding success. The rice polishings he used were thereafter called vitamin B (for beriberi?) and thought to provide a single essential chemical. Today known to be a team of vitamins, the B complex (as well as vitamin C) are all water-soluble, indispensable, and generally not stored by the body.

Thiamin proved to be the cure, and the only cure, for beriberi. It is designated vitamin B_1. (One of its parts is a *thia*zole ring, and it is a vita*min,* hence the name.) Thiamin helps form a coenzyme needed in glucose oxidation to either get energy from glucose or to produce fat (which is called lipogenesis). Without thiamin, these do not occur. At all. Hence, the fatigue and wasting away of beriberi. The mineral magnesium is another essential factor in this process.

Thiamin is not stored in tissues. You need it every moment of every day, and it plays a crucial role in carbohydrate metabolism, pregnancy, lactation, and muscular activity. Less well known is that more thiamin is needed by the body's tissues during fevers.

205

A long-standing inadequate thiamin supply may cause severe neurological effects, most significantly nerve irritation, diminished reflex response, prickly or deadening sensations, pain, damage to or degeneration of myelin sheaths (the fatty nerve cell insulation material), and ultimately paralysis. Dr. Klenner, aware that this could well describe multiple sclerosis, went to work trying megadoses of thiamin. On the principle that it takes a lot of water to put out a well-established fire, Klenner ignored the RDA of 1 to 2 mg per day and gave MS sufferers thousands of milligrams of thiamin per day. He administered other vitamin megadoses as well. Patients improved.

So when you inform your physician that Frederick Robert Klenner, M.D., was curing multiple sclerosis back in the 1950s and '60's, you will not be easily believed. And who in their right mind would? An MS patient in a wheelchair, perhaps. Like the one who was wheeled into my office one day by his private R.N.

I shared the details of Dr. Klenner's protocol with them. They went home and did it. It worked. In little over two weeks, the man was out of his wheelchair, walking with a walker or cane. It was beautiful to see. Why did it work? Because Dr. Klenner's experience in treating MS taught him to understand it as a vitamin deficiency disease.

Not only is Lendon Smith's *Clinical Guide to the Use of Vitamin C* available without a prescription, it is available online without charge. For readers who have long been hunting for copies of this amazingly valuable 68-page book, their wishes have been answered. It is posted in its entirety at www.seanet.com/~alexs/ascorbate/198x/smith-lh-clinical_guide_1988.htm. The multiple sclerosis protocol takes up about five pages. An Internet search may locate it online elsewhere as well.

Additionally, an important, dosage-specific paper by Dr. Klenner on the nutritional treatment of neurological diseases is posted at www.tldp.com/issue/11_00/klenner.htm. Similar information is also included in Dr. Klenner's megavitamin protocol for MS, published in "Treating Multiple Sclerosis Nutritionally," *Cancer Control Journal* 2(3):16–20.

I've just given you your first semester's education in heresy. People embrace health heresies not because they are stupid, but because nothing else worked, and counterculture healing often does. And, despite the huge shadow of monopolistic medicine, we still live in a more or less free-market economy. This is America, and you have the right to remain sick. Or not.

That book again? *Clinical Guide to the Use of Vitamin C.*

"Two maggots were fighting in dead Ernest."
—CHEAPER BY THE DOZEN

When I reflect back on the bugs, worms, pond snails, bullheads, dead frogs, desiccated fox carcasses, and other carrion that we handled as children, I am amazed that any of us made it to adulthood. One of our self-appointed youth projects was the rescue and rehabilitation of wounded and sick animals, and we specialized in pigeons. We routinely found them, bleeding, flapping and helpless, mired in mud and their own droppings, under a nearby railroad overpass. Parents, think before you give your kid a BB gun.

The common pigeon has been called the "feathered rat" because of the lice and other undesirables that it is known to carry. But to us, filthy or not, they were beautiful, iridescent birds that needed a home. When they were inevitably evicted from my parents' garage, the pigeons ended up convalescing in our treehouse. I would like to tell you that we all donned masks, gowns, and gloves when we handled them, but we did not. Pigeons perched on our fingers. We hand-fed them bread and graham crackers. They ate our lunches with us. Their droppings surrounded us. I doubt if we even washed our hands half of the time. My great-grandmother often said, "You have to eat a peck of dirt before you die." She almost certainly meant this metaphorically, but we took it pretty much literally.

Foolish or not, we had no fear of parasites, seen or unseen.

Years later, as a masters student, I studied the common dog tapeworm, *dipylidium caninum*. It is rather odd to learn that you can literally eat this tapeworm, or its eggs, and you will not get infested with it. This is because the animal needs an intermediate host, such as a flea, to complete its life cycle.

Therefore, do not eat fleas. More on this later.

Periodically I receive questions from folks worried they might be toting around a veritable menagerie of nameless internal parasites inside their body. The answer is, yes, you are literally loaded with little critters. Most are harmless, and a few are beneficial. There are tiny mites that live in the roots of each of your eyelashes. If you saw yogurt, bread, or cheese under the microscope, you would never eat it again. There are far more bacteria on your skin than there are people on the earth. Your bowels are full of bacteria: nearly one-half of the dry weight of a bowel movement is nothing but bacteria.

The notion of parasites is so creepy that it cannot help but get your attention. It can also be great way to sell a product. Beware.

Truly harmful parasites are the biggest problem for the world's poorest people. If you have a sanitary food and water supply, your worries are few. For most of us, household pets are probably our biggest potential source of unwanted fellow parasitic passengers. Fleas from your dog or cat can carry tapeworm larvae. If you eat a flea, you can get a tapeworm. So don't. Eliminate fleas by frequent vacuuming and an occasional steam cleaning of any carpeting. Bathing a dog (lots of luck bathing your kitty) will also kill fleas. Regular use of a flea comb (on the animal, not yourself) will trap the little arthropodia as you groom your pet.

If you find yourself obsessing about parasites at 3 AM, go and get tested. Better yet, go and have your dog or cat tested. They are much more likely to have them than you are. For the vast majority of people, I think the fear far surpasses the danger.

As a biologist, I know that a population's existence is dependent on its environment. Habitat and food supply are absolute limits to *any* population. This is why, to the overfed Westerner, undereating and periodic fasting can be so effective in preventing and often reducing overgrowths of fungi, bacteria, worms, and what have you. I also think that near-vegetarians, who get abundant dietary fiber, drink a lot of vegetable juice, and megadose on vitamin C, will have a particularly clean internal environment that parasites cannot abide.

So here's the plan: Eat right, and make parasites' lives miserable. Let's drive the little buggers right out of town.

I recognize that serious microbial diseases may require serious medication. Don't be a martyr: when in doubt, see a physician.

"The best way to have a good idea is to have a lot of ideas."

—LINUS PAULING

Medical scientists have spent the last few hundred years carefully describing diseases that are in reality the end results of chronic malnutrition. Researchers have expended colossal amounts of time and money searching for drug cures for nutritional disorders. And they have dismissed out of hand even the possibility that pharmaceutical therapy for malnutrition might be the dead end it has so frequently been shown to be.

Parkinson's disease is a case in point. L-dopa (levodopa) is a commonly prescribed treatment for Parkinson's. The human body can make this substance without drug intervention. Vitamin C in very high doses greatly stimulates L-dopa production, as well as enabling your body to naturally and safely produce its end product, the neurotransmitter norepinephrine. A depletion of norepinephrine may result in poor memory, loss of alertness, and clinical depression. The chain of chemical events in the body resulting in this substance is:

L-phenylalanine (from protein foods) $\longrightarrow$ L-tyrosine (made in the liver) $\longrightarrow$
dopa $\longrightarrow$ dopamine $\longrightarrow$ norepinephrine $\longrightarrow$ epinephrine (also known as adrenaline)

This reaction chain looks complex but actually is readily accomplished, particularly if the body has plenty of vitamin C, which facilitates the process. Since one's dietary supply of the first ingredient, L-phenylalanine, is usually adequately provided by protein foods, more likely a shortage of vitamin C is what limits production of norepinephrine. Physicians giving large doses of vitamin C have had striking success in reversing depression. It is a remarkably safe and inexpensive approach worth trying for Parkinson's.

Here's another: lecithin. Lecithin contains a lot of choline. Parkinson's patients are known to have low choline levels in their nervous systems.[1] Giving various forms of choline seems to help.[2–5] Choline works well with L-dopa medication, improves efficacy of the drug, and therby reduces the necessary dose.

But designer-cholines are not necessary. Research has shown that plain old lecithin granules can work, too. Added bonus: lecithin reduces the side effects of L-dopa therapy. One study reported that "we have given 10 levodopa-treated parkinsonian patients with dementia a regimen of lecithin (average 20 g/day). A clear improvement in Kohs block design test of constructive ability was noted with a decrease in the toxic symptoms of confusion, hallucinations and nightmares. In another study lecithin produced a decrease in levodopa-induced abnormal movements. . ."[6]

I have personally observed hand tremors go away in three days with large (5 tablespoons/day) lecithin intake. As Abraham Lincoln said, quoting a child putting on her sock, "It strikes me that there is something in it."

References

1. Manyam BV, Giacobini E, Colliver JA. Cerebrospinal fluid choline levels are decreased in Parkinson's disease. *Ann Neurol*. 1990 Jun;27(6):683–5. See also: Nasr A, Bertrand N, Giroud M, Septien L, Gras P, Dumas R, Beley A, Bralet J. Cerebrospinal fluid choline levels in Parkinson's disease. *Ann Neurol*. 1993 Jul;34(1):114–5.

2. Levin OS, Batukaeva LA, Anikina MA, Yunishchenko NA. [Efficacy and tolerability of choline alphoscerate (cereton) in patients with Parkinson's disease with cognitive disorders]. Zh Nevrol Psikhiatr Im S S Korsakova. 2009;109(11):42–6. [Article in Russian]. English translation: O. S. Levin, L. A. Batukaeva, M. A. Anikina and N. A. Yunishchenko. Efficacy and safety of choline alphoscerate (cereton) in patients with parkinson's disease with cognitive impairments. *Neuroscience and Behavioral Physiology,* 41(1): 47–51.

3. Cubells JM, Hernando C. Clinical trial on the use of cytidine diphosphate choline in Parkinson's disease. *Clin Ther.* 1988;10(6):664–71.

4. Agnoli A, Ruggieri S, Denaro A, Bruno G. New strategies in the management of Parkinson's disease: a biological approach using a phospholipid precursor (CDP-choline). *Neuropsychobiology.* 1982;8(6):289–96.

5. Tsubaki T, Kase M, Ando K, Manaka N, Sato Y. [Therapeutic effects of Nicholin (CDP-choline): Parkinson's syndrome—a double-blind study]. *Nihon Rinsho.* 1974 Nov 10;32(11):3435–50. [Article in Japanese].

6. Barbeau A. Lecithin in Parkinson's disease. *J Neural Transm Suppl.* 1980;(16):187–93.

I realize this is a mighty short section for such a severe illness. I am neither physician nor neurologist, and that is all the more reason to try vitamin C and lecithin. If they have not suggested it, it is time for you to.

"Doctors are the same as lawyers; the only difference is that lawyers merely rob you, whereas doctors rob you and kill you too."

—ANTON CHEKHOV, WHO WAS HIMSELF A PRACTICING PHYSICIAN

She was a really cute, really curly-haired ten-year-old girl, and she was really dying. She knew it, her Mom knew it, and her doctors told them so. Her name was Patty. Patty's body was destroying her platelets faster than she could make new ones. Platelets are specialized blood cells that are responsible for clotting blood. Hospitals full of specialists had studied this girl and her rare problem. They concluded by telling her mother that they had tried everything, and there was nothing else to do.

So, Patty's mom brought her to see me. That guy; the health nut.

Patty knew more about her illness than I did. I still don't know the proper medical name for it, and it doesn't much matter. She was a cheerful, calm, bright, personable little thing, and this was in tremendous contrast to her gaunt, wired mother. The mother had passed the point of mere panic long ago; she was desperate.

"We've tried everything," the mother said. "She's had all the tests. She's seen all the specialists. Nothing helps. Her platelet count is less than one-tenth of normal, and keeps dropping every week. What can be done? Can you help her?"

I didn't know. So I sat down and talked to Patty. "Do you understand your illness, Patty?" I asked. She nodded. Then she proceeded to tell me all about it. I listened, and came up with an idea. "There is at least one thing the doctors have not tried," I said. "Vitamin C and vitamin K are necessary for platelet production. It is a long shot, but maybe Patty's body needs more of these vitamins—far more—than other people do. You can megadose her on vitamin C easily enough, as it's nonprescription, cheap, and safe. You can get vitamin K from alfalfa sprouts, like the ones you see at salad bars and supermarkets."

They looked back at me. The mom eventually asked, "How much does she need to take?"

"I'm not sure, but probably a lot. It's pretty hard to hurt yourself with sprouts, and guinea pigs have been given the human dose equivalent of half a million mg of vitamin C a day without harm. You could try 10,000 mg a day. If Patty takes too much, she'll get loose bowels. If she were my daughter, I'd have her eat all the sprouts she can hold. If she eats too much alfalfa, her blood will clot too easily."

"That would be a nice problem to have!" Patty said, and her mom actually smiled.

I heard from the mother about two weeks later, and I was nervous when she started speaking. "Patty has been eating one to two jars full of alfalfa sprouts a day. She's been real good about it. And she's been taking the 10,000 mg of C every day as well."

"And?" I asked.

"The doctors have seen her several times, and her platelet count is now 85 percent normal. She is going to live! I'm so thrilled!" And off she went for a while, talking of how wonderful this all was. Inevitably, she came to the question that I've heard a thousand times. "So why didn't the doctors try this?"

It's a good question, isn't it? You can usually find only what you are looking for. There are famous exceptions, and Columbus comes immediately to mind. He was looking for India and bumped into an entirely different continent. At least explorers are usually listened to when they return with their first-hand accounts of discovery. You should see what happens to unorthodox health practitioners, and scientists, and medical doctors too, when they "discover" that vitamins cure real diseases. One of the first things that happens, as they gracefully lose their reputations, is that they are forever labeled quacks.

Patty does not care about any of that. She lived, and that's enough.

"Be good, and you will be lonesome."

—MARK TWAIN

Do you remember when there wasn't even a name for what we now know as PMS? It wasn't that many years ago that doctors considered it to be all in a woman's head. Long before that, "hysterical" women were considered to have it all emanating from their uterus. The solution? Surgery to remove the uterus (and with it the hysteria), hence the term *hysterectomy*. Half a million hysterectomies are still performed annually, most of them medically unnecessary.

Even twenty years ago, I do not recall much serious discussion about PMS. A lot of angry ladies changed that. Now TV ads discuss PMDD (Premenstrual Dysphoric Disorder). What's a dysphoric? A person exhibiting dysphoria, of course. Now for the real answer: a person with anxiety, depression, and restlessness.

So now I've got dysphoria to read. (That was subtle, but did you get it? If you didn't, I'll get datphoria next time.) But seriously, folks, many cases of PMS/PMDD can be relieved through vitamin B_6 and magnesium supplementation. Let's explore each.

Vitamin B_6

PMS/PMDD symptoms are greatly relieved by vitamin B_6 supplementation. Depressed persons are commonly deficient in this vitamin, which is necessary for your body to make the neurotransmitter serotonin. Serotonin is that wonderful feel-good substance that SSRI drugs such as Prozac try to maximize in your brain. If B_6 can do the same thing, at a fraction of the price, it is no surprise that there have been attempts to discredit its use.

B_6 dosage to the tune of 500 mg per day is generally very safe. Probably tens of millions of women suffer PMS symptoms; very few cases of B_6 overdose have been reported. High daily dosage (usually over 2,000 mg) has occasionally caused temporary neurological symptoms in some people. But as a rule this only happens if it is given alone, or way out of proportion to the other essential B vitamins. Taking all the B vitamins together (as B complex) is the safest and most effective therapeutic approach. When a balance is maintained, B-vitamin toxicity is virtually nonexistent. Is there a safe harbor? I think so. Use the entire B complex, taken every two to three hours. Consider adding perhaps 50–100 mg of pure B_6 to each dose if dysphoric symptoms are really awful.

You can get some (probably less than 5 mg) B_6 from food, if you really like to eat whole grains, seeds, and organ meats. A slice of beef liver contains a whopping single milligram of B_6. Other dead animal parts contain less (turkey and chicken breasts are pretty good, but chicken liver is only 0.6 mg per serving), while most other foods contain very little. Avocados (0.5 mg each) and bananas (0.7 mg each) lead the pyridoxine league for fruits. Potatoes (0.7 mg each) and nuts (especially filberts, peanuts, and walnuts) are relatively good veggie sources.

The RDA for B_6 for women is 1.6 mg daily, which is ridiculously inadequate. A strong case can be made for increasing this to at least 25 to 65 mg per day for people without PMS symptoms. But don't hold your breath for a raising of standards anytime soon. It seems to be hard enough to get people in the United States just to met the RDA. Consider that about three-quarters of children ages 2–12 do not get the RDA of B_6. That's pretty terrible, but it is worse for adults 19 and over: 99 percent get less than the RDA of B_6. That goes a long way to explaining the prevalency of the PMS problem.

Magnesium

Increasing dietary magnesium often decreases menstrual cramping associated with PMS. While calcium is also important for normal muscle function, magnesium can specifically help them to relax. Lots of women take extra calcium, which may help relieve cramping, and certainly has bone benefits. However, supplemental calcium alone effectively depletes the body of magnesium and ensures cramping will occur in the following month if magnesium is not replenished.

If you do not suffer from kidney disease, consider taking an oral daily magnesium supplement. For generally healthy people the only significant side effect from taking too much magnesium is diarrhea. Your body continuously discards excess magnesium through urine and feces.

The RDA for magnesium is 420 mg per day for men and 320 mg for women. This standard may be inadequate, and, what's worse, the majority of people do not get even that much. Magnesium is necessary for the normal functioning of more than three hundred enzymes in your body. If you do not have enough available magnesium (magnesium deficiency), it slowly degrades your general health in a variety of ways. Magnesium deficiency is directly linked to heart disease. Moreover, because of the many ways your body employs magnesium, it plays a role in preventing diabetes, cancer, stroke, osteoporosis, arthritis, asthma, kidney stones, migraine, leg and menstrual cramps, eclampsia, PMS, chronic fatigue syndrome, tetany, and a variety of other problems.

Magnesium supplements are inexpensive and readily available without prescription. Women might try starting with 200 mg per day, divided up into two or three separate doses. After two weeks, you can increase your daily dose by a convenient increment, say 100 mg per day (tablets are easily snapped in half). If frequent bowel movements or gas become a problem, reduce the amount.

Recommended Reading

Dean, C. *The Magnesium Miracle.* New York: Ballantine Books, 2006.

Seelig M. *Magnesium Deficiency in the Pathogenesis of Disease.* New York: Plenum, 1980.

Pneumonia and Severe Acute Respiratory Syndrome (SARS)

"No man is a good doctor who has never been sick himself."

—PROVERB

New strains of one of hundreds of flu, common cold, or other viruses appear constantly. Our fears are that they will go absolutely berserk in a person with a low immune system. But few viruses are worse than, say, polio. Even polio can be stopped by megadoses of vitamin C. Please look at this book's section "High-Dose Vitamin C Therapy for Major Diseases."

A "new" opportunistic virus is a big surprise to no one. History is full of them. About 10 million soldiers were killed in World War I, charging machine guns and getting mowed down month after month. There were nearly a million casualties at the Somme and another million at Verdun. A terrible slaughter went on for four years. Yet, in just the two years following the war, over 20 million people died from influenza. That is more than twice as many deaths from the flu in one-half the time it took the machine guns.

Preventing is obviously easier than treating severe illness. Immediate use of half-hourly gram (1,000 mg) doses of vitamin C, up to saturation, will usually stop a cold from escalating to pneumonia. But if it has, *treat serious illness seriously:* in the very young or the very old, pneumonia can kill. Do not hesitate to seek medical attention.

And while you are so doing, here is a second opinion. Dr. Robert Cathcart advocates treating pneumonia with up to 200,000 milligrams of vitamin C daily, often intravenously (IV). You and I can simulate a 24-hour IV of vitamin C by taking it by mouth very, very often. When I had pneumonia, it took 2,000 mg of vitamin C every six minutes, by the clock, to get me to saturation. My oral daily dose was over 100,000 mg. Fever, cough, and other symptoms were reduced in hours; complete recovery took just a few days. Bronchitis clears up even faster. That is performance at least as good as any pharmaceutical will give, and the vitamin is both safer and cheaper.

I suggest consulting the *Journal of Orthomolecular Medicine* for additional support for megavitamin therapies. The research is done, the write-ups are out there, and you can read forty years' worth of *JOM*s for free. The archive is online at www.orthomed.org and at http://orthomolecular.org/library/jom. Treating respiratory infections with massive amounts of Vitamin C is not a new idea at all. Frederick R. Klenner, M.D., and William J. McCormick, M.D., used this approach successfully for decades beginning back in the 1940s. All who think that, though vitamin C generally has merit, massive doses are ineffective or somehow harmful will do well to read the original papers for themselves. Clinical evidence confirms the powerful antiviral-antibiotic effect of vitamin C *when used in sufficient quantity*. I realize that this is a very short chapter for such a big, and important, topic. That's because I'd like you to refer to the vitamin C chapters in this book.

Speaking as a parent, I can confirm that vitamin C works. Vitamin C can be used alone or right along with medicines if one so chooses.

Each year, nearly 50,000 Americans die from pneumonia (National Vital Statistics Reports, Vol. 58, No. 19, May 20, 2010). That is over 135 deaths *every day*. That means prescription drugs are not doing the job. There is no question that aggressive use of vitamin C would lower that figure a great deal. There is no excuse for excluding it.

"Disease is the censor pointing out the humans,
animals and plants who are imperfectly nourished."

—G. T. WRENCH, 1941

Imagine that you are a junior high school science teacher. Scary thought though it be, I was one. Now let's say you want to try nutritional experiments with animals in a seventh-grade biology class. Let me clue you in: you can forget about any hopes you might have for either control or objectivity. Take two cages of hamsters, mice, Guinea pigs, or what have you, and feed one group a really good diet and the other group a really bad diet. You, the teacher, know exactly what results to expect. So do the students. The moment you are not looking, they will smuggle nuts, raw vegetables, and probably vitamin tablets into the "deficient diet" cage. They cannot stand to see those little mammals suffer the ravages of malnutrition, and they will make quite certain that it does not happen.

Junior high students, like everyone else, including even the youngest of children, know that junk food leads to junked bodies. Yet these very same kids will eat the most gosh-awful food they can find in the school cafeteria, if they eat anything there at all, when so many schools still have competing snack- and drink-vending machines.

Knowing clearly does not make it so. Consider food preparation. We know that animals in the wild never eat cooked food, yet we feed nothing but that to our dogs and cats. If it's in a can, pouch, bag, or box, that pet's food has been cooked.

And along with it, perhaps its goose as well.

Between 1932 and 1942, Francis M. Pottenger Jr., M.D., conducted his now classic ten-year, multigeneration nutrition study on cats. This decade of data has been neatly condensed into a concise, inexpensive 119-page book entitled *Pottenger's Cats: A Study in Nutrition,* also incorporating summaries of some two dozen of the doctor's nutrition papers.

Pottenger's cat experiments were, in a nutshell, a decade-long, scientifically controlled "Supersize Me" experiment. Basically, there were two groups of cats: the cats who daily ate the kitty equivalent of Burglar King and McNothing foods—that is, nothing but cooked food. The other group was fed raw food.

What do you suppose was the result?

OK, class; let's not always see the same hands.

Yes, you're right. The raw food cats thrived. The cooked food cats did not, and there were no merciful middle-schoolers there to save them.

I have a cat; her name is Dolly. She is asleep on my lap as I write this. Dolly was cast off in a rural store parking lot. We brought her home hungry, and to this day she retains the most amazing kitty appetite I have ever seen. We have repeatedly discovered that she is inexplicably partial to fresh Italian bread. She will energetically eat cooked green beans, zucchini squash, and beets. As for raw vegetables, she is moderately famous in cyberspace as the Carrot Cat (photos at www.doctoryourself.com). The Carrot Cat will eat raw carrot pulp left over when I make carrot juice. (Of course, she is also fed a variety of animal foods.) As I write these very words, she is using her forehead to lift my hand away from the keyboard and go feed her.

Even for the cat-lovers among us, the larger question must be, to what extent do the Pottenger cat experiments apply to people? I am particularly intrigued with Pottenger's observations that cats fed on cooked meat and milk develop "all kinds" of allergies and hypothyroidism. When fed raw foods, the cats' symptoms go away (p. 33). I personally have seen a case where a sixty-seven-year-old woman, who was on a prescribed low dose of Synthroid, no longer needed it after just a few weeks of raw vegetable juicing. She is eighty-seven now, and her doctors have confirmed that still does not require any thyroid supplement.

At the very least, the Pottenger cat experiments show what an unsupplemented lifetime diet of cooked meat can do to a carnivore. But the more important message of the experiments is that they also show recovery on a raw-food diet. I think we can reasonably infer that this applies to people. And for those bound and determined to go Atkins, well, maybe you'd better consider eating your meat raw.

Repellant though this thought be, I'd better be careful what I say. Once I had a reader who took an offhand comment like this seriously. He wrote to me that he'd started eating wild game, uncooked. While, in truth, he also claimed he'd never felt better, I cringe at the bacterial and parasite load one might incur in eating raw animals.

Ugh.

Though Pottenger does recommend "raw beef hors d' oeuvres three times weekly" (p. 105), it would be inaccurate to imply that Dr. Pottenger expected people to eat meat raw. His instructions for cooking brains are on page 108; recipes for cooking kidneys on p. 109; preparing heart and tripe on p 110. He advocated minimal cooking (p. 103), but even that is difficult to avoid seeing as a philosophical inconsistency in his writing. Minimally cooked is still a far cry from raw.

More to my taste is raw bean and grain sprouting, of which Pottenger said, "To enhance their protein value, sprout before cooking" (p. 106). There it is again: cooking. However, he also recommended uncooked sprouts for salads (p. 111). Dr. Pottenger advocated clean, raw milk. As a former dairyman and college clinical nutrition instructor, so do I.

Just how lifeless is cooked food? Well, Dr. Pottenger even tested the value of cat excreta as fertilizer. Guess what? He found that plants would not grow in the presence of waste from cooked-food cats and cooked-milk cats.

Evidently, neither did bones, jaws, and teeth. Malocclusion was prominent among the defects and disorders Pottenger saw in cooked-food fed cats. The problem has not gone away. A MEDLINE search for "malocclusion cats" brings up two dozen papers on the subject . . . and 153 papers on the condition in dogs. Try an Internet search , and you can see more than you probably want to at a number of Web locations. Orthodontics for housepets is a big and growing business.

Transferring this knowledge when it comes to people, I strongly support Pottenger's stance in favor of a whole-food, whole-grain, low-sugar diet. However, I do have a bone to pick with the good doctor, and here it is:

In recommending his High Protective Diet, Pottenger calls for an adult human to consume 225 grams of fat per day, and an equal amount of protein (p. 103). I am tempted to try to dismiss this as a misprint, but it is not, as he has previously presented this opinion on page 94. Pottenger states (p. 99) that "Fat is the energy fuel of the body." There are many complex-carbo fans who would sharply disagree with this statement, especially to the tune of 225 grams of fat per day. For an adult, 60 to 80 g/day total dietary fat is usually recommended. According to the US government, even an eating machine such as a teenage boy, chowing down a 3,000 calorie/day

217

diet, should get no more than 100 g/day. Dr. Pottenger would seem to suggest that we should eat well over twice that amount of fat, every day.

There is, in fact, no US RDA for fat. Technically, we do not need to eat much fat at all; we do need some to help absorb fat-soluble vitamins like vitamins A, D, and E. What we absolutely must have are the essential fatty acids: linolenic and linoleic acid. To his credit, and to my relief, Pottenger says, "The primary source of man's fats is vegetable; the secondary source is animal" (p. 98).

My interpretation of Pottenger's work is this: It is not about eating more meat and fat; it is about eating more raw food. Raw for cats and carnivores means raw meat. Raw for people, who cannot be reasonably expected to eat raw meat, must emphasize foods other than meat.

Differences aside, I submit that Pottenger's essential message might best be expressed in his own words:

> Those kittens that receive cooked meat instead of raw develop all types of malformations of the face, jaws and teeth. . . . (When) cats put on the cooked meat diet and are allowed to become pregnant, their kittens' skulls show marked variations from the normal. . . . (O)nce such deficiencies are produced and maintained by a faulty diet, they become progressively worse through the second and third generations. . . . Deficient cats exhibit progressive allergic symptoms from generation to generation. They show most of the common respiratory, gastrointestinal and constitutional problems as well as various skin disorders. (*Pottenger's Cats*, pp. 39–42).

Surely these observations demand our most serious consideration. They are a powerful argument in favor of minimal food processing, maximal raw-food intake, and in my opinion, the use of vitamin supplements. I would like to see a new ten-year cat study in which one multigenerational group of cats gets cooked food with supplements, another group raw food with supplements, another cooked and no supplements, and another raw and no supplements.

In a way, this experiment is already underway, and you and everyone you know are part of it. But in our unintended, uncontrolled, worldwide version of the study, we find that even Pottenger's all-cooked-food test animals had advantages over us: 1) they did not eat junk food; 2) they did not eat sugar; and 3) cats (like practically all other animals) make their own vitamin C. We have none of these advantages.

What this means is that the unsupplemented human race's health can be expected to be even poorer than Pottenger's sickest cats.

And it is. The lesson of Dr. Pottenger's work, over seventy years ago, is yet to be learned.

Reference

Pottenger Jr., FM. *Pottenger's Cats: A Study in Nutrition.* Elaine Pottenger, editor, with Robert T. Pottenger Jr. Lemon Grove, CA: Price-Pottenger Nutrition Foundation, 1995. (www.price-pottenger.org)

"A vegetarian diet can prevent 97% of our coronary occlusions."

JAMA, Vol. 176, No. 9, June 3, 1961, p 806.

Vegetarian or Carnivore?

Cornell University's extensive nutrition studies in China have shown that people eating little or no animal protein are less likely to get either cancer or heart disease. "These diets are much different from the average American diets, containing only about 0–20% animal-based foods, while the average American diet is comprised of about 60–80% animal based foods. Disease patterns in much of rural China tend to reflect those prior to the industrial revolution in the U.S., when cancers and cardiovascular diseases were much less prevalent." (www.nutrition. cornell.edu/ChinaProject/results.html)

Decades earlier, researchers such as Dr. Francis Pottenger and Dr. Weston Price had repeatedly shown that "primitive" peoples or laboratory animals eating a natural, not-too-much-meat diet simply do not have serious diseases. (See www.price-pottenger.org/articles .htm and www. westonaprice.org/splash_2.htm.)

I do not mean strict vegetarianism, not by a long shot. The Cornell China studies clearly support near-vegetarianism ("0–20% animal-based foods"), which is my preferred long-term dietary maintenance plan. And I would be pleased if everyone followed Pottenger's dictum and ate pretty much raw everything, especially raw milk, which I have long advocated. My reading of Price's work says to me, "eat unprocessed foods." If people want to eat the seafood and organ meats that Dr. Price advocated in his book *Nutrition and Physical Degeneration,* they will do well nutritionally to do so.

Dr. Pottenger's emphasis was on the nutritional value of raw foods, and he got it right. Pottenger knew that carnivorous animals, normally, would never be in a position to hunt a cooked meal. His studies were primarily on cats, and most felines are carnivores. But even "carnivores" are not strictly carnivorous. Lions and similar predators gobble up the predigested vegetable material from an herbivorous prey animal's digestive organs in preference to any other part of the kill. I caught my cat up on the kitchen counter the other day. She was eating carrot pulp left over from the morning's juicing. Plain carrot pulp. Years ago, I had a cat that would stand up on her hind legs and beg for cooked green beans. But this is in addition to an appropriately meaty kitty diet.

For humans, if a vegetable, fruit, or dairy food can be eaten uncooked, then it should be. As for raw meat, well, no thank you. The natural hygienists have what is at heart the same message: eat fresh and raw. I admire and seek to emulate such knowledge to the maximum practical extent. However, I do not apologize for having a stove. A whole-food, good-food diet including legumes (peas, beans, lentils), grains, and potatoes clearly needs some cooking. But there is definitely no need to make one's home on the range.

Meat: Lots, Some, or None

Americans consume at least twice as much protein as they need. Worldwide, 30 grams of protein daily is usually adequate. The USRDA of protein is about 60 grams daily for a man and about 50 grams daily for a woman. We generally eat over 100 grams of protein daily, mostly from meat. Chronic protein excess can overload and irreversibly damage the kidneys by middle age (Williams, S. [1993]. *Nutrition and Diet Therapy,* 7th ed, Mosby).

When in doubt, eat like other primates do. Chimps, gorillas, orangutans, and that crowd are very strong, very smart, and mostly but not entirely vegetarian. By moving *toward* a vegetarian diet, you automatically reduce your too-high intake of protein, fat, and sugar. It is just that simple. There is no diet plan to buy. I think dairy products and eggs and fish must remain occa-

219

sional options for most of us. My kids did so well as lacto-ovo-vegetarians that they never had a single dose of an antibiotic, not once. Had they *not* been healthy, the state and the school board would have been on our backs instantly.

To avoid all animal products makes one a vegan. I am most certainly not a vegan, and I do not universally advocate it. I have many good friends who utterly and totally reject animal products. For this I admire them. I also observe that their conviction is, at times, more admirable than their health is. Ethical issues aside, veganism truly is an excellent transition diet. As limited-term treatment for overweight, constipated, drug-soaked people, veganism cannot be beat. I think a few months without animal products is worth a therapeutic trial for most illnesses. But long term, for most people, I think some animal foods are necessary as the decades pass.

The majority of vegetarians are actually near-vegetarians, eating some animal products, such as milk products. My readers know I am something of a cheese and yogurt fan. As a former dairyman, what do you expect? I also use eggs now and then for cooking, and I make a mean broccoli quiche. But I am not really much of a milk-drinker, and typically do not go through even half a dozen eggs in a month.

Albert Einstein wrote, "Nothing will benefit human health and increase the chances for survival of life on Earth as much as the evolution to a vegetarian diet." Evolution, a key word, means gradual change with time. "Vegetarianism" is a process, not an absolute.

For my children, the process began in infancy. Okay, so they were not fed meat. But "meat-less" most certainly does *not* mean "zero animal products." The two are far, far apart. And when considering the moral arguments on the dialectics of dietetics, we are humbled when we recall that Mahatma Gandhi ate dairy products, and Jesus ate fish.

In truth, I cannot even be described as a lacto-ovo-vegetarian (eggs and dairy), for I also eat seafood. Not often, and usually not directly in front of my aquarium. But I maintain, in the face of animal-rights adversity, that fish and their oceanic roommates are valuable nutrition sources. After millennia of changes to human civilization, the world's number-one animal protein source is still seafood. By the time we come up with a definition of "fishatarian," we are very close to the natural animal-products percentages that Dr. Weston Price found again and again in his travels amongst "primitive" (aka "healthy") cultures back in the 1930s. I have no shame whatsoever in eating like a South Sea island native.

Weston Price and Native Diets

I am quite willing to eat along the dietary lines of other traditional cultures that Dr. Price visited and wrote of. Price found that isolated, healthy Swiss communities ate cheese and raw milk daily, plus a lot of whole-grain bread. But they only ate meat once a week. The basic foods of the islanders of the Outer Hebrides, Price wrote, "are fish and oat products with a little barley. Oat grain . . . provides the porridge and oat cakes which in many homes are eaten in some form regularly with every meal" (p. 44). Even traditional Eskimos, often held up as the ultimate example of human carnivorism, also eat nuts, "kelp stored for winter use, berries including cranberries which are preserved by freezing, blossoms of flowers preserved in seal oil, (and) sorrel grass preserved in seal oil" (p. 71).

In short, most vegetarians are not, and most carnivores are not. Optimum human diet is not to be found at either extreme. The issue is *natural food,* more than where it comes from. Unprocessed foods, whether animal or plant origin, are the healthiest. This is the enduring message of Price and Pottenger.

220

A Poem

Dunderbeck, oh Dunderbeck
Oh how could ye be so mean
To ever have invented
The sausage-meat machine.
Now all the rats
And puddy-cats
Will never more be seen;
For they'll all be ground
To sausage meat
In Dunderbeck's machine.

(AUTHOR UNKNOWN, FORTUNATELY)

"I firmly believe that if all medicines could be sunk to the bottom of the sea, it would be all the better for mankind and all the worse for the fishes.

—OLIVER WENDELL HOLMES

It was 1979. The nurses were practically lined up at my wife's hospital room door. You could hear them down the hallway: "Her baby was 10 pounds, 2 oz, the mother's pre-pregnancy weight was 110, and she has no stretch marks!"

All true. I was there, the proud dad of my newborn daughter. Her brother had been born two years previously.

That was three and a half decades ago. So here's a welcome update: after my granddaughter was born, my daughter didn't have any stretch marks, either. I think we may be on to something here, and that something is vitamin C.

It takes vitamin C to make collagen and strong connective tissue. That fact is in every nutrition textbook ever written. It has also been shown that vitamin C supplementation enhances collagen synthesis.[1] And does so rapidly, too.[2] But few know that, over sixty years ago, it was Toronto physician William J. McCormick, M.D., who pioneered the idea that poor collagen formation, due to vitamin C deficiency, was the principal cause of stretch marks.

In 1948, Dr. McCormick[3] wrote: "[T]hese disfiguring subdermal lesions, which for centuries were regarded as a natural sequence of pregnancy, are the result of increased fragility of the involved abdominal connective tissue, secondary to deficiency of vitamin C."

The strength of a brick wall is not truly in the bricks, for a stack of bricks can easily be pushed apart. Collagen is the "mortar" that binds your cells together, just as mortar binds bricks together. If collagen is abundant and strong, body cells hold together well. It is possible to see how this property would prevent stretch marks.

References

1. Chan, D, Lamande, SR, Cole, WG, and Bateman, JF. (1990). Regulation of procollagen synthesis and processing during ascorbate-induced extracellular matrix accumulation in vitro. *Biochem J.* 269(1):175–81.

2. Franceschi, RT, Iyer, BS, Cui, Y. (1994). Effects of ascorbic acid on collagen matrix formation and osteoblast differentiation in murine MC3T3-E1 cells. *J Bone Miner Res.* 9(6):843–54.

3. McCormick, WJ. (August 1948). The striae of pregnancy: A new etiological concept. *Medical Record.*

FOLIC ACID AND PREGNANCY

"What Took the FDA So Long to Come Out in Favor of Folic Acid?"

by William Kaufman, M.D., Ph.D.

Folic acid (or folate) is frequently referred to in the news media, so I will make some comments about it. Folic acid is an artifact of chemical isolation, pteroylglutamic acid. This active molecule is a partially degraded, fully oxidized derivative of the folates. Virtually no folic *acid* exists in either plant or animal tissues. But the folates do.

Folic acid is an inexpensive chemical with a vitamin-like action. One can buy it anywhere for a few pennies cents per tablet..

Who is most susceptible to general folic acid deficiencies? Pregnant woman, fetuses, premature infants, and elderly people. Women with folic acid deficiency can develop precancerous changes in the uterine cervix. In addition, some women (users of oral contraceptive agents or smokers), who do not have a systemic folic acid deficiency, can develop areas of localized folic acid deficiency in the uterine cervix, which. may then become precancerous or actual cancer. Administration of adequate amounts of inexpensive folic acid can stop this before it starts. Changing the diet to include foods rich in folates helps sustain such a cure. But it is often hard for a woman to make a sustained improvement in diet; poor women simply cannot afford the fresh produce. Either way, it would seem wise to use inexpensive, adequate pill-a-day folic acid maintenance therapy in addition to as good a diet as they can afford and get themselves to eat.

In a pregnant woman, folate deficiency may cause a special kind of anemia, a premature separation of the placenta, spontaneous abortion, bleeding, an abnormal fetus including those with a neural tube defect, anacephaly, spina bifida, and low-weight babies. Not only do these sad events cause misery to the mother, father, and family, but they simultaneously cause a large drain on medical resources as well as an enormous economic drain on Medicaid and on other sources for financing medical care. These complications of pregnancy can be largely prevented by good nutrition and appropriate folic acid supplementation for the entire duration of the pregnancy, from conception onward.

Nutritional substances such as vitamins and minerals are not drugs. Folic acid is a vitamin. However, FDA regulations that state that any substance can be considered to be a drug if a claim is made that it can improve function or structure in an individual or prevent illness. Because of this, folic acid once was legally characterized as a drug. FDA had previously rejected a new drug applications for the use of folic acid intended to prevent neural tube defects in the fetus of a pregnant woman who had such a tragic event in a previous pregnancy. This went on for years. In the meantime, women who had the misfortune to have had a fetus with a neural tube disorder in a previous pregnancy could not, for a long time, legally be prescribed folic acid with the view of reducing her future risk of having another baby with a neural tube defect, such as spina bifida.

SAFETY OF FOLIC ACID

Folic acid has been used for over half a century as a vitamin, and has been found safe in the treatment of men, nonpregnant women, and in pregnant women who have had folic acid deficiencies. Even a very high daily oral dose (10 milligrams, which is 10,000 mcg) that is 50 times the present RDA (Recommended Daily Allowance) taken by 27 nonpregnant women for four months was safe and there were no adverse side effects.

There are no folic acid adverse side effects excepting the following:

1. folic acid in huge doses administered to epileptic persons may block the anti-epileptic action of their drugs and cause them to have an increase in epileptic attacks (this is unlikely to occur with lower doses of folic acid);

2. it may rarely decrease absorption of zinc but this does not lower blood zinc levels because of decreased urinary excretion of zinc; and

3. the patient has concurrent deficiency in both vitamin B_{12} and folic acid, a condition that requires concomitant treatment with both vitamin B_{12} and folic acid. Therefore, folic acid alone cannot be effective.

223

Thus, folic acid is safer than most of the drugs, if not all the drugs, that FDA has approved for prescription use.

FOLIC ACID IN THE PREVENTION OF NEURAL TUBE DEFECTS IN THE FETUS

Many published reports in the medical literature indicate that giving such a woman folic acid in sufficient amounts can greatly lower the risk of recurrences of birth defects. In addition to taking folic acid, I recommend:

1. that the nonepileptic woman who has had a previous fetus with neural tube defects start the agreed upon dose of folic acid before conception and continue it throughout her entire pregnancy

2. that she will agree not to indulge in alcohol before conception and throughout her entire pregnancy and if she does, she will inform her physician how much and how often she partakes of alcohol (alcohol will negate folic acid action)

3. the obstetrician or nurse-midwife who delivers the infant will make a full record of the pattern of folic acid oral usage, whether or not alcohol has been indulged in during the pregnancy, and the amounts and frequency of intake, and the condition of the infant on birth.

This information combined with the prospective information reported to the FDA on the incidence of neural-tube-defect babies occurring in women treated with folic acid, in turn, would make it possible to assess accurately how effective folic acid is in lowering the risk of occurrence of such tragedies.

(Editor's note: FDA did ultimately approve folic acid as preventive for neural tube defects such as spina bifida. It took them almost ten years to do so. In each of those years, at least 1,200 babies were born with neural tube defects. That makes some 12,000 birth defects that FDA failed to prevent because of unwarranted caution over a substance that is vastly safer than any drug that they have ever approved.)

(Abridged and reprinted with the kind permission of Charlotte Kaufman.)

Vitamin C, Viruses, and Pregnancy

Marta, age 30, was in her sixth month of a long-desired pregnancy. She came to see me specifically because of genital herpes. Her obstetrician had correctly told her that she could not deliver vaginally as long as there were active lesions. Exposure to herpes constitutes a real danger to a newborn. The doctor had said that if the lesions were inactive, and preferably gone, for a period of so many weeks, he'd OK a natural delivery. Otherwise, it would be a Cesarean for her.

Her question was expected.

"Is there any way to get rid of the lesions with nutrition?" Marta asked.

Conformist, party-line dietitians will vigorously deny such a possibility, but then, they don't read their own journals, and certainly not Linus Pauling's books or the *Journal of Orthomolecular Medicine*.

So the truthful answer, the one I'd have to give if under oath, is: Yes, there probably is: very large doses of vitamin C.

I ran this past Marta, and her concern was, once again, entirely predictable.

"Are megadoses of vitamin C safe for the baby?"

I knew that Frederick R. Klenner, M.D. (the trailblazer of vitamin C therapy) gave large doses to over 300 pregnant women and reported virtually no complications in any of the pregnancies or deliveries (Irwin Stone, *The Healing Factor,* chapter 28). Indeed, hospital nurses around Reidsville, North Carolina, the region where Dr. Klenner practiced, noted that the infants who were healthiest and happiest were in Klenner's care. The hospital staff dubbed them the "Vitamin C Babies."

Specifically, Klenner gave: 4,000 milligrams during the first trimester, 6,000 mg during the second, and 10,000 milligrams of vitamin C a day—or even 15,000 mg—throughout their third trimester. This was his routine prescription for healthy women. He would respond to any sickness with daily vitamin C injections totaling many times that.

Over a nearly forty-year practice, Klenner (and previous animal studies) rigorously ascertained the safety and effectiveness of vitamin C during pregnancy. Specifically, there were no miscarriages in Klenner's entire group of 300 women. There were no postpartum hemorrhages at all. There was no cardiac distress and there were no toxic manifestations (Stone, p. 191). Among Klenner's patients were the Fultz quadruplets, who, at the time, were the only quads in the southeastern U.S. to survive. Upon admission to the hospital for childbirth, Klenner gave all mothers-to-be "booster" injections of vitamin C.

So my answer to Marta's question of safety was an unfettered yes.

"Additionally," I added, for the ladies who had all the vitamin C, labor was both shorter and less painful."

Soon to be facing her first delivery, Marta had a vested interest in that little side benefit. "I've never given birth myself," I went on, "but my wife's two deliveries confirmed what Klenner said. Her first labor was two hours and forty-five minutes total, and her second labor was one hour and forty-five minutes from the very onset to 'It's a girl.' "

"Wow!" Marta said, happier than ever.

"I hesitate to keep this going, but there's still more. The obstetrical nurses at Klenner's hospital repeatedly verified that stretch marks were seldom seen on Klenner's postpartum patients. I can personally vouch for this being true with my spouse. After two kids, the second with a birthweight of 10 pounds, 2 ounces."

Marta's eyes grew large at the very idea.

"My wife had a single, half-inch stretch mark. Pretty neat, eh?"

Marta nodded several times.

"Well, I really want to get rid of this herpes thing so I can have a natural childbirth," She went on. "I know that herpes is most certainly not safe for the baby. And from what I've read, Cesarean delivery, like all operations, carries risk, too. It seems that my balance sheet favors trying the vitamin."

"Well," I said, "if you are going to do it, Marta, you might as well do it right. This means building up your C level to saturation. That's bowel tolerance, remember?"

She did.

"And you mean that I might have to take much more than I'd expect to, right?" Marta added.

"Yes," I said. "You do not take the amount of vitamin C you think you should take; rather, you take the amount of vitamin C that the body responds to. When your symptoms leave, that's the right level for you at that time. As you get better, you will not be able to hold as much of the vitamin. The dose is self-adjusting, and you need no equipment to monitor it.

225

Just take as much as you can comfortably hold, just enough to be symptom-free, but not so much as causes loose bowels."

Marta said, "How long will it be before I see any progress?"

"It depends on how much vitamin C you take, and how much vitamin C you need. A dry sponge holds a lot of water. The body seems to have an enormous capacity for vitamin C when infected with a virus. We'll all find out how much you need when we see how much you can comfortably hold. It is not a contest; just do what gets the healing. But it will take time to get to your saturation level."

"What can I expect along the way?" she asked.

"The first thing you will notice is: nothing. There is a latency period, a lag-time, while you load the body with the vitamin. It's a bit like waiting for your computer to load a new program."

"Can you try another analogy?" Marta said.

"Look at it this way," I responded. "Let's say you were in a plane taking off from Buffalo International Airport in the middle of winter. It is snowing, dark, gray, stormy and windy. Your jet takes off, and begins to climb. The wind rocks the plane, the snow and sleet and hail come down, and it's all dismally gray outside. The plane keeps climbing. All you can see out the window is snow, darkness and the wings shaking from the wind. The person next to you is turning a bit green. Up you go, still in the winter storm. Then, all of the sudden, the airplane breaks out on top of the clouds, and like magic, there's bright sunlight and blue sky every-where. Look down: far below you is the storm. It's like it never happened, like you were never in it.

"That is exactly what it is like when you reach saturation of vitamin C. At a certain altitude, higher than you expected, your symptoms go away. This characteristically occurs with such ease that it is hard to believe it until you experience it for yourself. Precious few medical pro-fessionals have learned this. The medical-dietetic industry has a real fear of flying if vitamin C is the aircraft. Too bad, when it is the safest and fastest plane in the air.

Marta was nobody's fool, and worked closely with her obstetrician. She had heard about something termed "rebound scurvy," and now asked me about it.

"Rebound scurvy, or the rebound effect, is when a person takes a lot of vitamin C, usually with great success, and then abruptly stops taking it. At that instance, symptoms come back, sometimes including a few classic vitamin C deficiency signs. Research shows that such an effect does not occur in the vast majority of situations.

"However, pregnancy is a special case. If the mother takes a lot of C while pregnant, Klen-ner and others confirmed that her labor and delivery will be shorter, easier and free of compli-cations. If the vitamin helped while Mommy was pregnant, it should most certainly be given to the baby. During gestation, the baby got all the C he needed. But now, baby is on his own: no more C through the placenta and umbilical cord. If the baby is used to, and benefiting from, abundant vitamin C, it obviously should be provided for him individually after birth. Klenner gave newborns about 50 milligrams a day. Not doing that results in a scorbutic baby."

"But doesn't that just mean that the baby is dependent on vitamin C?" Marta said. I told you she was nobody's fool.

"No," I answered. "No more than the baby is dependent on oxygen, or water, or food. Con-sider this: If you have a really high-paying job, and expenses to fit it, and you are suddenly fired, you have a problem. Your problem is not money. Your problem is a lack of money."

Marta smiled comfortably.

"So don't stop a good thing, then," she said.

"That's it," I agreed. "If vitamin C is important enough for the woman to take before giving birth, then it is important enough for the baby to get after it has been born."

"I can see that," she said. "But I'm going to breastfeed my baby. Is there vitamin C in breast milk?"

"There is some, but we do not know how much at any given feeding. Keep in mind that the nursing woman is healing up and stressed out. Along with recovering from childbirth, she is adapting to really momentous changes in her lifestyle and sleeping schedule, and everybody knows that taking care of a baby is a tremendous demand on a person. Mom needs a lot of vitamin C herself. So her amount of available surplus C is small. For this reason, breast milk is an unreliable source of vitamin C for babies. However, mother's milk otherwise is the perfect food for infants. You absolutely, positively are making the right decision when you breastfeed. Just slip the child a little C each day as you do it. Even a newborn can gum down a tiny bit of a finely-powdered chewable children's C tablet. You can put a little right on the baby's tongue. Vitamin C drops are also available. My own kids got supplemental C from the very first days of their lives."

"What if a baby is formula-fed?" Marta asked.

"Then supplemental C is ever more essential," I said. "Very little of the vitamin is found in formula, especially after it is manufactured, packaged, opened, heated, poured, and oxidized during bottle feeding."

"OK," said Marta. "I guess I should get started."

She did.

It was not that long afterward that I had a follow-up conversation with her.

"The delivery is on," Marta said. "The herpes lesions are all gone, and have been gone since I got to saturation with the C. Do you want to know how much it took?"

"You bet I do."

"44,000 milligrams a day!" she hooted. "Can you believe that? And at that much I hardly had any bowel signs at all. So I dropped it to about 35 to 40 thousand and stayed there. That's it!"

Not quite. A couple of months later, Marta had one of the most adorable baby girls I've ever seen. That Dr. Klenner fellow. I'd have liked to have met him. (For more about Dr. Klenner visit www.doctoryourself.com/klennerbio.html.)

Right now there are a whole lot of researchers searching for a good new antiviral drug. They are the blind leading the blind. They already have one. The pharmaceutical industry's mercenary scientists and their medical doctor clones will, in fact, try everything but megadoses of vitamin C. I think of them as birds that are willing to land on any branch except one. Too bad, because that one branch is the best in the tree.

Poignant Pregnancy Pointers

Good nutrition for a female's entire life is the best possible preparation for pregnancy. This is especially true during the years immediately preceding conception. In a manner of speaking, a baby is nearly a year old at birth. Many women only begin to eat right and take necessary vitamin supplements once they know they are pregnant. This is weeks or even months too late. The first few weeks of pregnancy are especially crucial to the embryo.

Let's steel ourselves to take a quick look under the bed at what every parent-to-be is most terrified of: the uncomfortable subject of birth defects. Here is a grim fact from the National

Institute for Drug Abuse: Fully 11 percent of all babies born in the United States are born to drug-abusing mothers. Here's another: Mothers who smoke tobacco are hurting their unborn child. The carcinogens and other harmful chemicals that a pregnant woman takes in when she smokes cigarettes are transmitted to the unborn baby. Many chemicals in tobacco products, such as benzene and formaldehyde, are known teratogens (causes of birth defects).

Maternal alcohol use also hurts the developing child. Two out of three adults use alcohol, and one in ten adults is a heavy drinker. The Surgeon General has stated that *there is no safe minimum level of alcohol consumption during pregnancy*. Fetal alcohol syndrome is the most severe expression of what alcohol can do to a baby. There must be millions of infants with less obvious but still handicapping alcohol-related congenital damage.

In addition, environmental pollutants and on-the-job exposure to chemicals are causes of birth defects. And we have not even considered pharmaceutical side effects (remember thalid-amide?) Then there is malnutrition, or undernutrition, which may be the greatest factor of all. I would be willing to say that the majority of pregnant women strictly avoid harmful behaviors. But there are others who persist in doing multiple dangerous behaviors well into, or throughout, pregnancy. This constitutes child abuse, and it must stop immediately, before it is too late.

Along with chemical abuse, poverty, adolescence, and advanced age traditionally make up the other three common problem pregnancy areas. Bottle feeding, unnecessary overmedication, and marginal nutritional deficiency diseases make up three additional problem areas. For a really bone-chilling summary of the consequences of vitamin deficiency during pregnancy, read the papers by Howard Hillemann referenced at the end of the chapter.

Nutrition needs rise during pregnancy, of course. Even the RDAs are higher. This may be obvious to you, but many women eat poor diets in general. They then tend to eat more of the same lousy foods in an attempt to "eat for two" and "to get all the nutrition they need from a balanced diet." This is a genuine tragedy, for which the medical and nutrition professions cannot easily be excused. At the very least, pregnancy increases the need for protein, calcium, iron, and all of the vitamins. The same for lactation. And don't forget Dad: conception is more likely if Dad takes supplemental vitamin C, zinc, lecithin, and a little Korean ginseng extract (*Panax ginseng*) each day. See my chapter on fertility for more information.

Ten Ways to Avoid Most Birth and Baby Problems

"The only way to win is not to play."
—QUOTING THE FICTIONAL DEFENSE COMPUTER IN THE MOVIE *WARGAMES*

The only sensible approach to nuclear war is to never have one. The only sensible approach to birthing problems is to prevent them.

1. A pair of really hip obstetrical nurses taught me that pain is a function of tension, particularly during childbirth. Try meditation to reduce stress and tension. (See my chapter "Stress Reduction.")

2. Avoid drugs of all kinds: alcohol, cigarettes, illegal drugs, and all but the most essential medications.

3. *Nurse your baby from day one!* Did you know that breast milk actually changes composition to meet the needs of the developing baby? For example, preemies actually get a higher-protein,

higher-fat milk than full-term infants. There is apparently a very sensitive and complex relationship between the physiology of the mother and baby after birth as well as before. Colostrum immunity is an important part of this. Breast milk changes again during later nursing and during weaning, supplying still more protein and, yes, some iron. Do not supplement with formula: the breast, or the udder for that matter, makes more milk when demanded of it. If you use formula "also," you will start to make even less milk. A spiral will develop, resulting in no more breast milk. I am forever grateful to my sister-in-law for telling my wife to just "put the kid on the breast and suffer with it for a day or two. There will be more milk, don't worry." She was right. I remember the baby virtually drowning in milk after that. Make a point to read *The Womanly Art of Breastfeeding,* by the La Leche League International. This is a good, good book.

4. Take vitamin A as carotene. What about vitamin A safety? Let's talk polar bears, shall we? Since three-quarters of a pound of polar bear liver contains 7 or 8 *million* units of preformed vitamin A, this food is rightly forbidden by Eskimo tradition. If it is of any satisfaction to you, polar bears themselves are at risk for vitamin A overdose since they routinely eat entire seals at one sitting. Seals, as we all know, are a very good source of vitamin A, yielding 30 to 100 million units per seal. Believe it or not, 6 million units of A have been taken by humans at once—in fact, five times in a row—without fatality. Naturally, this is idiotic, and especially so during pregnancy. Large prenatal doses of preformed oil (retinol) vitamin A can produce birth defects. However, deficiency of vitamin A also can, and is much more likely. Human fetuses and newborn infants generally have low stores of vitamin A. Back in 1946, the AMA approved doses of 25,000 IU, but in the *Physicians' Desk Reference* you will find cautions beginning at 6,000 IU during pregnancy. But it must be emphasized that this refers to the preformed oil form of vitamin A, such as in fish oil or liver. ***These cautions do not apply to carotene***, which the body only makes into vitamin A as it needs to. Occasional intake of large quantities of preformed vitamin A oil is probably quite safe during pregnancy, bearing in mind that a three-ounce serving of liver contains over 50,000 IU as retinol. I have yet to spot a pregnancy warning on supermarket packages of liver. Using carotene-rich green and orange vegetables and vegetable juices provides a vastly larger margin for error. These foods cannot possibly do any harm to mom or baby.

5. Take vitamin C. Because it is water-soluble, vitamin C is very safe at all times, including pregnancy. As mentioned above, Frederick Klenner, M.D., gave large doses to three hundred pregnant women and reported virtually no complications in any of the pregnancies or deliveries. Other physicians have similarly reported that they have observed a complete absence of birth defects in babies born to vitamin C–taking mothers-to-be. Klenner also gave booster injections of vitamin C to 80 percent of the women upon admission to the hospital for childbirth. The results? Wonderful, indeed: First, labor was shorter and sweeter. (My children's mother, with her three-hour and two-hour total labor times, can vouch for this.) Second, stretch marks were seldom seen. Third, there were no postpartum hemorrhages at all. Fourth, there were no toxic manifestations or cardiac distress. Fifth and most important, there were *no* miscarriages in the entire group of three hundred women.

Among Klenner's patients were the Fultz quadruplets, who at the time were the only quads in the Southeast to have survived. These were each given 50 mg of C daily at birth. This is an important point: if Mom is taking vitamin C, it has to be continued for *both* mother and baby afterward as well. Failure to do this will result in the well-publicized "rebound effect." There-

229

fore, don't stop a good thing. If C is important enough for the woman to take before giving birth, then it is important enough for the baby to get after it has been born.

Varying amounts of vitamin C will be found in breast milk. If Mom takes a lot of C there will be C in the breast milk, too. If Mom is healing up and stressed out, there will probably be less C available to the baby. And if Mom is sick (or eating hospital food), there will almost certainly be a diminished C supply in her breast milk. The solution, again, is for both mother and baby to supplement with vitamin C.

We did exactly this with our babies, and were impressed with the results. You can finely powder a tasty chewable C tablet and put it on your finger or the baby's tongue. This should be done at every feeding. Infants do not need a lot of supplemental C, but they do need it frequently each day for maximum success. "Success" is easy to define: a healthy, happy baby that eats and sleeps well.

Very little vitamin C is found in formula, especially after it is packaged, opened, heated, poured, and oxidized during bottle feeding.

6. This is a tough order, but make time for your spouse so your baby will have two parents even after the novelty wears off. Fortunately, almost all authorities indicate that sex during pregnancy does not harm the baby. Common sense is needed, certainly, during the times immediately before and immediately after giving birth. But make a point to not neglect each other.

7. Avoid caffeine! It is America's most widely used and abused drug. Caffeine can enter the fetus's blood supply. Even two cups of coffee contains up to 250 mg of caffeine, a pharmacological dose. Five cans of cola have the same total amount, plus a lot more sugar (or, even worse, aspartame).

8. Concerned about high blood pressure? Then monitor your blood pressure, yourself, at home. It's easy and, because you avoid "white coat anxiety," it's actually more accurate than in a physician's office. You therefore reduce your chance of unneeded worry, unnecessary doctor interference, and resultant overprescription. If you are diagnosed with high blood pressure, consider taking a B-complex supplement before resorting to a drug. I know of a woman who was diagnosed with mild pre-eclampsia and chose to try a natural approach first. She took a B-complex tablet three to five times a day. She also cooked with the unfortunately-named "black fungus," a delicious mushroom found in many Oriental dishes. She used about two teaspoons of the dried mushroom, reconstituted in a cup of hot water before cooking, daily. Her blood pressure was normal in a few weeks. There were no further problems with the pregnancy.

9. Take vitamin E—at least 200 and perhaps 400 IU daily. This greatly reduces the chance of miscarriage. This is no myth: by the end of World War II, there were already dozens of medical studies confirming this. The cardiovascular benefits are excellent as well. Contrary to what many dietitians' textbooks say, getting foods containing other fat-soluble vitamins does NOT guarantee adequate vitamin E intake for pregnancy . . . or at any other time, for that matter.

10. Timing: age-wise, it is best to be pregnant when you are an adult woman (especially since adult men seem to have such trouble getting pregnant). Better not to be an old woman or a girl. Risks to mother and child are greatly increased among very young and very old mothers. However, many of the risks are due to age-related nutritional deficits. A good diet, properly

supplemented with folic acid (folate) and appropriate quantities of the other vitamins, will go a very long way to reduce birth defects.

Prevention of Miscarriage

Several friends, who are Catholic missionary sisters, asked me if vitamin C supplementation would help the people they work with in the South American rainforests. Since I think supplemental C is valuable for all humans, my answer was an unqualified yes. They took it from there, and for several years now have been giving multithousand-milligram doses of ascorbic acid powder to the natives daily. The result is that miscarriage and infant mortality rates have plummeted.

Lemons are more acidic than ascorbic acid. Lemons are properly known to science as *Citrus medica*. Since medieval times, "lymons" (as they were once known) have been known and prized for their ability to ensure healthy pregnancies and easier deliveries. Could it be that they are the original, renewable, portable vitamin C supplement?

Vitamin C

One reader asks:

"Some women's websites talk about vitamin C being somehow used as an abortifacient. Any input would be greatly appreciated as I am concerned about the health of my unborn baby."

It is simply incredible what people have been told about vitamins, isn't it?

Well, then, what are ascorbic acid's biological effects on the developing baby? Far from being an abortifacient, vitamin C in fact helps hold a healthy pregnancy right from the start.

Earlier we mentioned F. R. Klenner, M.D., who made it a rule to give very large doses to over 300 pregnant women and reported virtually no complications in any of the pregnancies or deliveries. Indeed, the hospital nurses around Reidsville, N.C., noted that the infants who were healthiest and happiest were the "Vitamin C babies."

Lendon Smith, M.D., said, "Vitamin C is our best defense and everyone should be on this one *even before birth*. Three thousand mgs daily for the pregnant woman is a start. The baby should get 100 mg per day per month of age. (The six-month-old would get 600 mg, the one-year-old gets a thousand mgs daily, the two-year-old-would get 2,000 mgs., etc.) A daily dose of 2,000 to 5,000 mg would be prudent for a lifetime."(From the doctor's former website, smithsez.com/AlivearticleonCancer.html)

That would make ascorbic acid one singularly lousy abortifacient, don't you think?

Not only that, but vitamin C also helps with conception.

Try having the man take megadoses of vitamin C for a few weeks prior. At least 6,000 milligrams a day, and as much as 20,000 mg/day guarantees very high sperm production. Divide the dose throughout the day for maximum effect. And that effect is what, exactly? More sperm,

231

stronger sperm, and better swimming sperm all occurred, at even lower daily C doses, in a University of Texas study. Gentlemen, take more C and you'll make vast quantities of superlative spermatozoa. You think this won't work? Have I shown you my baby pictures?

It was Dr. Klenner's experience, with the hundreds of babies that he delivered, that vitamin C was not only safe but especially beneficial in early pregnancy. Klenner gave "booster" injections of vitamin C to 80 percent of the women upon admission to the hospital for childbirth. The results? Wonderful, indeed:

First, labor was shorter and less painful. My children's mother, with her $2^1/_2$- and $1^3/_4$-hour labor times, can confirm this. Second, stretch marks were seldom to be seen. (I can vouch for this; after all, I was there.) Third, *there were no toxic manifestations and no cardiac distress. And, there were no postpartum hemorrhages at all.* (Stone, *The Healing Factor*, p. 191.)

This is exceptionally significant. For centuries, postpartum hemorrhage was a leading cause of death in childbirth. (Postpartum infection was another, usually caused by doctors that did not wash their hands. This rejection of the teachings of Dr. Ignaz Semmelweis and other "quacks" is legendary.)

Hemorrhage does very often occur in scorbutic (vitamin C deficient) patients (www.doctoryourself.com/mccormick.html). Klenner-sized doses of vitamin C prevent hemorrhage and save women's lives. One way it may do this is by strengthening the body's large and small blood vessels. Believe it or not, the press tried to make that out to be a problem, claiming that vitamin C's "thickening" of artery walls would reduce blood flow. It does not. (www.doctoryourself.com/hoffer_factoids.html)

And finally, here is what I consider to be a definitive statement from the *Journal of the American Medical Association (JAMA)*: "Harmful effects have been mistakenly attributed to vitamin C, including hypoglycemia, rebound scurvy, infertility, mutagenesis, and destruction of vitamin B(12). Health professionals should recognize that vitamin C does not produce these effects" (Levine, M., et al. [1999]. *JAMA* 281(15):1419).

Vitamin C does not cause birth defects, or infertility, or miscarriage. (It does not cause kidney stones, either.) What vitamin C *does* do is deliver healthier babies.

Read Dr. Lendon Smith's *Clinical Guide to the Use of Vitamin C* for free at www.seanet.com/~alexs/ascorbate/198x/smith-lh-clinical_guide_1988.htm.

PREEEMIES AND PROZAC

Pregnant women taking antidepressants such as Prozac (fluoxetine, a selective serotonin reuptake inhibitor) are nearly five times more likely to have premature babies (Chambers CD, et al. [1996]. Birth outcomes in pregnant women taking fluoxetine. *N Engl J Med* 335 (14):1010–5): "The 73 infants exposed (to the drug) during the third trimester had higher rates of premature delivery (relative risk, 4.8), admission to special-care nurseries (relative risk, 2.6), and poor neonatal adaptation, including respiratory difficulty, cyanosis on feeding, and jitteriness (relative risk, 8.7). Birth weight was also lower and birth length shorter in infants exposed to fluoxetine late in gestation."

Vitamin E

1922 was the year the USSR was formed and "Little Orphan Annie" began. Trumpeter Al Hirt and future heart transplant pioneer Christiaan Barnard were born. Alexander Graham Bell died. And vitamin E was discovered by H. M. Evans and K. S. Bishop. In 1936, Evans' team had isolated alpha-tocopherol from wheat germ oil and vitamin E was beginning to be widely appreciated, and the consequences of deficiency better known. *Health Culture* magazine said in January 1936, "The fertility food factor (is) now called vitamin E. Excepting for the abundance of that vitamin in whole grains, there could not have been any perpetuation of the human race. Its absence from the diet makes for irreparable sterility occasioned by a complete degeneration of the germinal cells of the male generative glands. (T)he expectant mother requires vitamin E to insure the carriage of her charge to a complete and natural term. If her diet is deficient in vitamin E . . . the woman is very apt to abort. . . It is more difficult to insure a liberal vitamin E supply in the daily average diet than to insure an adequate supply of any other known vitamin."

Since the word *tocopherol* is taken from the Greek words for "to carry offspring" or "to bring forth childbirth," it is easy enough to see how Evan Shute and other obstetricians were drawn into the work. As early as 1931, Vogt-Moller of Denmark successfully treated habitual abortion in human females with wheat germ oil vitamin E. By 1939 he had treated several hundred women with a success rate of about 80 percent. In 1937, both Young in England and the Shutes in Canada reported success in combating threatened abortion and pregnancy toxemias as well. A. L. Bacharach's 1940 statistical analysis of published clinical results "show quite definitely that vitamin E is of value in recurrent abortions."

Yet when the MDRs (Minimum Daily Requirements) first came out in 1941, there was no mention of vitamin E. It was not until 1959 that vitamin E was recognized by the U.S. Food and Drug Administration as necessary for human existence, and not until 1968 that any government recommendation for vitamin E would be issued. (From Vitamin E: A cure in search of recognition, by Andrew W. Saul. Reprinted with permission from the *Journal of Orthomolecular Medicine*, 2003; 18(3,4):205–212.) All references and the rest of the above quoted paper are at www.doctoryourself.com/evitamin.htm.)

And, as attributed to Ed Sullivan, "And now you know. . ." Taking vitamin E (at least 200 and perhaps 400 IU daily) greatly reduces the chance of miscarriage. This is no myth: by the end of WWII, there were already dozens of medical studies confirming this. They are reviewed in a 1953 medical textbook, *The Vitamins in Medicine*, by Bicknell and Prescott (William Heinemann Medical Books Ltd.; Third Edition.).

Other Problems During Pregnancy and Lactation

Morning Sickness

1. Try a natural multivitamin, not an artificially colored one. Paint can be nauseating to eat.

2. Take all supplements on a full stomach, or better yet, in the middle of each meal.

3. Avoid ferrous sulfate iron supplements. Many doctors still prescribe this cookie-tossing form of iron in too large an amount, and without enough supplemental C for absorption. Constipation is almost guaranteed with ferrous sulfate. Use ferrous fumerate, ferrous gluconate, or especially carbonyl iron instead.

233

4. Try the homeopathic remedy Natrum Phos 6X for simple morning sickness, and possibly Kali Phos or Natrum Sulph.

5. You could also try some fresh, tasty juice first thing to get off to a good start in the morning. Fluids are always good, and it is a light, nutritious, natural way to get the blood sugar up.

6. Severe and prolonged vomiting requires medical attention.

Constipation

Constipation is quite common during gestation. It is also quite easy to avoid, as my thrilling chapter on hemorrhoids explains. Also see the above recommendation about avoiding ferrous sulfate iron supplements. When pregnant, do not take medication for this or any other condition if you can possibly avoid doing so.

Weight Gain or Loss

Weight gain is natural, necessary, and desirable during pregnancy. A woman does *not* have to "get fat," however! My wife gained 25 pounds to deliver a 10 pound, 2 ounce baby girl. Though a slightly larger weight gain is normal and fine, it really should be no more than 35 pounds or so; under thirty is better. No fasting or weight loss attempts during pregnancy or lactation! Eat right and exercise appropriately, and the weight will take care of itself.

Hemorrhoids

Constipation can cause hemorrhoids, so see the constipation recommendations above. Also, avoid gulping unchewed cheese pizzas. Bear in mind that babies and amniotic fluid are heavy, which puts a lot of pressure on your rectum. Supplemental vitamin C will often help here, because C strengthens connective and vascular tissues. Topical application of vitamin E will also definitely help.

Heartburn

1. Eat frequent, small meals. In other words, "graze" rather than feast.

2. Chew your food especially well. This simple measure really works.

3. Combine your foods especially well. No need to obsess over this, but from your own experience, you can tell that some foods do not mix well in your stomach.

Recommended Reading

Bicknell F and Prescott F. *The Vitamins in Medicine,* 3rd edition. Milwaukee, WI: Lee Foundation, 1953.

Billings E and Westmore A. *The Billings Method.* New York: Ballantine, 1983.

Case HS. *Vitamins and Pregnancy: The Real Story.* Basic Health Publications, in press.

Davis A. *Let's Eat Right to Keep Fit.* New York: Signet, 1970, 61.

Hillemann HH. *Developmental Malformation in Man and Other Animals.* [A Bibliography]. Milwaukee, WI: Lee Foundation, undated.

Hillemann HH. "Maternal Malnutrition and Fetal Prenatal Development Malformation" [Address at Oregon State College] (9 November 1956).

234

Hillemann HH. "Maternal Malnutrition and Congenital Deformity" Address at Grants Pass, Oregon] (17 March 1958).

Hillemann HH. The spectrum of congenital defect, experimental and clinical. *Journal of Applied Nutrition* 14 (1961): 2.

Klein D. A coroner's-eye view of drug babies. *Los Angeles Times* (3 March 1991). [Cited in Farrell W. *The Myth of Male Power.* New York: Simon and Schuster, 1993, 413.]

Mendelsohn R. *Confessions of a Medical Heretic.* New York: Warner Books, 1979.

Mendelsohn R. *How to Raise a Healthy Child in Spite of Your Doctor.* Chicago: Contemporary Books, 1984.

Mendelsohn R. *Malepractice: How Doctors Manipulate Women.* Chicago: Contemporary Books, 1982.

Shute WE. *The Vitamin E Book.* New Canaan, CT: Keats Publishing, 1978.

Shute WE. *Your Child and Vitamin E.* New Canaan, CT: Keats Publishing, 1979.

Smith L, ed. *Clinical Guide to the Use of Vitamin C: The Clinical Experiences of Frederick R. Klenner, M.D.* Tacoma, WA: Life Sciences Press, 1988.

Stone I. *The Healing Factor.* New York: Grosset and Dunlap, 1972.

The Womanly Art of Breastfeeding, revised edition. Franklin Park, Illinois: La Leche League International, 1963.

Williams SR. "Nutrition During Lactation and Pregnancy" in *Nutrition and Diet Therapy,* 6th edition. St. Louis: Mosby, 1989.

"Drugs make a well person sick.
Why would they make a sick person well?
—ABRAM HOFFER, M.D.

At the time, I had never encountered a case of psoriasis before. So I looked it up in the *Merck Manual* while Frank sat there and waited as patiently as he could.

"It says here that there is no cure for psoriasis, Frank," I said hesitantly.

"That's what everybody has told me," he said. "But I think nutrition is worth a try."

I couldn't fault that reasoning.

"I've got to do something," Frank continued. "The doctors, and I've seen plenty of 'em, say there isn't anything they can do except give me these ointments and lotions. I said the ointments and lotions don't help. They said I should learn to live with it."

"How do you feel about that?" I asked.

"You can imagine how I feel!" Frank answered. "There is no way I'm going to spend the rest of my life itching and looking like this." Frank's psoriasis came and went periodically, but at that time it was back with a vengeance, and where the world could plainly see it: on his arms, neck, forehead, and face.

"What would you be willing to do to get well?" I responded.

"Anything," he said. "Anything at all, and I'm not kidding."

Frank was in his late twenties, energetic and prematurely bald. And resolute though he was, I expected that he was about to have his resolve sorely tested by what I suggested next: a complete change of diet to a naturopathic regimen of fresh foods and loads of vegetable juices, plus lecithin and assorted vitamins, including some extra vitamin D.

He didn't bat an eyelash.

I sensed that, unlike most people, Frank not only wanted it all but was willing to get his hands dirty to get it. He might therefore be willing to earnestly try the classic health-nut cure-all: fresh vegetable juice fasting. Really hard-core, nature-cure quacks uniformly hold to the doctrine that whatever is wrong with a body, systemic toxemia is the root cause and fasting is the real cure. I presented the idea to Frank, who embraced it at once.

"So I could alternate a week of just vegetable juices with a week of a mostly fresh-and-raw diet," Frank concluded. I agreed. "How long do I keep it going? Oh, I know: until I'm symptom-free, of course."

"Provided you are feeling good doing it, yes."

So off he went to juice like crazy.

Right off the bat, Frank's psoriasis began to fade. He was much better within days. In little over a week, there was no trace whatsoever. But Frank's symptoms had gone away on their own before, so we all decided to bide our time.

Week after week, month after month, Frank stayed completely free of anything even remotely resembling psoriasis. He also felt better in unexpected ways: he said he was happier, sleeping better, thinking more clearly, had more energy, and hadn't a trace of a cold or any other sickness since he'd begun the program. He had lost a few pounds, but then his weight had leveled off automatically. He was one fit and trim, clear-skinned, happy guy.

Years passed, and Frank kept juicing on a regular basis. He never had psoriasis again. Of course, there is no cure for psoriasis, so this cannot be. Frank must have been deluded.

Yet I've seen this approach work on other people, too. Part-time vegetable juice fasting, employed intelligently, is safe and effective for reasonably healthy, nonpregnant people. Those who ridicule it should first meet Frank, who will confirm what it did for him.

Or his dermatologist, who now will, also.

Probably.

"No amount of evidence can persuade anyone who is not listening."

—ABRAM HOFFER, M.D., PH.D.

Duck and Cover

As schoolchildren, we were actually taught in school, and practiced in class, how to duck under our little desks in the event of a nuclear attack. Quaint now, perhaps, but it was no joke at the time. I was a very little boy during the very heart of the times of US atmospheric testing. When I was three years old, **the US did sixty-two atmospheric nuclear tests in just one year**. I was eight when Linus Pauling and other scientists finally put a stop to it in 1963.

According to the Natural Resources Defense Council, governments have conducted over 2,000 nuclear tests worldwide since 1945 (www.nrdc.org/nuclear/nudb/datab15.asp). The United States conducted over 1,000 of them . . . and **215 of those were in the open atmosphere**.

No one asked me or anyone else if we wanted any of those 215 atmospheric exposures. 215 in 18 years. Hard to imagine, but it happened. Somehow we got through it. And we will get through recent nuclear accidents (first in Chernobyl, then in Japan) too, in part simply because the Ukraine and Japan are so far away. That is not a satisfying answer, is it? With 104 active nuclear power plants in the US, there is one near you.

If you will pardon me, the real cure, the long-term solution, is widespread use of solar and geothermic power. But for now, take your nutrients.

RADIATION RELEASES:
WHAT YOU CAN DO TO PROTECT YOURSELF

Linus Pauling[1], Andrei Sakharov[2], and other scientists estimated that there would be an extra 10,000 deaths worldwide for each megaton nuclear test in the atmosphere. A nuclear reactor can contain much more radioactive material than a nuclear weapon. The 2012 Fukushima disaster involved six reactors, plus stored additional radioactive material and nuclear waste.

Ionizing radiation acts to damage living tissue by forming free radicals. Essentially, electrons are ripped from molecules. Removing an electron from an atom or molecule turns it into an ion, hence the term ionizing radiation. X-rays, gamma rays, alpha- and beta-radiation are all ionizing. Most of the damage occurs from ionizing radiation generating free radicals in water, as water molecules are by far the most abundant in the body.

Free-radical scavengers, as the name suggests, mop up the damaging radicals produced by radiation. The more common term for free radical scavenger is antioxidant. Antioxidants replace the electrons stripped from molecules by ionizing radiation. Antioxidants have long been used in the treatment of radiation poisoning.[3-7] Most of the harm from ionizing radiation occurs from free radical damage which may be quenched by the free electrons antioxidants provide. Fortunately, safe antioxidants are widely available as nutritional supplements.

Vitamin C is of particular importance and should be included at high intakes for anyone trying to minimize radiation poisoning. High dose vitamin C provides continual antioxidant flow through the body. When it is used up, it is excreted in the urine. Importantly, it can chelate, or grab onto, radioactive heavy metal atoms and help eliminate them from the body. Large doses of vitamin C (about 3,000 mg, taken 4 times a day for a total of 12,000 mg) would exemplify antioxidant treatment. Higher doses (25,000 mg intravenously) have been used by Dr. Atsuo Yanagisawa and colleagues.[8–9] Dr. Gert Schuitemaker has provided a review of vitamin C as a protectant against radiation damage.[10]

The Japanese College of Intravenous Therapy has released a video for people wishing to learn more about how to protect themselves from contamination by taking large doses of vitamin C. It can be found online with an internet search, or at http://www.youtube.com/ watch?v=Rbm_MH3nSdM and related links.

References

1. The Nobel Foundation (1962) *The Nobel Peace Prize 1962, Linus Pauling Biography,* http://www.nobelprize.org/ nobel_prizes/peace/laureates/1962/pauling-bio.html.

2. Sakharov A. (1975) *The Nobel Peace Prize 1975, Andrei Sakharov, Autobiography,* http://www.nobelprize.org/ nobel_prizes/peace/laureates/1975/sakharov-autobio.html.

3. Brown SL, Kolozsvary A, Liu J, et al: Antioxidant diet supplementation starting 24 hours after exposure reduces radiation lethality. *Radiat Res,* 2010; 173: 462–468.

4. Zueva NA, Metelitsa LA, Kovalenko AN, et al: Immunomodulating effect of berlithione in clean-up workers of the Chernobyl nuclear plant accident [Article in Russian]. *Lik Sprava,* 2002; (1): 24-26.

5. Yamamoto T, Kinoshita M et al. Pretreatment with ascorbic acid prevents lethal gastrointestinal syndrome in mice receiving a massive amount of radiation. *J Radiat Res* (Tokyo) 2010; 51(2):145–56

6. Gaby A. Intravenous Nutrient Therapy: the "Myers' Cocktail". *Alt Med Rev* 2002; 7(5):389:403

7. Narra VR, Howell RW, Sastry KS, Rao DV. Vitamin C as a radioprotector against iodine-131 in vivo. *J Nucl Med* 1993; 34(4):637-40

8. Yanagisawa A. Orthomolecular approaches against radiation exposure. Presentation Orthomolecular Medicine Today Conference. Toronto 2011. Free download of the presentation at http://www.doctoryourself.com/Radiation_VitC.pptx.pdf)

9. Green MH, Lowe JE et al. Effect of diet and vitamin C on DNA strand breakage in freshly-isolated human white blood cells. *Mutat Res* 1994; 316(2):91–102

10. Schuitemaker GE. Vitamin C as protection against radiation exposure. *J Orthomolecular Med* 2011, 26: 3; 141–145. [Also in Dutch: Schuitemaker G.E. Radioactiviteit in Japan: Orthomoleculair antwoord. *Ortho* 2011:3, June. http://www.ortho.nl]

Iodine and Fallout

Radioactive iodine from a nuclear event is taken up by the body from air, food, and water. Preventively consuming normal iodine helps prevent your body from taking up radioactive iodine. I first learned this way back in 1976 from Michael Ash, M.D., of Cornwall, UK. More on him later. The United States Environmental Protection Agency basically agrees. (Scroll down at www.epa.gov/rpdweb00/radionuclides/iodine.html.)   Your thyroid gland soaks up most of the iodine it can get, and does not care whether it is radioactive or not. But you do. If the thyroid has ample normal iodine, it is less likely to take up radioactive iodine. A wet paper towel absorbs little water. Excess iodine is excreted in the urine; a saturated paper towel drips. The analogy isn't perfect, but you get the idea.

Radioactive iodine has a half-life of only about eight days. That means that a milligram of it will be only half a milligram in just over a week. That half-mg decays to one-quarter in another eight days, and decays to one-eighth in another eight days, and at the end of just over a month, you'd only have one-sixteenth of a mg left. With radioactive substances, even a little is far from good. A radioactive substance is generally considered trouble for ten to twenty half-lives. But at least this stuff does not endure for thousands or millions of years. As Marty Feldman quipped in the movie *Young Frankenstein,* "Could be worse."

The iodine you take to block radioactive iodine uptake may be virtually any kind, taken any way. You get iodine from sushi, because the "seaweed" wrap, nori, is actually an algae that contains iodine. No, you do not have to eat raw fish. That is sashimi. Sushi can be cooked (in some states, crab and shrimp sushi has to be cooked). You can have vegetarian sushi as well: cucumber, carrot, avocado, celery, and such. But then there is an onion in the ointment, so to speak: most nori comes from China and Japan.

Sea vegetables are the foods that are naturally highest in iodine. Kelp and seaweeds are not as bad as they sound. I had a plateful of them at a really out-there veggie restaurant decades ago. I still remember the meal. First of all, it looked weird. Green, brown, and dark red limp leaves filled entirely too much of my plate. But I was with food-fanatical friends, it was a set lunch, and I did not want to be a wet blanket. So I braced myself, closed my eyes, and ate the wet leaves. Surprise: they tasted good. Better than most "normal" American canned vegetables, at the very least. I ate the lot. Cooking does not destroy iodine. Just as well: raw sea veggies is probably best for sea otters. No wonder they are so cute and playful: they aren't mineral deficient like most Americans are.

Kelp powder, kelp granules, and kelp tablets are also good sources of iodine. Read the label to see how good.

If you do not want anything to do with any of the above delicacies, you can simply rub tincture of iodine on your skin and take it in that way. My favorite non-tastebud vector for taking in iodine is to put a drop or two of iodine tincture in a half-gallon of juice. Shake and consume as you normally would. Now, you have an iodine-fortified beverage. I drink several glasses daily.

A note on skulls and bones: You have doubtless learned that iodine tincture is a poison. If you drink it straight, it most certainly is. Don't do it. However, a couple of drops diluted in a half-gallon (that's nearly two liters) is without the slightest danger. And, a mere drop (or two) will do ya. The government says you only need about 150 micrograms per day. A microgram is very tiny: one millionth of a gram, and a gram is about a quarter-teaspoon. The highest health-nut daily iodine recommendation I have seen is 12 milligrams per day. A milligram is one-thousandth of a gram, but a thousand times a microgram. I haven't lost you yet, have I? This means that 12 mg is 12,000 mcg, and that is 80 times the RDA. I do not know how much iodine is bioavailable from a drop of iodine tincture. It is somewhere in the middle of the range.

Is this worthwhile? Yes. After two atomic bombs were dropped on Japan at the end of WWII, there was a lot of radiation sickness. Unsurprisingly, the further away from the blast area, the less severe the sickness. There was one notable exception: people living near or at the seashore had less radiation poisoning than inland residents . . . even if the seaside residents were actually closer to ground zero. Their seaweed-rich diet is likely the reason for their advantage.

Niacin and Fallout

I recall from Dr. Michael Ash's 1976 lecture that he had actually applied for a patent for a "Radiation Sweet" (that's "candy" to us Yanks). The active ingredients were to be iodine and niacin.

Why niacin? Because niacin is needed for your body to make nicotinamide adenine dinucleotide (NAD). NAD helps protect and repair DNA. Radiation damages DNA, causing malfunction and mutation. More niacin means plentiful NAD, and that is a good thing. NAD helps prevent cancer. There is no debate on that. (Scroll down at http://lpi.oregonstate.edu/infocenter/vitamins/niacin/.)

However, there is debate on just how much niacin is needed to have a protective effect against cancer. The US RDA is less than 18 mg/day. That is almost certainly too little for optimum protection from radiation. I think a minimum of 500 mg/day, in divided doses, is a good idea. Personally, I take several thousand mg/day of niacin, and so did Dr. Abram Hoffer, the world's premiere niacin researcher. If the customary "niacin flush" bothers you, you can take either niacinamide or inositol hexaniacinate. Neither of these forms causes flushing.

What Else?

Vitamin E has been shown to reduce tissue damage from actual radiation burns. This is very different from fallout exposure. I suspect that high-fiber diets would help, and drinking more liquid would as well. Raw fresh vegetable juices provide both, with carotene antioxidants that are almost always protective. Avoiding food from contaminated areas is an obvious step. Eating home-grown organic produce is ideal. Extra antioxidant supplementation, especially vitamin C, would certainly be a good idea.

RADIOACTIVE FALLOUT: CAN NUTRITIONAL SUPPLEMENTS HELP?

by Damien Downing, M.D.

241

The Fukushima nuclear accident has already been described as "the largest accidental release of radiation we have ever seen,"[1] and it's not over yet.

Already, radioactive plutonium, strontium, and iodine have reached the continental USA.

SO SHOULD WE WORRY? AND, WHAT CAN WE DO ABOUT IT?

When the earthquake and tsunami hit northeast Japan on 11th March, it disabled all the multiple safety mechanisms at the Fukushima nuclear power plant. Fires started in three of the six reactors, and 24 hours later a large hydrogen explosion caused the collapse of part of the structure. From then on, radioactive material would have been released to the atmosphere. This is reasonable to assume, despite the usual assurances from the operators, TEPCO, and the Japan Atomic Energy Agency. Six days later, after all, traces of radioactive material were detected in Washington State[2] and then right down to California. This material can only have reached the USA by the airborne route.

Fukushima is now off the media map, replaced by dramatic political events. Contrast this with the coverage that was given to the Chernobyl disaster. Perhaps at that time there was a sense that the destruction of a nuclear power plant in the Ukraine was a metaphor for the failure of the Soviet Union. But Fukushima is, or will eventually prove to be, a far worse disaster. It is one that will be underplayed. The world is committed to nuclear power, and we will not be shown its true dangers. Do not expect to be told the whole truth when reading reassuring statements from industry or governments. Fukushima is affecting us all.

Radioactive elements released from Fukushima include plutonium, strontium, cesium, and iodine. Ten days after the tsunami, Japanese scientists reported increased radioactive cesium and iodine in seawater offshore of Fukushima, and they rapidly reached levels "more than 1 million times higher than previously existed."[3] More serious radiation levels are likely in the USA when this polluted seawater reaches the west coast, which is estimated to take from 18 months to 3 years.

MORE SERIOUS? WHY?

Because:

- there will be radioactive elements that are ingested or absorbed by people, animals, and plants

- they will biomagnify, concentrating up the food chain, as do all pollutants

- they won't go away; once inside us they will stay there.

There are two different kinds of radiation: external, when you are exposed to radiation sources around you (the Fukushima clean-up workers are currently getting a lot of that), but which stops when you are no longer near the source; and internal, when a source of radiation gets into your body and stays there. This is much more serious because you are constantly exposed for much longer. Former Russian agent Alexander Litvinenko was killed in London that way in 2006—by being given, probably swallowing in a beverage, some highly radioactive polonium. Traces of the same polonium were found on some airline seats, but nobody seems to have been harmed by sitting in them.

You may already have been exposed to (mostly) depleted uranium back in 2003. Despite official denials, it does seem to be true that increases in uranium were detected in Berkshire, England, nine days after the start of Shock and Awe[4]. To get there it must have traveled across the whole of the USA.

By the time it reaches the continental USA the radiation from Fukushima will be very spread out, so individual doses will be very small. But they will be on top of the radiation to which we are all exposed already: from X-rays, from flying at 30.000 feet, from radon in the ground, and on top of all our other toxic exposures such as mercury, pesticides, and thousands of other chemicals. This is the "Who killed Julius Caesar?" phenomenon; the answer is at least 23 people, stabbing him at least 36 times. None of them could have been proved to have caused his death, but they all contributed to it. All the poisons to which we are exposed add up to harm us, too.

Epidemiologist Dr. Steven Wing makes the useful point that whether a dose of radiation is spread thickly across just a few thousand people, or much more thinly across tens of millions, around the same number of cancers will result. So although the increase in individual risk from Fukushima is likely to be tiny for any individual in the USA, it will still amount to a major public health problem.

- The Chernobyl nuclear disaster certainly caused thousands of premature deaths in a sweep across northern Europe, and may have caused more than a million deaths[5]. But Fukushima is worse in several ways;

- At Chernobyl there were only 180 tons of nuclear fuel on-site, whereas at Fukushima there are thousands of tons.

- Chernobyl is 250 miles from the nearest sea, but Fukushima is on the coast. Already the radiation released to sea from there is 10 to 100 times worse than Chernobyl.

- Chernobyl was sealed into a "sarcophagus," although too late to prevent some airborne release. Fukushima is and will likely continue releasing radiation into the sea for some time.

Best-case scenarios (from the nuclear industry, of course) are saying it will take nine months to shut the reactors down and seal them. Skeptics say that you truly cannot "seal" a reactor with concrete, because the radioactive material will then go downwards, into the soil and the water table, and end up in the sea anyway.

You may say; "Surely the government has this all in hand?" Well, the strange thing is that the EPA is set to revise its Protective Action Guides—the levels of radiation that it deems safe for us to be exposed to, from food, water, air or soil. Some of the upper limits are rising more than 1,000-fold, into the "will definitely give cancer to some people" zone. You can read more about this here,[6] which also gives useful e-mail addresses in case you want to express your views to the EPA. I know it looks like another one of "those" websites, but this is corroborated many times over elsewhere.

The European Union has moved fast to respond; on March 25 EU Regulation 297/2011[7] came into force. Although this looks like a sensible precaution, requiring testing of foods from affected areas of Japan for radioactivity, it in fact introduces upper limits for radioactivity that are significantly higher than previous ones. Baffling.

WHAT CAN YOU DO?

For each radionuclide there is a different risk and a different set of measures. The US Department of Homeland Security funded a guidelines' paper in 2006.[8]

Radioactive iodine-131: For this threat, we take regular iodine, to minimize the amount of the bad stuff that gets taken up by the thyroid. Various forms, such as potassium iodide, do work, but only if given before or within 12 hours of exposure. And since I-131 has a half-life of eight days, by the time it gets from Fukushima to the USA there won't be much radioactivity left. So don't worry about that one.

Uranium (half-life: thousands of years) is there in Fukushima in large quantities in the fuel rods. No reports of it being found in the environment yet, but there's plenty of time. And even depleted (nonradioactive) uranium is a highly toxic heavy metal, and one to which anybody who served in Gulf I or II, or in Bosnia or Kosovo, has probably been exposed. So a Fukushima exposure would just add to that toxicity. For uranium there are protocols worked out by the US military. Large doses of sodium bicarbonate (baking soda, in the orange box) minimize the damage caused by uranium and encourage its excretion in the kidneys. You can buy bicarb in bulk for less than a dollar per pound. It is certainly worth stocking up on. You can absorb it through the skin, so a good fistful in a warm bath, which you sit in for 15–20 minutes, is the simplest way to take it in.

Cesium-137 has a half-life of 30 years, and like uranium is still a toxic metal even when not radioactive. The US government stockpiles the chemical Prussian Blue for removing cesium.[9] Prussian Blue is ferric ferrocyanide—$Fe_7(CN)_{18}$ plus a load of water. It is not absorbed from the gut; it can only trap cesium (and also thallium) as it is recycled through the bile to gut to blood again. It works by cutting the biological half-life (time to get rid of half the total body burden) from about 80 days to 25. But that would still take three months to bring the level below 10 percent of starting, which is plenty of time to do harm. Prussian Blue was used in photography before we went digital, so there might be some left in your garage. Leave it there and DO NOT try this at home. Prussian Blue contains cyanide, a strong poison.

Plutonium: When uranium is used in a reactor it converts to plutonium, which is a big worry. Plutonium is extremely dangerous. It is estimated that one gram could kill ten million people. This is what the CDC has to say[10]:

243

Because it emits alpha particles, plutonium is most dangerous when inhaled. When plutonium particles are inhaled, they lodge in the lung tissue. The alpha particles can kill lung cells, which causes scarring of the lungs, leading to further lung disease and cancer. Plutonium can enter the blood stream from the lungs and travel to the kidneys, meaning that the blood and the kidneys will be exposed to alpha particles. Once plutonium circulates through the body, it concentrates in the bones, liver, and spleen, exposing these organs to alpha particles. Plutonium that is ingested from contaminated food or water does not pose a serious threat to humans because the stomach does not absorb plutonium easily and so it passes out of the body in the feces.

What can you do about it? There are no grounds for thinking iodine or bicarbonate will work. The medical recommendation at present is DTPA, which is a version of EDTA—a chelating agent, specific to transuranic elements.

In each of the above exposures, of course you should get to a doctor, fast, and get the appropriate treatment. But an exposure coming from Fukushima is likely to be a dirty mix of any or all of these, so we need some universal measures. There are three worthwhile ones, all of which you can do for yourself:

ANTIOXIDANT VITAMINS

It's easy to get down to the health store and buy some bottles of these, and in these circumstances an overdose is the last thing to worry about. While the shelves are full of nutritional and herbal products that might help, my personal advice would be to take:

- Vitamin C (the body's main water-soluble antioxidant) approximately 3,000 to 5,000 milligrams, three times daily; option to combine water-soluble and oil-based forms.

- Vitamin E (the main fat-soluble antioxidant) mixed tocopherols and tocotrienols, around 400 IU, once daily.

- R Lipoic Acid (operates in both water and lipid compartments, spares both vitamins C and E) 100-plus mg, three times daily.

GLUTATHIONE

This amino acid is known to chelate certain minerals, but there's no evidence that it works on radioactive ones. Some experts say nothing does. However, it's a crucial antioxidant, which will protect against radiation damage and help to mop up the toxic molecules produced. Take loads; say 1,000 mg three times daily. And because it can be tricky to absorb, consider using the oil-based version that you rub into your skin.

PHOSPHATIDYLCHOLINE

If you turned up in the ER in an eastern bloc country with acute radiation exposure, they would give you an IV shot of phosphatidylcholine. It is found in egg yolk, organ meats, and lecithin supplements and is easily absorbed into our membranes as a phospholipid. There are no human experiments I know of, thankfully, but this is backed up by some doctors: "Ionizing radiation first disturbs the phospholipid metabolism, then provokes severe inflammatory reactions, and finally leads to death . . . The survival of rats exposed to lethal doses of radiation was clearly prolonged with phospholipid supplementation."[11]

You can get liquid or capsules; take at least a tablespoon or equivalent daily, with food.

If you've got the time, it's wise to build all of these up slowly, or they may give you loose bowels for a few days. If you haven't got the time, you have bigger things to worry about.

(Dr. Damien Downing is president of the British Society for Allergy, Environmental and Nutritional Medicine. He practices orthomolecular medicine in London.)

References and Links

1. Ken Buesseler, marine radiochemist at Woods Hole Oceanographic Institution;

http://articles.cnn.com/2011-04-26/opinion/buesseler.fukushima.radiation_1_radioactive-contaminants-chernobyl-nuclear-plant-waters?_s=PM:OPINION.

2. www.epa.gov/japan2011/.

3. http://ex-skf.blogspot.com/2011/03/fukushima-i-nuke-plant-radioactive.html.

4. http://blog.imva.info/medicine/danger-concern-sanity.

5. Yablokov, AV.(2009). Mortality after the Chernobyl catastrophe. *Ann N Y Acad Sci.* 1181:192–216.

6. www.collapsenet.com/free-resources/collapsenet-public-access/item/723-fallout.

7. http://eur-lex.europa.eu/LexUriServ/LexUriServ.do?uri=OJ:L:2011:080:0005:0008:EN:PDF.

8. www.acnmonline.org/docs/MMRSManual-Carol_Marcus.pdf.

9. www.remm.nlm.gov/prussianblue.htm.

10. http://emergency.cdc.gov/radiation/isotopes/plutonium.asp.

11. Gundermann, KJ. (1993). The "essential" phospholipids as a membrane therapeutic. Institute of Pharmacology and Toxicology, Szczecin, Poland.

References

Boyonoski AC, Spronck JC, Gallacher LM, et al. Niacin deficiency decreases bone marrow poly(ADP-ribose) and the latency of ethylnitrosourea-induced carcinogenesis in rats. *J Nutr.* 2002;132(1):108–114. (PubMed)

Franceschi S, Bidoli E, Negri E, et al. Role of macronutrients, vitamins and minerals in the aetiology of squamous-cell carcinoma of the oesophagus. *Int J Cancer.* 2000;86(5):626–631. (PubMed)

Gensler HL, Williams T, Huang AC, Jacobson EL. Oral niacin prevents photocarcinogenesis and photoimmunosuppression in mice. *Nutr Cancer.* 1999;34(1):36–41. (PubMed)

Hageman GJ, Stierum RH. Niacin, poly(ADP-ribose) polymerase-1 and genomic stability. *Mutat Res.* 2001;475(1–2):45–56. (PubMed)

Jacobson EL. Niacin deficiency and cancer in women. *J Am Coll Nutr.* 1993;12(4):412–416. (PubMed)

Negri E, Franceschi S, Bosetti C, et al. Selected micronutrients and oral and pharyngeal cancer. *Int J Cancer.* 2000;86(1):122–127. (PubMed)

Jacobson EL, Shieh WM, Huang AC. Mapping the role of NAD metabolism in prevention and treatment of carcinogenesis. *Mol Cell Biochem.* 1999;193(1–2):69–74. (PubMed)

Weitberg AB. Effect of nicotinic acid supplementation in vivo on oxygen radical-induced genetic damage in human lymphocytes. *Mutat Res.* 1989;216(4):197–201. (PubMed)

For Further Reading

Downing, D. Radioactive fallout: Can nutritional supplements help? Orthomolecular Medicine News Service, May 11, 2011, http://orthomolecular.org/resources/omns/v07n04.shtml.

Rectal Bleeding

"It's time to take the bull by the tail and face the situation."

—W. C. FIELDS

Bleeding is scary, and rectal bleeding is the scariest. Marjorie, age fifty-three, came to visit. She was losing half a cup of blood a day rectally. That is a lot of blood; a woman's entire five-day menstrual flow is only about that much in total. Marjorie was worried, and rightly so. She had seen an assortment of doctors and was currently under the care of a proctologist who could find nothing really wrong with her bowel. He found some slight, general inflammation during a sigmoidoscopy, but no lumps, bumps, polyps, or lesions of note. He told her that there was nothing to be done except keep an eye on it.

Keep looking. Not a nice thought under the circumstances.

Marjorie's question to me was the obvious one: what can be done? My standard answer, and it is also the truth, is that I wasn't sure, but natural therapies are generally worth a full and fair trial.

Years ago I had read an article from *California Medicine* about a doctor who treated bleeding peptic ulcers with cabbage juice, of all things. It was just crazy enough to get my attention: he gave one hundred hospitalized patients four glasses (yes, that's one full quart) of raw cabbage juice daily. The doctor, Garnett Cheney, M.D., reported pain relief in a few days, and healing in one third of the customary time. All this, not with medicines, not with surgery, but with cabbage juice. And he published his findings in a medical journal, no less. In 1953!

Figuring that it would be hard to hurt yourself with cabbages, unless you dropped them on your toe, I told Marjorie about the study. She was a lot more interested than a healthy person would have been, and said she'd do it. She had little to lose that she wasn't already losing.

Marjorie called back a week and a half later. She hadn't bought a juicer, but was putting fresh cabbage through her blender, and then straining it through cheesecloth to get the juice. She was drinking four glasses a day this way. Her bleeding had been reduced to a teaspoon on most days, and no blood at all on others. She was delighted. Then the really odd part of the conversation began: she had been to her proctologist, and told him of the improvement. He was pleased, of course; nothing odd about that. She then asked him if he'd care to know what she'd been doing lately. He said, certainly, he was a doctor, and was always interested to know what helps his patients. So she told him that she'd been drinking a quart of fresh, raw cabbage juice every day. He stared back at her for a long moment, and then said, "No, that couldn't be it."

Marvel at this: to the specialist, it just couldn't have been due to the cabbage juice; it couldn't have been something that she had done on her own. Truth is, she got better in spite of him. He still got paid his specialist fees, of course.

"One of the first duties of the physician is to educate the masses not to take medicine."
—SIR WILLIAM OSLER, M.D.

To stop nighttime twitching, shaking, and kicking of the legs, try taking some niacin. Doses vary from person to person, ranging anywhere from a low (50–100 mg) to high (500–1,000 mg). By trial and experience, you learn just how much to take. While doing so, you are likely to experience a warm flushing sensation, described in the Niacin chapter. I take just enough to gently flush. Personally, I like that warm feeling, and at bedtime, it settles me right out. Here is a reader's report:

> My husband has never been officially diagnosed, but has a lot of trouble sleeping. This year when the work season started again, he began kicking me all night. It got so bad that I wasn't going to be able to sleep in the same room. Every few seconds, his legs would move and it was driving me up the wall. I persuaded my husband to try niacin with vitamin C right before bedtime. Works like a charm. In fact, when he missed his vitamins the other night, I could tell within minutes. What a great solution to a problem that so many suffer with!

Others, including my own family members with the problem, have tried this, and they have had success. Some persons will still need relaxant medication. But with the niacin, the medication dose may be, and generally is, less. Or even zero.

Taking a tablespoonful of lecithin may also help, as it provides choline. The benefits of choline from lecithin were discussed in the Alzheimer's chapter. The trick is to not take lecithin at bedtime, as it can "come up on you" in the form of a slightly oily indigestion. Take it with a meal, and that occurrence is far less likely. Take it at lunch or breakfast, and the benefits will be there that night . . . and the burping won't.

I think eating less salt may help. It certainly cannot hurt to cut down; many a physician will tell you that. Additionally, more potassium might be good to try. No supplement needed: fruits and veggies are loaded with potassium. A single banana, or a few plums or prunes, an apple, an orange: these are all good for you and equally good for the muscles and nerves in your legs.

One more hint: try the Schuessler cell salt Kali Phos. It is available in many health food stores, or on the Internet, usually in the homeopathic 6X potency.

"For schizophrenics, the natural recovery rate is 50%.
With orthomolecular medicine, the recovery rate is 90%.
With drugs, it is 10%. If you use just drugs, you won't get well."

—ABRAM HOFFER, M.D.

Psychosis is spooky. Jim, a twenty-one-year-old, was brought to me by his mom and dad. They looked uncomfortable, and he looked miserable. Jim was a diagnosed schizophrenic. He was so violent that he had been—get this—kicked out of the state hospital and sent home to his parents. You've got to love that logic.

Jim had been completely unmanageable. He threatened his parents' lives on a daily basis and punched holes in the walls. He slept one hour per night, and roamed the city streets the other seven or eight. Jim is one of the premier reasons to not be out too late yourself. His skin was scaly and his face severely broken out with acne. His dietary and digestive habits were appalling, and he was, to quote *Far Side* cartoonist Gary Larson, just plain nuts.

I faced this unhappy trio and felt helpless. The good part of it all was that they'd caught Jim on a good day (as far as I could see) and he wasn't going to tear up the place. From somewhere I recalled the three Ds of pellagra, that "extinct" niacin deficiency disease: dermatitis, dementia, and diarrhea. It was a reasonably close textbook match to the walking, talking Jim in front of me. I was also aware of the work of Abram Hoffer, M.D., a Canadian psychiatrist. Beginning in the early 1950s, Hoffer cured a vast number of psychotic patients with megadoses of niacin and vitamin C. The success of such vitamin treatments had earned him a quack's label too, of course.

But three feet away from me was a psycho with two terrified parents. Medical science had not helped him, and had, ironically, discharged him in the face of its own impotence. I told them about Dr. Hoffer's approach.

"We'll try anything," the father said, and the mother nodded energetically.

"Jim, how about you?" I asked.

"Yeah, I'll take the stuff," Jim said.

"I'll settle for that. Dr. Hoffer would have you take about 3,000 mg of niacin a day, and you'll want to take about 10,000 mg of vitamin C daily as well. Niacin deficiency actually causes psychosis, as well as the skin and GI problems that Jim happens to be experiencing. He may just need more niacin than the average person. Probably a lot more. At really large doses, niacin has a profound calming, sedating effect. Yet it is a nutrient, not a drug. The safety margin is huge. Dr. Hoffer has prescribed as much as 20,000 mg a day. 3,000 mg is not a particularly high dosage."

"And the vitamin C?" the father asked.

"Niacin's side effects, such as some possible changes in liver function, are minimized when you take at least the same amount of C," I answered. "As an added precaution, I think you should take even more C than that. Linus Pauling considered 10,000 mg for a man to be just an everyday dose. By body weight, it is about the same amount that a goat, cow, dog, cat, or rat would make each day. We cannot manufacture vitamin C because our livers lack a necessary enzyme, L-gulonolactone oxidase, and no, you cannot purchase and swallow that enzyme to do the job for you. Ask yourself: why would nature have these animals make that much for nothing? I think we should copy their example. These vitamins, at worst, are much less risky than any of the prescriptions Jim's ever tried."

Jim was silent and looked at his sneakers.

"How will we know if that's enough niacin?" his mother asked.

"If he behaves better, it's enough," I said. "If he takes too much niacin, he'll flush. That means his skin will get pink, or even red, especially the face, ears, and forearms. Sort of like a half-hour hot flash. You'll feel like you have a sunburn, Jim."

"That's okay with me," Jim said. "I like to be out at the beach."

They left, and I wondered how they'd managed to get by this far.

About two weeks later, Jim's father called for a follow-up conference. "Let me tell you what happened," he began. "You know Jim only sleeps maybe an hour a night? Well, the first night on the niacin, he slept eighteen hours. He's been sleeping about seven hours a night since."

"That's terrific," I said.

"That's not all," he said. "Last Friday morning, for the first time in I don't know how many years, Jim came down for breakfast. He walked into the dining room and said 'Good morning, Dad.'" Even on the phone I could hear the tears in the man's voice. It was wonderful.

There's more. Weeks later, Jim came in alone for an appointment. We sat down, and he told me that the niacin had worked, and that he'd stopped taking it.

"But why?" I asked. "It was helping you!"

"Yeah. Yeah. But I sort of like my sickness," Jim said.

I tried not to show my shock. This was nearly twenty years ago, and I hadn't yet learned that some psychotics simply prefer the psychotic state. As they get well, they may back away from the cure in favor of the disease.

Jim continued. "Whenever I get too far gone, though, I soak in a hot bath for a while and down a bottle of niacin. Then I feel fine." A whole bottle of niacin? That is literally what he said; I remember the line like it was uttered this morning. But if that's what he did, it seemed to work.

Here's the footnote: when a raving, dangerous patient can manage his illness and actually select the degree of psychosis he wants in his life, you have something unlike your standard idea of "cure." You have empowered a person to take responsibility for his life. And with the freedom that includes, you can get odd results.

Quick, how many psychoanalysts does it take to change a light bulb? One, but the light bulb has to really want to change.

Sick humor aside, we now are at a time when shrinks are breaking ranks. Some continue to say that the emotionally ill just need someone to talk to, to understand them and reason with them, but most want to drug patients into oblivion. Modern psychiatry has moved away from the Freudian couch and closer to Huxley's *Brave New World*. Prozac, Paxil, Thorazine, and their kin are our nonfictional soma, the mood-elevating wonder drugs that make psychoanalysis seem like the slow boat to China. Odd, really, that with a climate favoring medication over analysis, Abram Hoffer's niacin protocol is so unappreciated. After all, if "a gram is better than a damn," why not use grams of vitamins? Why not? Perhaps because niacin therapy is really, really cheap. There is no profit for the pharmaceutical companies, so why should the medical schools they fund teach upcoming doctors to use it?

Niacin, or vitamin B_3, has two forms: niacin and niacinamide. Both are water-soluble white powders. Your body obtains a small amount of niacin from metabolizing the essential amino acid tryptophan, found in protein (60 mg of tryptophan yields about 1 mg of niacin).

249

Pellagra is the classic niacin-deficiency disease. It was once common in the rural South, where the poor had little else to eat except tryptophan-poor foods like milled corn. The symptoms are the three Ds I mentioned earlier: diarrhea, dermatitis, and dementia. More specific pellagra symptoms include weakness, anorexia, lassitude, indigestion, skin eruptions, skin scaling, neuritis, nervous system destruction, confusion, apathy, disorientation, and insanity.

Does this sound a bit like schizophrenia to you?

A few physicians thought so, too. They noticed that psychotics frequently had assorted pellagralike symptoms in addition to their mental problems. In the early 1950s, an insightful young psychiatrist named Abram Hoffer began clinical trials to see if there was a connection. He used very high doses of niacin, with very good results. He and his colleagues discovered that, whereas pellegra is a vitamin deficiency, schizophrenia is a vitamin dependency. For a while, niacin was used as a treatment for psychosis, but the convenience and relentless advertising of later "wonder drugs" diminished niacin's popularity. Then, the American Psychiatric Association unscientifically trashed megavitamin therapy in the 1970s. So now we have legions of nutritionally challenged, mentally malnourished Americans who don't know it. And we pay out big bucks for behavior-modifying drugs that come factory-equipped with dangerous side effects.

Some additional and interesting therapeutic uses of niacin include Ménière's syndrome (chronic ringing in the ears plus nausea) and high-tone deafness. In long-term therapy, improvement was obtained with only 150–250 mg daily. Resistance to X-radiation was greatly improved at 500–600 mg daily. Nausea was also reduced. Supplemental niacin could therefore be of much value for cancer patients undergoing radiation therapy. Even healing after surgical shock and other trauma, including burns, hemorrhage, and infection, is more rapid with niacin administration.

Niacin is very safe. "No toxicity has ever been shown for humans," Dr. Hoffer says. "For animals, it is about 5 grams per kilogram." This means that for an animal that weighs what an average human does (165 pounds, or 75 kg), a fatal dose would be about 375,000 mg/day. The most psychotic person you are ever likely to meet could probably not hold more than 15,000 mg per day, and most people, healthy or not, would never exceed a fraction of that. Physicians frequently give patients 2,000–5,000 mg of niacin to lower serum cholesterol. The safety margin is large. There is not even one death from niacin per year. The most common side effects of niacin therapy include flushing, skin itching, and, upon large overdose, nausea. Such symptoms vary with dose, the body's need, and volume of food consumed with the vitamin. I have noticed that taking large doses of vitamin C diminishes the side effects of very large doses. I think that patients should take at least twice as much C as niacin, and more C works even better.

Measurable side effects, such as changes in liver function tests, tend to be a significant problem primarily in people with a history of alcohol abuse. But doctors citing such test variations as a reason why patients should not take megadoses of niacin are jumping to conclusions, Dr. Hoffer says: "Doctors confuse the elevation of liver function tests with underlying liver pathology, but this is wrong. It merely means that the liver is more active. And such changes can be prevented by taking some lecithin twice daily." People cannot take enough niacin to hurt themselves because they first would become nauseated, according to Dr. Hoffer. He adds. "It is important that the working dose always be less than the nauseant dose."

It is a lack of niacin that is the real public health problem. The RDA is only about 20 mg. Half of all Americans will not get even that much from their diets. Niacin's special importance is indicated in that the RDA for niacin is twenty or more times higher than the RDA for other B vitamins, and that's just for everyday, healthy people.

Dr. Hoffer gave immensely higher doses, and it worked. I copied him with Jim, and that worked as much as Jim wanted it to. To continue your knowledge of niacin therapy, consult the books found in the recommended reading for this chapter. I would actually go so far as to advise reading everything Dr. Hoffer has ever written.

Recommended Reading

Bicknell F and Prescott F. *The Vitamins in Medicine,* 3rd ed. Milwaukee, WI: Lee Foundation, 1953, 379.

Hawkins D and Pauling L. *Orthomolecular Psychiatry* David Hawkins and Linus Pauling, eds., W. H. Freeman, San Francisco, 1973.

Hoffer A. *Hoffer's Law of Natural Nutrition.* Kingston, ON: Quarry Press, 1996.

Hoffer A. *Putting It All Together: The New Orthomolecular Nutrition.* New Canaan, CT: Keats, 1996.

Hoffer A. *Vitamin B$_3$ and Schizophrenia: Discovery, Recovery, Controversy.* Kingston, ON: Quarry Press, 1999.

Hoffer A. and Foster HD. (2007) *Feel Better, Live Longer With Niacin.* Toronto: CCNM Press.

Hoffer, A and Saul AW. (2011). *Niacin: The Real Story.* Laguana Beach, CA: Basic Health Publications.

Hoffer, A and Saul AW. (2008). *Orthomolecular Medicine for Everyone.* Laguna Beach, CA: Basic Health Publications.

Williams RJ, ed. (1979). *A Physician's Handbook on Orthomolecular Medicine.* New Canaan, CT: Keats.

Sciatica, Spinal Stenosis, and Other Painful Back Problems

"There is a principle which is a bar against all information, which is proof against all argument, and which cannot fail to keep man in everlasting ignorance. That principle is condemnation without investigation."

—HERBERT SPENCER

SCIATICA

Here is what a reader, Robert McClain, had to say about curing a severe case of sciatica:

"In 2004, I was disabled to the point of being unable to put on my own socks and underwear. My four- and eight-year-old sons had to help me get dressed everyday. For three months, my wife had to help me get off the floor in the morning, because I was unable to lie down in our bed. I couldn't drive, fly in a plane, or even sit in a chair. I had lost the ability to function normally. My condition was diagnosed as sciatica, which in my case was the result of a bulging disc in my lower back pressing on nearby nerves. This pressure inflamed the nerves. As a result, I experienced debilitating pain in my lower back, legs, and feet. Bluntly speaking, I was disabled.

"During this time, two of the Cleveland area's finest neurologists performed a 'walletectomy' to the tune of $4,000, not counting money paid by my insurance company. They hooked me to electrodes; they tapped, poked, and prodded; they bathed me in X-rays and the magnetic fields of an MRI. They tried drugging me with Bextra, but two doses of that now-withdrawn COX-2 inhibitor made me violently ill. All this was nearly as expensive as it was painful. I faced the very real possibility of losing my career, my life savings, and even the family home.

"When these two doctors met with me for the last time, the taller of the two stood next to me, put his arm around my shoulder, and said, 'You're just going to have to learn to live with this condition.'"

"So, that was it. The best minds in medicine decided I was hopeless, and I was just supposed to support a wife and two kids on whatever I could make standing up. By the time I hobbled to my wife's car and crawled across the back seat, I was genuinely angry. I left that clinic determined that there had to be a better way to regain my health than trust it to overpaid pill-pushers.

"Determined to find a way to heal, I searched the web for anything related to inflammation and how to cure it naturally. Quite by accident, I stumbled across www.doctoryourself. com, and began my education as a student of orthomolecular medicine. I learned how nutrition could be used to treat and cure an amazing array of diseases that make up the cash cows of modern medicine.

"Well, it all looked simple enough: drown the inflammation in vitamin C, and I might start to feel better. To be fair, I've never been the type of person to go into a program half-heartedly. I crawled back into the car and my wife took me to the health food store. For about $8, I bought an eight-ounce jar of ascorbic acid powder. We drove home, and using the Klenner

protocol for vitamin C, I started on a regimen of 3 grams (just under 1 tsp) in a glass of water . . . 10 times a day, for a total of 30,000 mg daily.

"By the end of the first day, nothing had changed. On the morning of the second day, I got up off the floor by myself. It was difficult, but I did it. My back and legs still felt like there were ropes of pain burning inside my legs.

On the morning of the third day, I dressed myself, socks and underwear included, and that night I slept in my own bed for the first time in months. The pain in my legs and back was still there, but not a constant irritant as before.

"On the morning of the fourth day, I was in a state of health. I dressed myself for outdoor work, grabbed the chainsaw, and set to the task of cutting up a load of slab wood that I'd neglected for the last three months. When she heard the chain saw fire up, my wife came running out of the house. 'What are you doing?' she shouted above the rumbling saw in my hands. Shutting off the saw, I assured her that I was completely cured, had no pain, and couldn't wait to get back to work.

"Over the next two weeks, I continued the regimen, astonished at the amount of C that my body seemed willing to absorb. Eventually, I reached bowel tolerance, cut the regimen by 50 percent, and continued to add other forms of supplementation to my diet.

"Exactly four years later, I find myself amazed at the difference in my life using the information on the Doctor Yourself website. I've helped myself, and I've been able to assist friends, relatives, and my own family in ways I never thought possible.

"One special example of this is my own mother. In 2006, we lost Dad to lung cancer and a staph infection. On the same day as my father's passing, we were told that Mom had stage 3A colon cancer that would require surgery. After the operation, Mom was moved to a rehab facility where she was told she would have to stay for six to ten weeks. By using supplementation from the very first day in rehab, Mom was home in eighteen days, and driving her own car within another month.

"We now believe in the value of orthomolecular medicine because we live it. Standing on the shoulders of giants, we have seen the way to health."

Vitamin C

A lack of vitamin C is specifically involved in the cause and progression of chronic back problems such as sciatica and spinal stenosis. The premise is basic: *long-term inadequacy of vitamin C causes weak spinal disks.*

Without enough vitamin C, the body is unable to make collagen, the protein glue that holds cells together. When the cells of a cartilaginous intervertebral disk are not holding together, the disk will degenerate, rupture, herniate, or "slip." There is a lot of body weight on the bones of your lower back. When you flex and move, and the disks are weak or worn down, the bones can compress nerves emerging from the sides. If only one or two disks are involved, it may result in the characteristic back and leg pain called sciatica.

SPINAL STENOSIS

It is worse if multiple vertebrae are involved. Without healthy disks to prevent it, the center spinal channel can gradually stenose, or narrow. This channel is very important: it is the hollow through which your nerve superhighway, the spinal cord, runs. Squeezing or kinking the spinal

253

cord means pain and problems. Try watering your garden when a cow is standing with its hoof on your garden hose.

While spinal stenosis is sometimes congenital or caused by a tumor, by far the most common form is acquired stenosis. The usual way one "acquires" it is through injury, or osteoarthritis, or both.

OTHER PAINFUL BACK PROBLEMS

Injury

Inadequate vitamin C weakens ligaments and connective tissue, making injury easier, inflammation likely, and healing much more difficult.

Osteoarthritis

Inadequate vitamin C also causes the cushioning cartilage in your joints to deteriorate, roughen, and wear ever thinner. As the cartilage degenerates, bone scrapes on bare bone with each movement. That is osteoarthritis.

Bone Spurs

In the absence of cartilage padding, bone may begin to grow (spur) in the joints of the spine. This is probably the body's attempt to brace up and splint the vertebrae and limit the movement that is causing pain. Unfortunately, bone spurring can narrow the spinal canal and painfully squeeze the spinal cord in the center. If bone spurs form in the little joints (facets) of the sides of the vertebrae, the nerve roots at the sides get pinched.

Spondylolisthesis

Without enough vitamin C to maintain their strength, ligaments can degenerate, thicken, and lose their elasticity. This too may narrow the spinal canal. If disks and ligaments are especially weak, lower-back (lumbar) vertebrae can slide over each other and squish nerves.

All of the above conditions have a common causal factor: inadequate vitamin C. The good news is that they can all be significantly helped by administering large quantities of the nutrient.

Vitamin Treatment

Doctors have seen many research studies on drug therapy but very few on megavitamin therapy. This does not mean that vitamin therapy will not help; it means that vitamin therapy has not been applied.

Well, not quite. One of the great proponents of massive-dose vitamin C therapy was Dr. Robert F. Cathcart III, an orthopedic surgeon. One might want to think on that for a long moment. Cathcart, the inventor of a widely used hip replacement prosthetic, advocated doses of vitamin C, often in excess of 100,000 mg per day, to reduce severe inflammation. In decades of practice, he safely and effectively administered such treatment to tens of thousands of patients. Many had arthritis, back pain, or injury; some had ankylosing spondylitis.

254

In scanning Cathcart's work, one notices that none of his papers are expressly devoted to "treatment of chronic back problems with vitamin C." Patients and doctors may therefore be tempted to walk away from this line of inquiry. Yet vitamin C is an important and overlooked key to understanding spinal stenosis and doing something nonsurgical about it.

One question, of course, is whether vitamin C can actually rebuild cartilage. The answer is this: cartilage cannot be made without it. The odds greatly favor taking Dr. Cathcart's advice over the "just eat a balanced diet for your vitamin C" line that you so often hear.

There is more good news about vitamin C:

Pain Relief

Very high doses of vitamin C provide prompt and profound pain relief. Low doses will not work.

One of the biggest surprises in analgesia occurred during the 1970s in Scotland at the Vale of Leven Hospital. There, Ewan Cameron, M.D., was giving ten grams (10,000 milligrams) of vitamin C intravenously each day to terminally ill patients. In Great Britain at the time, it was acceptable to provide terminal patients with any and all pain relief available, including addictive narcotics such as heroin.

Cameron and Baird reported (in 1973) that the first five ascorbate-treated patients who had been receiving large doses of morphine or heroin to control pain were taken off these drugs a few days after the treatment with vitamin C was begun, because the vitamin C seemed to diminish the pain to such an extent that the drug was not needed. Moreover, none of these patients asked that the morphine or heroin be *given to them—they seemed not to experience any serious withdrawal signs or symptoms* (Cameron and Pauling, *Cancer and Vitamin C*, 1981; revised 1993, p. xii)

Any vitamin that approaches the pain-relieving power of opiates must be considered some kind of analgesic indeed. Although quite a lot of vitamin C is needed for results, it is a remarkably safe and rather simple therapy.

Tobacco Smoking

Smokers are in a constant state of vitamin C deficiency. Do not let anyone tell you differently.

William J. McCormick, M.D., found that just three cigarettes a day robs your body of the RDA of vitamin C. Therefore, even smokers without any obvious illness symptoms require daily vitamin C supplementation. Effectively treating illness requires far more.

It is not difficult to see why smokers are much more likely to have serious disk and back problems. What really is difficult to understand is:

1. how few physicians order their back-surgery candidates to stop smoking

2. how very few physicians order their smoking patients to take vitamin C supplements

3. how almost no physician offers high-dose vitamin C therapy as a treatment option

More patients would stop cigarettes, and start vitamin C, if they knew why they absolutely had to.

How Much Is Needed

For results, vitamin C needs to be taken to bowel tolerance. That means exactly what you think it means.

The dose varies widely from person to person, but the effective amount is in the range of tens of thousands of milligrams per day, taken in frequent divided doses. Serious cases may require vitamin C initially be given intravenously. *High daily oral amounts, divided into every-half-hour doses all day every day, may substitute if IV C is not available.*

In massive doses, vitamin C (ascorbic acid) strengthens cartilage, reduces inflammation and relieves pain. Your doctor may not believe this, but unless you consult a shaman, your health care should not be a matter of belief.

About "Objections" to Vitamin C Megadoses

Many people wonder why the medical professions have not embraced vitamin C therapy with open and grateful arms. Probably the main roadblock to widespread examination and utilization of this all-too-simple technology is the equally widespread idea that there *must* be unknown dangers to tens of thousands of milligrams of ascorbic acid. Yet, since the time megascorbate therapy was introduced in the late 1940s by board-certified chest specialist Fred R. Klenner, M.D., there has been a surprisingly safe and effective track record of physician reports for one to follow.

When an experienced orthopedic surgeon such as Dr. Robert Cathcart chose to give patients huge amounts of vitamin C, it is time to ask why your physicians have not. There are many possible excuses, none of which should be accepted without examining the evidence.

A search of the medical literature shows that vitamin C does not cause kidney stones. It is safe even at very high doses. Other mistakenly believed "side effects" of vitamin C have been found to be completely mythical. According to a NIH report published in the *Journal of the American Medical Association* (April 21, 1999), **none** of the following problems are caused by taking "too much vitamin C":

- Allegations of Hypoglycemia
- Allegations of Infertility
- Allegations of Rebound scurvy
- Allegations of Destruction of vitamin B_{12}

This, however, *is* verifiably true: national USA poison control center statistics show that there is not even one death per year from vitamins. On the other hand, pharmaceutical drugs, properly prescribed and taken as directed, kill well over 100,000 Americans annually.

Hundreds of thousands of Americans suffer from lower back (lumbar) spinal stenosis, which is now the most common indication for surgery for those over sixty. Vitamin therapy is safer than drug or surgical treatment. There is very little to lose, and very much to gain, by trying high-dose vitamin C therapy in advance of, or along with, conventional treatment.

Other Nutrients

Dr. Cathcart and other orthomolecular (nutritional) physicians usually give patients additional nutrients along with megadose vitamin C therapy.

Vitamin B$_{12}$

B$_{12}$ may help with injury and with spinal stenosis, although the dose probably needs to be much higher than the 0.5 mg given orally three times daily in this study: Waikakul, W and Waikakul, S. (2000). Methylcobalamin as an adjuvant medication in conservative treatment of lumbar spinal stenosis. *J Med Assoc Thai.* 83(8):825–31, in which the researchers report that "(N)eurogenic claudication distance [was] better in the M (vitamin)-group." See also: Petchkrua, W, et al. (2003). Prevalence of vitamin B$_{12}$ deficiency in spinal cord injury. *Arch Phys Med Rehabil.* 84(11):1675–9, and: Vitamin B$_{12}$ deficiency in spinal cord injury: a retrospective study. [*J Spinal Cord Med.,* 2003].

Chondroitin sulfate and glucosamine sulfate

Healthy cartilage contains a large amount of chondroitin sulfate, which helps strengthen it. Strong cartilage resists compression; weak cartilage means osteoarthritic changes. A common therapeutic dose is 1,200 mg/day.

Glucosamine sulfate also helps your body rebuild cartilage. And, it relieves pain about as well as ibuprofen does. 1500 mg/day is a common therapeutic dose. In another study, (Ruane, R and Griffiths P. [2002]. Glucosamine therapy compared to ibuprofen for joint pain. Br J Community Nurs. 7(3):148–52), researchers report that: "Glucosamine's pain-relieving effects may be due to its cartilage-rebuilding properties; these disease-modifying effects are not seen with simple analgesics and are of particular benefit. In practice glucosamine can be used as an alternative to anti-inflammatory drugs and analgesics or as a useful adjunct to standard analgesic therapy."

Both chondroitin and glucosamine have been shown clinically to be exceptionally safe.

257

It Is Not Just the Placebo Effect, Either

Since these substances work for horses, they might work for you. (See Forsyth, R, Brigden, C, and Northrop, A (2006). Double blind investigation of the effects of oral supplementation of combined glucosamine hydrochloride (GHCL) and chondroitin sulphate (CS) on stride characteristics of veteran horses. *Equine veterinary journal.* Supplement (36): 622–5. PMID 17402494.)

Additional References

Bassleer, C, et al. (1998). Stimulation of proteoglycan production by glucosamine sulfate in chondrocytes isolated from human osteoarthritic articular cartilage in vitro. *Osteoarthritis Cartilage* 6(6):427–34.

Bruyere, O and Reginster JY. (2007). Glucosamine and chondroitin sulfate as therapeutic agents for knee and hip osteoarthritis. *Drugs Aging* 24(7): 573–580.

Kwan Ta,t S, et al. (2007). Chondroitin and glucosamine sulfate in combination decrease the pro-resorptive properties of human osteoarthritis subchondral bone osteoblasts: a basic science study. *Arthritis Res Ther.* 9(6):R117.

Pavelka, K, et al. (2002). Glucosamine sulfate use and delay of progression of knee osteoarthritis: a 3-year, randomized, placebo-controlled, double-blind study. *Arch Intern Med* 162(18):2113–23. PMID 12374520.

Reginster, JY, et al. (2001). Long-term effects of glucosamine sulphate on osteoarthritis progression: a randomised, placebo-controlled clinical trial. *Lancet* 357(9252):251–6. PMID 11214126.

Sowers, M and Lachance L. (1999). Vitamins and arthritis. The roles of vitamins A, C, D, and E. *Rheum Dis Clin North Am.* 25(2):315–32.

Skin Problems

"He who lives by rule and wholesome diet is a physician to himself."

—CONCISE DIRECTIONS ON THE NATURE OF OUR COMMON FOOD
SO FAR AS IT TENDS TO PROMOTE OR INJURE HEALTH.
(PUBLISHED BY SWORDS OF LONDON: 1790, P. 7)

While in college, a friend of mind went to an expensive dermatologist because he had a slight rash. The specialist told him it was "dermatitis" and issued him a nifty cream to put on it. The visit cost my friend half a week's pay, and when he came to realize that "dermatitis" meant "itchy skin," he went ballistic. You might be able to save some space in your checkbook, and maybe even some time in the waiting room, with my very own "Ten Ways to Dodge Your Dermatologist."

1. Shampoo less often. If you are troubled by simple but annoying scalp conditions, this is really worth a try before you drop the big bucks on a doctor. A physician I go to for once-a-decade physicals prescribed not one but *two* antibiotics (one topical, one oral) for a chronic scalp irritation. He also recommended a very expensive shampoo and said to use it often. Nuts to that; the condition went away when I simply stopped shampooing every day and went to just once a week. Will this make your hair look all icky? Come on, now: do you shampoo your cat every day?

2. Use less soap. Not none, but less! I am not suggesting that you become the poster person for vagrancy; just use less of what everybody knows dries out skin. You use soaps and detergents to dissolve grease and oil when you wash your clothes and clean your dishes. We all know that soaps and detergents "cut grease." Right! They do the same to your skin, removing the natural oils that protect the skin—and the moisture and softness that no product can truly replace. A naturopath once told me that one should shower without soap, except for judicious application to personal areas that really need it.

3. Sunblock alone will not protect you from the sun. To avoid sunburn, wear a brimmed hat and loose, cool, comfy clothes instead. Simple, no? You'd be genuinely surprised just how many people still do not realize that the ozone layer is not what it was thirty years ago. More ultraviolet light (UV-B in particular) does in fact now reach us than was the case a generation or two ago. You can avoid practically all basal cell and squamous cell carcinoma, the two most common types of skin cancer, simply by putting on some clothes. I like a nice tan as much as the next person, but you simply have to use common sense here. Look: if you were diagnosed even with relatively easy-to-cut-out skin cancer, wouldn't you do just anything to be able to go back and prevent it? Even wear a hat and a shady shirt? Well, now is the time to start.

TOPICAL VITAMIN C STOPS BASAL CELL CARCINOMA

The most common form of skin cancer, basal cell carcinoma, often responds to a remarkably simple, safe, at-home treatment: vitamin C. Physicians and patients report that vitamin C, applied directly to basal cell skin cancers, causes them to scab over and drop off.[1] Successful use involves a highly-concentrated vitamin C solution, directly applied to the blemish two or three times a day. Vitamin C is selectively toxic to cancer cells, but does not harm healthy skin cells. This is also the basis for high-dose intravenous vitamin therapy for cancer.[2] Even higher concentrations of vitamin C can be obtained by direct application. The use of topical vitamin C to kill basal cell carcinoma has been known at least since 1971. Frederick R. Klenner, M.D., wrote: "We have removed several small basal cell epithelioma with a 30 percent ointment" of vitamin C.[3]

One person, who reported that a 2 mm diameter spot on the nose would not heal for months, had it disappear within a week with twice-daily concentrated vitamin C applications. Another patient reported that after dermatologist-diagnosed multiple spots of basal cell carcinoma were coated with vitamin C, the spots fell off within two weeks.[4]

Basal cell carcinomas are slow growing and it is rare for them to metastasize. This provides an opportunity for a therapeutic trial of vitamin C, provided one has proper medical diagnosis and follow-up.

Preparation of a water-saturated vitamin C solution is simple. Slowly add a small amount of water to about half a teaspoon of vitamin C powder or crystals. Use just enough water to dissolve the vitamin C. Using less water will make a paste. Either way, application with the fingertip or a cotton swab, several times daily, is easy. The water will evaporate in a few minutes and leave a plainly visible coat of vitamin C crystals on the skin.

Consult your doctor before employing this or any other self-care treatment. A physician's diagnosis is especially important, since other forms of skin cancer, such as melanoma, are faster growing and more dangerous. If the vitamin C-treated area is not improved after a few weeks, a doctor should be consulted once again.

References

1. William Wassell, MD. Skin cancer and vitamin C. Cancer Tutor, www.cancertutor.com/Cancer02/VitaminC.html.

2. Riordan NH, Riordan HD, Meng X, Li Y, Jackson JA. (1995). Intravenous ascorbate as a tumor cytotoxic chemotherapeutic agent. *Med Hypotheses* 44: 207–213. www.brightspot.org/cresearch/intravenousc2.shtml. See also www.seanet.com/ ~alexs/ ascorbate/199x/riordan-nh-etal-med_hypotheses_1995-v44-p207.htm and www.doctoryourself.com/riordan1.html

3. Fredrick R. Klenner, MD: Observations on the dose and administration of ascorbic acid when employed beyond the range of a vitamin in human pathology. *Journal of Applied Nutrition* Vol. 23, Nos 3 & 4, Winter 1971. http://yost.com/ health/klenner/klenner-1971.pdf and www.doctoryourself.com/klennerpaper.html.

4. Age spots, basal cell carcinoma and solar keratosis. www.doctoryourself.com/news/v5n9.txt.

259

A reader says:

"After reading Pauling and Cameron's book *Cancer and Vitamin C,* I decided to put what I learned to the test. For more than two decades, I've gone to the dermatologist two or three times a year to remove the spots on my face. Last May, I had about twenty spots on my face and was about to make an appointment with the dermatologist. Instead, I decided to start applying ascorbic acid topically. It works beautifully! I still apply ascorbic acid daily in solution, and keep the new spots under control. As an a extra benefit, the skin on my face has taken on a more youthful appearance and its clear to me that loose and wrinkled skin is not an inevitable result of aging, (I'm 73), but rather a symptom of anascorbemia of the skin."

Another says:

"For many years, I've mixed up vitamin C powder and vitamin E oil into a 'heavy' liquid. Put this on a wart or a skin cancer with a small bandage over it, and replace every day. The wart will drop off soon, and cancerous area will cure in about a week. We keep inventing the wheel."

And another:

"Many thanks for posting the information on this. I am only a week and a half into treatment and my basal cell is nearly gone."

4. Switch to more natural perfumes, soaps, and deodorants. For this, you may need to stop by your local health food store. There really are many natural, gentle alternatives to the cheap, caustic, common cosmetic chemicals that irritate our skin! (Has the Pulitzer Prize in Alliteration been awarded yet?) I know two people who used to have numerous, small polyplike growths on their neck and underarms. These were no more than slightly unsightly, yet they were hardly an improvement to the basic birthday suit. In each case, they went away when the one person stopped using antiperspirant deodorants, and when the other stopped putting perfume directly on her skin. Read the label; even some "natural" deodorants are not that natural. However, most are a big improvement for a small cash difference.

5. Build skin health from the inside out. To have healthy skin, grow it. Your skin is an organ, like your lungs or heart, but a lot more visible, and a lot bigger, too. Your skin is, in fact, your body's largest organ. Feed your skin nutrients by eating more fiber, trying a vegetarian diet; and how about a few days of juice fasting? See for yourself if a healthy inside equals a healthy outside.

6. Chocolate: Stop eating it. It is no myth but a matter of observable fact that if you eat a good bit of chocolate, your skin will break out. If you cut out the chocolate, your skin will likely improve. Part of this is due to dietary fat; part is due to the chemical makeup of cocoa itself. Try and see. Hershey's common stock will do fine without your help.

7. Use less skin and hair glop. You'll save a pile of cash, and if you follow the suggestions above, you won't need all that stuff anyway. I remember a neat "Nancy" cartoon where she bathed and showered and dried her hair, then covered it with all the sprays, gels, mousses, and what have you. She looked in a mirror, realized how yucky her chemical hair was, and went back into the tub to wash it all off again. Okay, it wasn't the most hilarious cartoon I've ever seen (that, of course, would be the "Far Side" take on "the real reason dinosaurs became extinct"). But the point was made nonetheless.

8. Take your vitamins. Your skin really loves vitamin E (internally and externally), the B-complex vitamins, and assorted other nutrients that modern diets so often lack.

9. Eat more lecithin. Lecithin contains linoleic and linolenic acid, the absolutely essential fatty acids. As adult Americans try to reduce their fat intake (generally a good idea), no one has told them that they may thereby be creating a fatty acid deficiency. Since the government, the medical profession, and most dietitians just cannot own up to the necessity of food supplements, we had better consider them ourselves. The irritable-skin, dry-skin, broken-skin

260

consequences of long-term linoleic and especially linolenic-acid deficiency are probably very common. I eliminated my own chronic dermatitis with just a few days supplementation of three tablespoons of lecithin per day. A few tablespoons per week keeps it away. No dermatologist needed.

10. Reduce stress. (See my chapter "Stress Reduction" for specific suggestions.) A personal observation: I was under high stress at one job for about four years, and I noticed four things:[1] my hair got gray;[2] my hair started to come out in the comb;[3] when I started taking more vitamins, the hair stopped coming out; and[4] when I started doing the work I love, my hair stopped graying. In my opinion, I am less gray than I was in 1989. You can look at my untouched photo on my website, marvel at my toupee, guess my age, and mail me your answer. The winner will receive absolutely nothing.

I am kidding about the toupee; it's all mine.

Getting into Your Outside: Healthy Skin Tips

Health nuts have long emphasized skin health for total health. Your skin is your body's largest organ, and virtually the only organ that you can watch. Since so many people have skin rashes, dryness, sores, blisters, corns, dandruff, and such, more attention needs to be given to what holds you together. Do you realize what you'd look like without skin? A heap of organs on the floor: how explicit! The skin also excretes wastes from the body. That's what sweating does, in addition to automatically cooling you.

Nature cure proponents hold that rashes, pimples, eczema, and illnesses like chicken pox or measles are attempts by the skin to clean itself out. This idea will never cease to come up as long as we talk of nature's way in health: the body will try, must try, to clean itself of toxins, foreign chemicals, and poisons. Nature eliminates wastes. You may not like it; it may not look romantic; it might even itch. However, the toxins must be expelled. Since the skin is your largest organ, it will by nature want to do a lot of cleaning out. The more it does so, the more you needed it to.

"So that's where all those hives and rashes come from," you might think, and you'd be essentially correct. Take a very common complaint: dandruff. An overabundance of mucus-producing items in the diet seems to be a basic cause. Persons with dandruff have found that if they reduce their consumption of milk, ice cream, yogurt, and eggs that their dandruff goes away. No medications, no special patent shampoos. I have seen this in my own experience, and if you will pardon me, on my own scalp. Yogurt and aged cheeses seem to be less involved in making up what comes off us as dandruff.

Overconsumption of cooked, processed foods in general seems to predispose a body for complaints like this. I even had a dog with dandruff . . . until I stopped giving him dry skim milk plus cream plus milk on top of all the dog food he could eat. When the dog's diet was cut in half, following a four-day cleansing fast, the dandruff was gone and never returned until the animal was overfed again.

Simple, proper diet eliminates so many complaints. Whole foods, raw or lightly cooked vegetables, grains and fruits, no meat, and no chemically doctored food will go a very long way to improving your skin in a short time. Unfortunately, many folks are inclined to and even encouraged to put creams, salves, ointments, and other patent remedies on their skin to "relieve the itching and scaling of the heartbreak of psoriasis" or to "restore moisture to dry, worn-out skin."

261

Let's "clear up" this skin medication question right here. First of all, there is no such thing as "worn-out skin." Fortunately for us, skin is perennial, self-repairing, and virtually indestructible. Now just think how many times you scraped, cut, or bruised your skin when you were a kid! Look at you now; look at your hands, arms, and knees. You're not covered with patches, are you? Nature repairs and mends skin beautifully. When you cut yourself, you might disinfect the wound with iodine or some other preparation. But does the iodine reknit the skin, make the new cells, or weave new tissue? No, nature does. When a surgeon stitches up an incision or a wound she brings the skin together and holds it in place with sutures. But if nature didn't reunite the cells, what good would the stitches do?

Vitamins C and E seem to be most important for proper healing and maintenance of your skin. Drs. Wilfrid and Evan Shute used vitamin E, both internally and externally, in their extremely successful treatment of third-degree burns. Vitamin C is well-known to be essential to holding the cells together and encouraging their normal growth (that's a reason why C is so desperately important to a cancer patient's body). Vitamin C compresses have been used on severe skin ulcerations with success surpassing that of antibiotics. Both of vitamin C and E can be given internally, plus applied topically, without danger of side effects. Recovery periods are rapid with each, and probably best with both. Show me a person with chronic skin problems and two times out of three I'll bet their diet is deficient in E or C.

For the other one time out of three, the person may benefit from Schuessler's Cell Salts, particularly if a needed mineral is missing. How can the skin function normally if it is lacking a raw material that it must have? The absence of any one nutrient is a problem for the whole system. A high-fidelity enthusiast once told me that a stereo system is only as good as its weakest part. You can spend a fortune on the best speakers, the finest amplifier, the highest quality CD player, and the greatest recordings. But if there's just one bad electrical connection, all the rest is useless to you. The Schuessler minerals in homeopathic potency are provided in minute but vital quantity and quality. "A little dab will do ya" if you'll pardon me. J. B. Chapman, M.D., lists over 85 different skin ailments that are helped by Schuessler minerals in *Dr. Schuessler's Biochemistry* (London: New Era, 1973).

Would you like to know what some of the indications for use are? Here are some of the conditions and their mineral remedies that Dr. Chapman suggests:

Cracks in hands: Calc. Flour. (calcium flouride)

Dry skin: Calc. Phos., Kali. Sulph. (calcium phosphate, potassium sulphate)

Excessive dryness: Natrum Mur. (sodium chloride)

Face full of pimples: Calc. Phos., Calc. Sulph (calcium phosphate, calcium sulphate)

Greasy scales on skin: Kali. Phos.(potassium phosphate)

Skin that heals slowly: Silicea, Calc. Sulph. (silica, calcium sulphate)

Hives: Natr. Phos. (sodium phosphate)

Itching, as from nettles: Calc. Phos. (calcium phosphate)

Itching of skin, with crawling sensation: Kali. Phos., Calc. Phos. (potassium phosphate, calcium phosphate)

Ivy poisoning: Kali. Sulph., Natr. Mur. (potassium sulphate, sodium chloride)

Rawness of skin in little children: Natr. Phos. (sodium phosphate)

Shingles: Kali. Mur., Natr. Mur. (potassium chloride, sodium chloride)

Warts: Kali. Mur. (potassium chloride)

And there are over 72 more suggestions in this one book alone.

Many of what we call "allergies" are probably just local or systemwide deficiencies of vitamins or minerals. I submit that one's body is often showing in symptoms what it needs in nutrition. Also, I believe in the body showing that it has received something it doesn't need. If you're "allergic" to prescription medications, consider yourself lucky . . . and normal. Drugs, and other ingested chemicals such as preservatives and food-coloring dyes, have to be high on the body's list of "things to excrete at first opportunity." These are foreign, toxic, and very commonly ingested although bad for us. How is it then, that we are surprised when the irritant starts a rash, fever, nausea, or sneezing? Wouldn't you expect your body to indicate poisoning in some way? If someone ate poisoned food and then developed fever or threw up, we'd agree that the body was reacting to get rid of the toxin in the best way it could. When a child eats preserved, colored food with the vitamins and nutrients processed out of it, and then develops food sensitivities, where is the surprise? Every computer geek I know knows that it's GIGO: garbage in, garbage out.

Injections are forced through our skin in an effort to get a drug or vaccine into our bloodstream. We should remember that the body may utilize that same path in trying to get foreign toxins and poisons out.

Think of that next time you see a rash or other skin symptom.

Your skin is a living, breathing, body-cleaning organ. If you stop it up, you're in trouble. In the James Bond story *Goldfinger,* people were spray-painted gold. Remember that they supposedly died? It's likely the author used a smidgeon of literary license, but still: your skin should be free from pore-clogging coatings. That's why commercial creams, ointments, and salves are not doing any more than removing the symptoms of skin excretion. In slowing down or blocking this excretion they are clogging the pores and, in and of themselves, adding to what has to be cleaned out. Why make the skin have to now excrete these added toxins on top of the old ones? It's like shaking the dirt out of your rugs . . . in the middle of the living room.

If you don't use any of the countless patent skin treatments for beauty or disease, your skin will be that much better. Treating symptoms is just trying to fool Mother Nature. Coating over the body's cleansing efforts does not make you or your skin well. I don't think it's wise to use chemical creams or antibiotic ointments or any of that. Keeping drugs, artificial colors, preservatives, alcohols, artificial fragrances, and those foot-long chemical names off your skin can only help it.

If nature had wanted us to use lots of synthetics on our body, she would probably have put triethanolamine, carbomer-934, methylparaben, propylparaben, dimethicone, titanium dioxide, sodium myristate, stearyl alcohol, FD&C Red #4, Yellow #3 and other "beauty necessities" within easy reach. As it is, these and other nostrums are key ingredients in today's best-selling lotions. I read right from cosmetic labels, including a "mysterious beauty fluid (that) works with your skin's own natural moisture to quickly ease away dryness" and "impart a new radiance and glow to your skin." Some are in "a unique conditioning lotion" that "keeps skin wonderfully soft and smooth." Would you care to tell me how they can do that? It's small wonder why peo-

263

ple think they've got allergies, or that there's something wrong with their skin. There's nothing wrong with the skin; there's something wrong with what's layered onto it.

As for my family, we use a lot of vitamin E. It's hard to beat when directly applied to rough, sore, or dry skin. For topical (external) application, simply take any E capsule and carefully puncture the end of the capsule. This is easily done with a push-pin or plastic-handled thumb tack. Then just squeeze the E directly where you need it. We keep a bottle of 200 IU capsules in the bathroom cabinet, and in the past kept another bottle near the baby's changing table, and use it almost daily for diaper rash, dry skin, chapped hands, burns, and so forth.

Unlike commercially concocted skin preparations, vitamin E is wholly natural as long as it's D-alpha-tocopherol. The "D" form is right-handed in molecular structure, and the "L" form is left-handed. As far as vitamin E is concerned, the body seems to have a preference for "right-handed" molecules". (On the other hand, your body can only use left-handed vitamin L-ascorbic acid, or vitamin C.) The natural "D" form of vitamin E is manufactured from vegetable oils. Fresh vegetable oil is a nutritional source of E as well, and the Biblical "anointing with oil" or "binding up wounds in oil" may be seen as very sensible.

Vitamin E promotes rapid, scar-free healing, prevents infection, feels a lot better on a kid's cut than iodine, and is almost unbelievably versatile. Please refer back to the appendix for a list of some of E's uses. Other entirely natural, simple skin aids are olive oil and cocoa butter. Both are just vegetable oils, although cocoa butter is not liquid in its natural form. It is more like a wax candle, like a stick. "Cocoa butter lotion" or "cream with natural cocoa butter" is not 100 percent cocoa butter. It may contain some cocoa butter and have wonderfully natural names, but the words "100 percent cocoa butter" should be on the label you look for if you want the real thing. Just apply the cocoa butter to skin like a stick deodorant or lipstick.

And Speaking of Lipsticks and Deodorants

Read the labels on cosmetics and anti-perspirants for a surprise. To think that people coat their lips, faces, and underarms with chemicals! Natural cosmetic products are fortunately available, but label reading is absolutely necessary. Don't let a company's natural reputation, natural label names and natural slogans substitute for a natural product. Please read the label.

Deodorants don't skimp on chemicals. The non-antiperspirants (talk about a double negative!) are less bad (again!) than most, but not as good as what health food stores generally carry. Antiperspirants are the worst kind of all deodorants because they contain aluminum and chemically block up skin pores and prevent natural sweating. Okay, so you don't want to sweat? Then dress more seasonally When I was in Sydney, Australia, I saw businessmen go to work in shirts and ties . . . and shorts. Good idea. Try wearing cottons more; cotton fabrics "breathe" more easily than polyesters, nylons, and other synthetics. Some people think and feel that their bodies prefer natural fiber clothing as they also prefer natural foods. When I was in high school, the guys in gym class used to spray their deodorants on their lockers. Took the paint right off them. Even back then we wondered, "If it does that to a locker, what's it doing to our armpits?" Perhaps it's enough to say that I'm glad my family uses something slightly more natural!

Concerning cosmetics, I can't really say that much from personal experience. Ahem. My better half uses some make-up, although I think she's very attractive without it. It would seem to me that moderation and natural ingredients would be the two things to look for in using cosmetics, if you choose to use them at all.

Loofas and Dry Towels

There's nothing like a good old-fashioned friction rubdown. A coarse, sponge-like "loofa" is great for this. A loofa is actually the dried center of a squash-like plant, which grows easily in a garden should you have the seeds and the inclination to grow bath sponges. Loofas are sold at many drugstores for a few dollars. Brittle and dry when you buy it, the loofa softens somewhat when wet but remains an excellent skin toner. While showering, just scrub with soap and the loofa and you'll see what I mean. Old, dry, and scaly skin is rubbed away and the friction will give you a healthy pink glow all over. If you finish your warm shower with a cool water rinse-off and then a dry towel rub-down, you will find it both relaxing and invigorating. If you scrub, and rub, towards the heart, you'll be giving yourself a valuable massage. Masseurs always work in the direction of the heart to stimulate blood flow in and below the skin. The direction would be up the arms and up the legs and then up the trunk.

Soaps

I think that simple, pure, plain-old soap is best. After all, all soaps are basically the same anyway, with added colors, fragrances, chemicals, fancy boxes, and higher prices. As the founder of the large Pear's Soap company said a century ago, "Any fool can make soap. It takes a clever man to sell it." The best soap on the market is unquestionably still plain, no-colors, no-perfume soap. You can use soap sparingly and still get very clean. This is especially beneficial if a person is prone to dry skin. Supplementing the diet with vitamin E may also help you as much as it has helped my family's complexions. Soap really doesn't harm healthy skin, but so many people don't know what it's like to have healthy skin because of—here it comes again—because of an unnatural diet that doesn't nourish the skin in the first place. Beauty is not only skin deep: it goes from your nose to your toes and from inside out.

Shampoos

If you've never read your shampoo label, now would be a good time to start. Have you wondered why babies cry when they get shampoo in their eyes? There are so many chemicals—in addition to simple detergent, including artificial colors, preservatives, and any number of unpronounceable chemicals. It had always been known for its "No More Tears" products, but in 1999 Johnson and Johnson really overreached. Their popular baby shampoo label in September of that year specifically stated that it was "As gentle to eyes as pure water." I guess I'd been reading only the front of their label for too long, so now I looked on the back to find, in addition to the usual detergents, these goodies: polyquaternium-10, tetrasodium edta, quaternium-15, D&C yellow #10, and D&C orange #4. I'm not saying that this stuff is dangerous. I actually used the product on my kids for years. I am surprised, though, that any company would claim it is *as gentle to the eyes as PURE water*. It might have a pH of 7, but those other ingredients *must* make it *just a little* different from H_2O.

So who can be surprised that natural, herbal shampoos are highly recommended by many health advocates. There are many brand names of natural-origin shampoos, and you'd want to read the labels before purchasing any, and reject any with bright colors, preservatives, or long names! One or two natural ingredients don't make a product natural unless the rest are natural, too. In case you think that natural shampoos and soaps must be expensive to use, please consider this: In terms of quality of ingredients, "bargain brands" may be the real waste of your

265

money and generate the biggest profit for manufacturers that don't care what's in their product. Natural products may not be the cheapest, but they do cost more to produce in the first place. Keeping these points in mind may help you compare quantity and quality and still save money in the long run. Good daily skin care is cheaper than a visit to a dermatologist.

In case you feel that natural ingredients are not important in your shampoo because synthetic ingredients are carefully tested and approved, please consider this quotation from "And Now A Word About Your Shampoo" by Harold C. Hopkins in the March 1975 *FDA Consumer:*

FDA (Food and Drug Administration) authority under the Food, Drug and Cosmetic Act to regulate synthetic detergent shampoos, along with other cosmetics, falls considerably short of the comprehensive kind of jurisdiction the Act authorizes for regulation of foods and drugs. The maker of a cosmetic is not required, as is the sponsor of a new drug, to obtain FDA approval before marketing to assure that the product is safe and effective. And cosmetics makers, unlike food processors, are not required to obtain FDA clearance to use new additives (except for color additives) in their products. The law does hold the manufacturer of a synthetic detergent shampoo or other cosmetic solely responsible for safety in its use. He is expected to use ingredients about which there have been no questions of safety, and to perform adequate studies . . . to make sure his product is safe before he puts it on the market. FDA must trust that the manufacturer has fulfilled his responsibility.

It is only if, or should we say when, an "adverse reaction" occurs that the consumer or the manufacturer is supposed to notify FDA and then FDA will "look into the matter." This does not seem like much of a safeguard to the millions of people who may have been using the product already.

FDA's enforcement of its regulatory powers over foods are weak enough. Think of all the chemicals, preservatives, dyes and other additives that are legally allowed, to contaminate our food. To think that FDA's authority over cosmetics and shampoos is actually less than its control over Kool-Aid, Twinkies, and Mello Yello!

And if you think that's bad, consider soap itself. This same article also says this:

"The Food. Drug and Cosmetic Act of 1938 defines a cosmetic. But the same law specifically excludes soap from this definition of a cosmetic and it is thus exempt from FDA regulation."

We'd better all read the package labels for everything we put on our bodies as well as for everything we put into them. The Food, Drug and Cosmetic Act of 1938 was a very watered down excuse for the original and very strict Food and Drug Act of 1906. The original 1906 law actually permitted only pure foods and drugs! It didn't last long, after industrial lobbying and government corruption started after it. If you want to read an account of this amazing and unlawful process, it is all in Dr. Harvey W. Wiley's *A History of a Crime Against the Food Law,* most recently republished only by photocopy. This is probably another job for your skilled librarian and an interlibrary loan. If you still think that the government protects us from toxic substances in what we eat or drink or put on our skin, it's time to reconsider.

There is little question that natural cosmetic products, soaps, and shampoos are nearly as important to us as natural foods. Nature is best for your inside and your outside.

"Joy, temperance, and repose slam the door on the doctor's nose."
—LONGFELLOW

One in ten adults takes sleeping pills. Those that do are *five times* more likely to die sooner from cancer and other causes than those who don't. In 2012, a study of nearly 11,000 adults concluded that this amounts to *half a million premature deaths every year* due to sleeping pills.[1]

In spite of the now-proven risks of sedative, hypnotic, or tranquilizing drugs, we are becoming a nation of nocturnal "users." With so many effective natural methods for falling asleep available, however, dependency on pharmaceuticals is often completely unnecessary. It is time for everyone to start "just saying no" to excessively prescribed drugs . . . and those over-the-counter drugs, too.

One of the best things about natural sleep aids is that they are safe and not habit forming. When your brain and body are well nourished, more restful sleep is a natural result. You are feeding your body, not drugging it. Here are some techniques that will help you get to sleep more quickly and without the assistance of the pharmaceutical industry.

How to Get a Good Night's Sleep. . . Tonight!

1. **Read** for a while. This will improve your mind while relaxing your body.

2. Get some **fresh air**. Open a window, walk the dog.

3. Try some moderate **exercise**, such as isometrics, yoga, or stretches. Couples have found that lovemaking works well, too. But you did not hear that from me.

4. Get more **L-tryptophan** in your diet. L-tryptophan is one of the amino acids your body uses to make serotonin, a neurotransmitter that helps your brain to shut down for the night—and be fully awake during the day. Seafood, the dark meat of chicken and turkey, milk, cheese, yogurt, beans, and cashews are good sources of L-tryptophan. More of the L-tryptophan in dairy products gets to your brain when you have a carbohydrate along with it. That's why cheese and crackers, or milk and a whole-grain cookie, are good evening snacks. Normal portions can provide the target dose of about a gram (1,000 mg) or so. After all, a palm-sized single portion of cashews contains 500 mg of tryptophan. Other nuts are nearly as good, and seeds too. Chew them thoroughly, of course. That's half the fun of snacking, anyway, isn't it?

5. **Niacin** in larger than RDA doses will help induce sleep. Taking between 50 and 200 milligrams about 20 minutes before bedtime usually works best. Some people need much more, but start small and discover for yourself. The amount required varies considerably from one person to another. Ideally, you take the least amount that makes you the most sleepy. Expect to experience a brief niacin "flush" (like a hot flash or blushing sensation), which is harmless and goes away in short time. The warm feeling is pleasant to most people, but may be avoided by simply taking less niacin at any one time. A bit of practice will tell you how much you need.

6. **Lecithin** makes up nearly a third of your brain's dry weight. This natural food substance is

found in soy products and egg yolks and is available as a supplement as well. Two or three tablespoons daily has consistently shortened the time needed for people to go to sleep.

7. **Prayer or meditation** may be very settling and help you sleep sooner and better. Certainly there are other benefits as well. The Transcendental Meditation technique has been shown to produce deep rest, reduced anxiety, and very effective relief from insomnia (Miskiman, DE. [1974]. The treatment of insomnia by transcendental meditation, Scientific Research on Transcendental Meditation: Collected Papers, Orme-Johnson, Domash, and Farrow, Eds., Vol. 1, MIU Press). The Trappist monastic tradition contains the phrase, "I lie down, and sleep comes at once." Psalm 127 says, "For he gives to his beloved sleep." That's a mighty good argument for prayer.

8. You may have heard about **melatonin**, the body's own natural sleep-promoting hormone. You can increase your body's melatonin production by keeping your bedroom as dark as humanly possible. You can also try 3 to 9 mg of supplemental melatonin (one to three tablets), taken about an hour before bedtime. Melatonin is very safe: studies using over 200 mg/day failed to show harm.

9. **For the kids**: Back when I was in grammar school, we actually got a grade on our report card that evaluated the extent to which we were "rested and ready for work." I cannot help but wonder why they didn't think a little more deeply about the fact that we also walked three-quarters of a mile each way to school, and home for lunch, for a total of three miles daily . . . at age seven. At day's end, I was as pooped as a farm boy. I'll bet your kids are more tired than they let on. Try getting them to bed earlier. They'll hate it. And probably you as well. But you will all sleep more, and that can be a very big payoff.

Ayurvedic Cycles

If you have tried all of the above and still find that you are one of those folks who fall asleep normally, but are wide awake at 3 A.M., and wonder what to do about it, I have an answer for you: get up. It may be perfectly normal for you to be awake then. It does no good to have someone tell you to get some sleep. It does no good to lie down and stay awake, either. Let's think outside the box, and take a few moments to see what Ayurveda, India's great heritage of natural healing, counsels us when it comes to sleep. I am one of many people who, once able to unlearn some very Western assumptions of proper sleep habits, have found a natural fit with Ayurvedic cycles.

In Ayurveda there are three time periods in every twelve hours, called vata, pitta, and kapha. Vata is from 2–6, kapha is from 6–10, and pitta is from 10–2. The cycle repeats itself in the next twelve hours, so there are two vata times, two kapha times, and two pitta times each day. In a nutshell, Ayurvedic beliefs about sleep can be summed up, to borrow from Ben Franklin, as "Early to bed and early to rise makes a man healthy, wealthy, and wise."

During vata time, a person's mind is at its peak. Mental alertness is high, but so is a tendency toward mental excess, stress, and anxiety. Vata time is a good time to study, but a bad time to worry. It extends, remember, from 2–6 P.M. *and* 2–6 A.M. Without knowing about this, I, as a college student, used to do all my studying from when afternoon classes ended up until supper. My body was perhaps tired then, but my mind was fully on. Trappist monks start their day at about 2 A.M., promptly commencing with study until dawn. This too is an Ayurvedic rhythm.

Pitta time, from 10–2, is a period of physical activity, appetite, and what we often call "getting our second wind." I know mothers and fathers who wait until the kids are in bed so they can get some work done. They tackle remodeling projects or clean the house starting at about 10 P.M. Once they get going, they can easily last until 2. Party-hearty college students are the ultimate pitta devotees. Their day is just beginning at 10 P.M., and goes great guns until 2 A.M.

If you want to stay awake, stay up for pitta time, but plan to be up for the whole 10–2 block. If you want to sleep, get to bed well before 10 P.M. This no doubt sounds unrealistically rigid to most people. That's too bad, because they are missing out on a good thing. The good thing is kapha time, 6–10. Kapha is slow, smooth, easy, heavy . . . and sleepy. How do you feel after your evening dinner? Yeah, just kick back and put your feet up. Many of us doze off in the early evening. It is easy to do, because nature is trying to tell us something: go to bed, you lummox! And the earlier, the better.

And then there is morning kapha: 6 until 10. Sleepyheads everywhere knows all about kapha time. When that alarm goes off at 6, and it's early, early dawn, and you cover your head with the pillow, or cuddle up with your blankets, sweetie, or Teddy bear, well, you know what I am talking about. Try to get a teenager up before 10. Not easy. Do you telephone your friends on weekends before 10 A.M.? Not if you want them to remain your friends.

When I was going through an unbelievably stressful period in my life, I could not sleep. No matter how tired I was, or how late I went to bed to get that tired, I would always wake up at the same time: very close to 2 or 2:30 A.M. This was driving me nuts, and in my desperation, I decided I had to try what you probably do not want to try: going to bed really early (again, like the Trappists do), around 8 P.M. I was surprised that I fell asleep so readily. I still woke up at 2, but by then I'd had six hours of sleep. With time, I was able to "sleep in" until 4 A.M. My life stresses were unabated, but I had a reliable eight hours of sleep each night with which to attack them. Sounds odd, of course, but it works.

Reference

1. Kripke DF, Langer RD, Kline LE. Hypnotics' association with mortality or cancer: a matched cohort study. *BMJ Open*, 2012 Feb 27;2(1):e000850. See also: Scripps Study: sleeping pills believed a cause of 500,000 premature deaths annually. March 1, 2012. http://www.pharma-watch.com

Recommended Reading

Chopra, D. *Perfect Health*. New York: Harmony Books, 1991.

Lad, V. *Ayurveda: The Science of Self-Healing*. Santa Fe, NM: Lotus, 1984.

"For every drug that benefits a patient, there is a natural substance that can achieve the same effect."

—CARL C. PFEIFFER, M.D., PH.D.

There is a nutritional alternative for most drugs. You have to dig a bit for the details, but the work has been done. You will find very few negative effects from vitamins in the *Physicians' Desk Reference (PDR)*, but you will see column after column and page after page of side effects, contraindications, and warnings for drugs.

For example, I give you Coumadin, the ubiquitous drug for thinning the blood. You can often use vitamin E instead. Vitamin E potentiates the effects of Coumadin, and at up to 3,200 IU or less daily, it can completely and safely substitute for the drug. That is just plain true. I've seen it again and again.

The case of the Big Trucker stands out in particular.

Bob was a big guy: tall, wide, and heavy. He had a lengthy history of thrombophlebitis and most of its possible complications. One day he came to see me, wondering what options he had to forever taking Coumadin.

"You need to lose weight, Bob," was the first thing I said. "You need to stop smoking, too. There's no way any therapy, drug, or anything else is going to really work for you unless you do those things first."

He listened thoughtfully. "OK," he said. "I'll try. What else?"

Pleased that we'd even gotten this far without his wiping the floor with me, I proceeded to tell this man of few words about vitamin E as a blood thinner. Doctors Wilfrid Shute and Evan Shute of London, Ontario pioneered such use of the vitamin back in the 1940s. Their medical society went berserk, blacklisted them from meetings, and expelled any doctor that even attended a lecture by the Shute brothers.

Vitamin E is vastly safer than warfarin, the generic name of Coumadin. Warfarin is the active ingredient in rat poison. Rats are pretty smart, by the way. They must be poisoned subtly and long-term, like patients. A cumulative moderate overdose of Coumadin causes their blood to be too thin, and the little bastards hemorrhage and die. A cumulative overdose of vitamin E, even extreme megadosing, has never killed anybody.

Bob's prothrombin (clotting) time was thirteen seconds without medication. His doc wanted twenty to twenty-two seconds, and got it with the drug. "Will I get the same results with vitamin E?" Bob asked.

"You might," I said. "Ask your doctor to try a gradual reduction dosage of the drug while gradually increasing the vitamin dosage. I've seen that work well before."

Weeks later I saw Big Bob again. He had stopped smoking and lost weight.

"How are you doing?" I asked him leadingly.

"Pretty good," Bob admitted. "Still on the Coumadin. Not taking the vitamin E yet."

"Why?" I asked.

The answer really surprised me.

"Well," Bob said, "I really don't want to talk to the doctor about it. He'll think I'm stupid. Says I've got to take it."

270

"You feel you can't talk to your doctor about this?"

"Nope. I didn't even finish high school," Bob said. "He'll just make me feel like a jerk for wanting to not take my medicine."

Witnessing a big strong man shrink childishly away from confronting his own doctor was a new one for me. "You can talk to your doctor, Bob. You've got to be able to discuss your own body with your doctor. What did he say to you when he observed that you'd lost weight?"

"He said just keep doing what I'm doing."

"And stopping the smoking?" I added.

"He said that was good, too," Bob answered. "He never brought that up before, but he said it was good that I'd quit." Incredibly, the great majority of patients who smoke have never been ordered to quit by their doctor.

"But our credit isn't good enough for vitamin E, huh?" I said with a half smile. "You know, you're not offering anything foolish when you ask for a tapering drug dosage schedule and willingly come in for regular monitoring. The safer alternative is always worth a therapeutic trial; any doctor should know that."

Bob shook his head. He paused, then shook it again. "No," he said. "Don't want to bring it up with him." There was a pause. "I'm just going to take the vitamin E anyway," Bob said quietly.

"I'd prefer the doctor was in on this," I responded, "but if you are going to do it, do it right. Increase the dose over a period of weeks. Most people start with 200 IU daily, and eventually get to between 1,200 and 2,400 IU daily. Do it gradually, and here's a way to tell how you're coming: go in to your doctor regularly, as you always do. Have him check your protime, as he always does. If you get the numbers he wants, he won't care how you got them."

"Could I increase the vitamin E and still stay on the Coumadin?" Bob wondered.

"More or less, but the more E you take, the stronger the Coumadin's effect. You'll probably get to the point where your protime is too long, and he'll have to cut back on the dosage of Coumadin."

Bob thought about that for a bit. "So I can just show him that I don't need the drug any more?"

"That's about it," I said. "If your protime is on the long side, he'll cut you back on the medicine."

A month later I saw Bob for a follow-up visit. "I did it," he said. "The last time I saw the doctor, my clotting time was a bit too long. So he asked me, 'What are you doing?' I told him I was taking vitamin E. He said, 'Stop taking that vitamin. It is interfering with the Coumadin.'"

Golly, Doc, we wouldn't want that, now would we?

> *"New opinions are always suspected, and usually opposed,*
> *without any other reasons but because they are not already common."*
> —JOHN LOCKE

Too Little: Hypothyroidism

One day, back in my middle-aged years, I was sitting in a doctor's examination room, waiting for a physical. Uncharacteristically, I had failed to bring a book with me. So, bored out of my gourd, I did what kids do at breakfast: I started "reading the cereal box." In this instance, without a magazine (or box of Wheaties) to be had, there was nothing to read except tongue-depressor jars, anatomical charts, and pharmaceutical advertising posters on the doctor's wall. One was a life-size representation of an unhappy looking woman. The poster lady was overweight, no pep, depressed, dry skinned, sad-eyed, and falling asleep all the time. The reason, said the poster, was underactive thyroid, or hypothyroidism.

It suddenly occurred to me that this was a very accurate and detailed description of a good friend of the family, Nina. Nina, in her early forties, was a poster girl for thyroid deficiency. Literally. She fell asleep driving home from work . . . on an interstate highway going 60 MPH. Not good. This dangerously chronic occurrence, plus my entreaties, got her to go to an endocrinoligist. It was a short visit. She outlined her symptoms, as previously itemized, and asked for a thyroid supplement (as they require a prescription). The endocrinologist responded by literally laughing her out of the office. That is not a figure of speech. It was all over in under five minutes, and that included "Please take a seat" and "Now what seems to be the trouble?" She plainly told him just what her symptoms were and what her reading led her to believe just might help. He never even offered to do a thyroid test. I guess he hadn't seen the poster.

I am glad I did, as I listened to Nina's rather humiliating story. I suggested she try a different doctor. To her credit, she promptly did so. This new doctor, a woman, was not a specialist but a general practitioner. She listened, heard the patient's request, and said, "Yes, we can certainly try some thyroid and see how it works for you." Beginning with a low dose, she said, would not require testing. If it helped, it was needed. That is a therapeutic trial. So-called evidence-based medicine scorns this approach. That is unfortunate: it worked. A grain of natural thyroid a day stopped her from falling asleep at the wheel. Two grains made her depression go away. Four grains prevented her from sleeping at night. Whoa, too much. Two grains it is, and that's what she continued with.

Although I saw this up close and personal, there was another case I saw at even closer range, years earlier. When I was a teenager, my mother suffered from assorted discomforts, including arthritis, depression, skin problems, fatigue, unexplained weight gain, and assorted other miserable symptoms. Nothing seemed to help, until she got a new, younger family physician. He promptly put her on thyroid medication, and she was a new woman. Surprisingly, her singing voice came back, along with her get-up-and-go. Her weight came down, her joy of living came up, and her skin looked great. No more bags under the eyes; no more three-hour daily naps. If either of these people sound all too familiar, then perhaps a thyroid supplement (by prescription) is for you.

TSH Test Is Inadequate

It certainly was the case for this reader. She writes:

"For thirty years I was a zombie with every low-thyroid symptom, but a "normal" TSH, so I was told my thyroid was not the problem. Finally, my body started shutting down (I started to feel dead), hair falling out and blood pressure skyhigh. I borrowed some Armour thyroid and started treating myself. Immediately I began to recover but the HMO refused to give me a prescription. They even wrote me a letter telling me to discontinue it! The mental and physical suffering were so great—as was realizing I had lost so many years. Eventually I got a prescription for Armour. I had to save my own life."

Others have shared similar stories with me. The biggest mistake a doctor can make is to disbelieve a patient. This goes triple for thyroid symptoms. Don't be a thyroid android! Stop "living with it." Speak up, and ask for a therapeutic trial of natural thyroid extract.

T-3 or T-4?

There is an important difference between T-3 and T-4 thyroid hormone. T-3 (triiodothyronine) would seem to be the one to watch. Doctors characteristically over-emphasize your T-4 (l-thyroxine, or "storage" thyroxine) level and effectively ignore T-3 (fast-acting or "active" thyroxine) levels. Physician fixation on test results' numbers, which are inadequate to detect borderline conditions, results in masses of people suffering the symptoms of low thyroid. These all-too-common symptoms include fatigue, depression, weight gain, insomnia, difficult menopause, endometriosis, and quite a variety of others including arthritis and rheumatic complaints, low sex drive, infertility, and skin problems. Many, many persons are therefore "uncomfortable but still normal."

What to do? First of all, if you feel crummy, insist on thyroid testing, and get a copy of your test results. By law, your doctor must provide them to you if you ask. So ask! Interpretation of the tests is likely to be better if you are in on it, and easier if you have done your homework.

Here's a start: it is important to know that a "normal" or even somewhat high T-4 can coexist with the symptoms of low thyroid function. Do not accept a test for T-4 alone. Insist on T-3 testing as well, and pay special attention to it. TSH (thyroid stimulating hormone) testing will almost always be done. High TSH levels indicate that your pituitary gland and brain want more thyroid hormone. If your TSH number is over 3.0, it is something of a warning. A number over 4.0 means "get on it now." If you still have low thyroid symptoms with a TSH of 2 or lower, you can order a TRH (Thyrotropin Releasing Hormone) test.

Be prepared to require your doctor to take action. Ask for and get a therapeutic trial. This statement will not endear me or you to the entire medical community, but who cares about that any more? Your health is not a popularity contest.

Side Effects

Remember my comment about "doing your homework"? Learn the side effects of too much thyroid. These include rapid heartbeat, unusual difficulty sleeping, sweating and otherwise feeling hot, hyperactivity, a racing mind, and twitching. Contrary to popular medical myth, thyroid medication does not cause osteoporosis; it helps prevent it. Excess iodine supplementation usually will not help low thyroid sufferers. Take thyroid medication on an empty stomach.

273

More Hints

My attitude toward thyroid-related issues essentially is this: If you have symptoms, there's something you can do about it. Other helpful tools include stress reduction, avoiding chemicals in both food and environment, choosing organic foods, and taking vitamin supplements. And don't forget your vitamin C (as if I'd let you, right?), which helps keep your adrenal glands happy. B-complex, vitamin E, plus calcium, magnesium, zinc, and chromium are also worth including in your supplemental program. You should also stop caffeine, tobacco, alcohol, and aspartame ("NutraSweet") use.

Read up. I suggest *Thyroid Power,* by Richard L. Shames and Karilee H. Shames.(NY: Harper Collins, 2001) The book provides a lot more information than I can, plus case histories, self-evaluations, and test numbers to look for.

Too Much: Graves' Disease (Diffuse Toxic Goiter)

Graves' disease is the largest single cause of hyperthyroidism, an overactive thyroid gland. Too much thyroid hormone causes protrusion of the eyeballs and a red rash and other skin lesions.

> ### A reader writes:
>
> "I have Graves' disease, diagnosed in February of 2000. I was put on various levels of propylthiouracil (PTU) to get my thyroxin levels under control. I'm supposed to be between 0–5. In March of 2002 I stopped taking my medicine (in two years I had never been below 9) and started vitamin and mineral therapy on my own. I had my blood tested a week ago and for the first time in two and a half years my levels are normal: 2.49 to be exact. My endocrinologist does not think it will last, of course, and wants me to get either radiation therapy or a thyroidectomy, but I feel better than I have in years.
>
> "I posted my story on a national Graves' disease bulletin board—the only story on the whole site about any type of vitamin therapy. Within twenty-four hours, all of my postings and responses and anything to do with vitamins were removed and my account was suspended.
>
> "I think Graves disease is a nutritional deficiency disease that is correctable with proper vitamin and mineral intake. Dosage is mostly something we have to research and figure out for ourselves, depending on one's own individual needs.
>
> It is so scary to me that the doctors are encouraging damaging medicine/radiation/surgery as treatments and completely ignoring the fact that vitamins and minerals have worked for other people."

Graves' disease organizations tend to take the view that only anti-thyroid drugs, radioactive iodine, and subtotal thyroidectomy are valid therapies, and that there is no "natural' alternative. But I think there are more options than these. Consider that Graves' disease may be triggered by stress, smoking, radiation, medication, and viruses. Genetics plays a small part, but there is no specific gene that causes the disease. If Graves' disease cannot be passed off as genetic and can be "triggered" by stress, smoking, radiation, medication, or even pregnancy, it sounds like a problem that therapeutic nutrition may help.

A *physician writes:*

"I usually approach Graves Disease by first giving standard solution potassium iodide (SSKI) to control the symptoms (and occasionally fix the problem right there). I don't like using kelp because you don't really know how much iodine you're getting. For the SSKI, I usually follow the PDR recommendation of about 30 drops a day (not all at once!) mixed in a healthy volume of water. You get tingling if you take it too fast. I'll do that for a week or two, depending on the response, then adjust or stop. Repeat later if needed. But do watch it, for too much iodine can be toxic. I go after the autoimmune aspects by using protocols similar to those from the Arthritis Trust (www.arthritistrust.org, click "Education" and then "Articles"). Of course, all patients start out with instructions for a healthy diet and supplements—after all, you must get the basics right before you can expect anything else to work. A basic multivitamin/ multimineral, plus omega 3 fatty acids are a good start for most folks."

Trigger Finger

*"Do not fear to be eccentric in opinion,
for every opinion now accepted was once eccentric."*
—BERTRAND RUSSELL

Thanks to the J. J. Newberry department store, I avoided hand surgery. Twice. Newberry's, in Batavia, New York, was a creaky, wooden-floored, iron-ceilinged five-and-dime. From the worn chrome lunch counter, selling hot dogs basted in grease, to the claustrophobic basement, where they kept the pet department (and the iguanas), every trip to Newberry's was a trip back into the forties. Friends and I made a pilgrimage to the store every time we were in town.

I'd been having some trouble with my left hand. A chiropractor friend of mine told me I was developing a trigger finger, and he sure had that right. Whenever I curled my hand, my ring finger locked in the down position. This was especially disturbing to me because both my mother and father had surgery for trigger fingers—in Dad's case, nine such operations! Oh, great, I thought. My turn now, at age thirty, in graduate school.

One evening, there I was in statistics class, trying to stay awake. My hand was aching and locking so that I wiggled and squirmed constantly. Class members probably thought I had to go to the bathroom. I flexed my hand, stretching and curling it. I cracked my knuckles (silently) and bent my wrist. Hmm. It all felt a bit better, but nothing remarkable. This went on sporadically, stimulated by the dullness of standard deviations, two-tailed t-tests, and chi squares.

Then I grabbed my wrist with my other hand, and applied some downward traction. I felt a pull, then a clunk, in my wrist. I grabbed a thicker part of my arm, closed my hand and curled my fingers around it and pulled, and it happened again. By then I'd nearly lost track of the lecture, just like everybody else had, but for a different reason. I left off my experimenting and hastened back to note-taking and question-asking.

So back to Newberry's, the five-and-dime, remember? It was a Friday evening, about 5:30. I was squeaking my way around the store, bargain hunting. Down one war-torn, metal-shelved isle, I spotted some three-inch diameter hard rubber balls. They were probably designed for playing fetch with your favorite medium-sized dog. They were solid rubber, unpainted, and three for a dollar. I summoned up unknown instincts, took the plunge, and bought two.

I still had the trigger finger problem. But I had pocketed the experience from statistics class that grabbing something, curling my hand, and stretching my wrists got me a clunk in the wrist and some relief. Holding one of the balls in my hand, I began to do the same procedure. I found that if I grabbed the ball with my fingers only (no thumb), I could roll the ball from finger tips to wrist, bending my hand more and more as I went. Furthermore, if I braced my wrist with the other hand, I could choose where the hand and wrist actually bent and stretched the most. The tangible rewards were straightforward: a clunk in the wrist and profound relief in the hand.

There are over fifty bones between your two hands. That's about one quarter of all the bones in your body. Your wrist is made up of many small bones through which a complicated robotic system of nerves, blood vessels, ligaments, and tendons must pass. The idea of physiotherapy for carpal tunnel syndrome and other repetitive motion disorders is hardly new, but such an approach for trigger fingers was never offered to anyone I've met.

Bottom line was that it was completely successful. Over a period of three weeks at most, all the triggering went away. No pain, soreness, or stiffness. No locking. Just a 34 cent (plus tax) ball from Newberry's, used a couple of times a day.

Newberry's has since gone out of business, but there's more. During my once-a-decade physical, I asked my doctor about a lump on my wrist. It was small and hard, on the outside wrist two inches south of my thumb.

"Ganglionic cyst," he said.

Ah yes, the "Bible" cyst. In the old days, doctors just whacked them out of existence with whatever big book was at hand. This guy referred me to a hand specialist instead.

The hand surgeon explained to me how he would set out my arm like this, use an anesthetic like so, cut off the blood supply here, and open an incision there. More details followed, which made me squeamish.

"What will happen if I don't choose to have the surgery?" I asked.

"It might get worse; it probably won't get better," he answered.

I was instructed to stop and schedule a date for surgery on my way out with one of a pack of office assistants, but I kept right on walking. I wasn't sure I wanted to go through all of that for a wrist lump.

I continued to use my exercise ball a few times a week to keep any chance of the trigger finger from returning.

Time passed.

One day I noticed that the wrist lump was gone. Nobody hit me with the Old Testament, and nobody operated, either. The lump has never returned, no it never returned, and its fate is still unlearned.

Newberry's saved my insurance company a pile of money, saved me two surgeries, and I get to keep the balls. Total cost of my therapy: 67 cents.

Plus tax.

"There is no such thing as freedom of choice unless there is freedom to refuse."

—DAVID HUME

Much of what I've shared with you throughout this book might be regarded as good common sense, and a rapidly increasing number of parents share the "vitamins yes, junk food no" point of view. Now for the really controversial part: my children did not get immunizations. My firstborn had two rounds of shots as an infant, but when his mother and I both saw that the vaccinations made him sick, we halted them. A lot of eyebrows may raise at this point, and that's fine. Let's raise them a bit further.

Criticism of vaccinations is by no means a new phenomenon. Some sixty years ago, William McCormick, M.D., of Toronto, published a series of papers (please see the Bibliography for an extensive list of McCormick's work) showing that inoculations have had very little, if any, influence on the history of these illnesses. In 1960, Howard H. Hillemann's lengthy paper, "The Illusion of American Health and Longevity," presented similar findings. Pediatrician Robert Mendelsohn was an outspoken critic of vaccination throughout the 1970s and 1980s. The debate continues to this day, with the Internet providing one of the major forums for discussion. (See the end of this chapter for web sites.) So before your heart stops at the thought of my meatless, shotless children, read these researchers' papers and start wondering not why my kids aren't "protected" but if yours really are. If you're a young parent with young children, the question of vaccinations for your family is an important one. You want what's best for your kids. We all do. So what's the right decision, then? Shots or no shots?

THE HEALTH HAZARDS OF DISEASE PREVENTION

by Damien Downing, M.D.

"No pharmaceutical drug is devoid of risks from adverse reactions and vaccines are no exception. Vaccination is a medical intervention and should be carried out with the informed consent of those who are being subjected to it."

—DR. LUCIJA TOMLJENOVIC, UNIVERSITY OF BRITISH COLUMBIA.

At a 2011 conference held in London by the British Society for Ecological Medicine, the main topic was vaccinations. Not one person speaking was anti-vaccination; most said they were in favor of vaccination, but even more so of vaccine safety. One speaker summarized it this way: "Most vaccines offer benefit to most children most of the time. Some vaccines do harm to some children some of the time."

Here are some of the surprising facts reported.

HOW SAFE ARE VACCINES?

- There are no studies comparing vaccine safety to a genuine placebo. The only study that claims to do so[1] compared active vaccines to a placebo containing all the adjuvants, including neomycin (a known neurotoxin).

278

- Adjuvants, a key component of all vaccinations, have been shown to predispose to auto-immune disease.[2]

- Aluminum is a serious neurotoxin but is used as an adjuvant in many vaccines; between 2 and 18 months of age children may repeatedly receive up to 50 times the FDA safety limit in vaccines alone.[3]

- A Cochrane review of MMR in 2005 found that "The design and reporting of safety outcomes in MMR vaccine studies, both pre- and post-marketing, are largely inadequate."[4]

- Recorded adverse events following HPV vaccine in the US, which are thought to represent less than 10% of the actual incidence, now stand at well over 21,000, including 93 deaths, 8,661 emergency room visits, 4,382 cases who have not recovered and 702 who have been disabled.[5]

DO WE NEED ALL THESE VACCINES?

- Why do we give rubella vaccinations to boys when the only people that rubella seriously affects are pregnant women and their babies?

- Mumps is very rare and only of serious danger to boys—so why give it to girls? Introduction of the mumps vaccine only served to shift the incidence of the disease from very young children, in whom it was harmless, to older children in whom it was not.

- Diphtheria had effectively disappeared by the time the vaccination for it was introduced.

- Catching measles in childhood reduces the risk of asthma by 80% and of allergy in general by 30%.[6]

- Chicken pox, caught under the age of eight, reduces the risk of eczema by 45% and of severe eczema by a dramatic 96%.[7]

WHO CAN WE TRUST?

Vera Hassner Sharav writes: "Public health officials on both sides of the Atlantic have lost the public trust because they have been in league with vaccine manufacturers in denying that safety problems exist. If vaccines posed no safety problems why has the US Vaccine Court awarded more than $2 billion dollars to settle 2,500 cases involving vaccine-related debilitating injuries in children?"[8]

When US FDA officials analyzed the data on autism and thimerosal-containing vaccines they found a clear link. Their response, detailed in transcripts of a meeting at Simpsonwood, VA in July 2000 was to "massage" the data to make the link go away.[9]

In the UK, JCVI (Joint Committee on Vaccines and Immunization) has known since 1986 that there were serious safety concerns around vaccinations, for measles in particular. JCVI has repeatedly responded to negative data by ignoring it or covering it up, and has downplayed vaccine safety concerns while overplaying benefits.[10]

CLEARLY NOT THE CDC

If you thought all that was bad, try out the proposal from the National Centers for Immunization and Respiratory Disease in CDC; a study found that the IgA antibodies in breast milk could reduce the potency of vaccines—especially in developing countries; American breast milk is not nearly as good[11]. Their proposal: delay breast-feeding. No, you didn't misread; the abstract says; "Strategies to overcome this negative effect, such as delaying breast-feeding at the time of immunization, should be evaluated."

Oh, right. That'll fix it. Not!

279

References

1. Virtanen M, Peltola H, Paunio M, Heinonen OP. Day-to-day reactogenicity and the healthy vaccinee effect of measles-mumps-rubella vaccination. Pediatrics.2000 Nov;106(5):E62.

2. Schoenfeld Y, Agmon-Levin N. 'ASIA' Autoimmune/inflammatory syndrome induced by adjuvants. Journal of Autoimmunity 2011; 36 4–8 doi:10.1016/j.jaut.2010.07.003

3. Tomljenovic L. Aluminum and Alzheimer's disease: After a Century of Controversy, Is there a Plausible Link? J Alzheimer's Dis 2010; 23: 1–32. doi: 10.3233/JAD-2010–101494.

4. Demicheli V, Jefferson T, Rivetti A, Price D. Vaccines for measles, mumps and rubella in children. Cochrane Database of Systematic Reviews 2005, Issue 4. Art. No.: CD004407. doi: 10.1002/14651858.CD004407.pub2.

5. VAERS; www.medalerts.org/vaersdb Accessed February 2011

6. Rosenlund H et al. Allergic disease and atopic sensitization in children in relation to measles vaccination and measles infection. Pediatrics 2009; 123[3]: 771–8

7. Silverberg JI, Norowitz KB, Kleiman E et al. Association between varicella zoster virus infection and atopic dermatitis in early and late childhood: A case-control study. Journal of Allergy and Clinical Immunology 2010; 126: 300–305

8. Alliance for Human Research Protection. www.ahrp.org/cms/content/view/765/9/

9. www.scribd.com/doc/2887572/Simpsonwood-Transcript20Searchable

10. www.dh.gov.uk/en/FreedomOfInformation/Freedomofinformationpublicationschemefeedback/FOIreleases/DH_4140335

11. Shane AL, Jiang B, Baek LJ et al. Inhibitory Effect of Breast Milk on Infectivity of Live Oral Rotavirus Vaccines. Pediatr Infect Dis J. 2010; 29(10): 919–923.

Certainly the U.S. government cannot say without qualification that shots are either safe or essential. After all, this is what was said about the infamous swine flu vaccine in a 1976 FDA consumer memo: "Some minor side effects—tenderness in the arm, low fever, tiredness—will occur in less than 4 percent of [vaccinated] adults. Serious reactions from flu vaccines are very rare." So much for blanket claims of safety, for many persons well remember the numerous and serious side effects of swine flu vaccine that forced the federal immunization program to a halt.

As far as being essential, in the same memo the FDA said this of the vaccine: "Question: What can be done to prevent an epidemic? Answer: The only preventive action we can take is to develop a vaccine to immunize the public against the virus. This will prevent the virus from spreading." This was seen to be totally false. After all, the public immunization program was abruptly halted and still there was no epidemic of swine flu.

Surely there are other factors involved in prevention of illness or epidemic. But try telling that to allopathically oriented health commissioners and doctors. You'd think that monks and nuns who work with the sick would frequently get their patients' diseases . . . but they seldom do. There is much more to wellness than just collecting shots. Real wellness is the result of healthful living: natural diet, whole raw foods, plentiful vitamins, internal cleansing through periodic juice fasting, ample rest, peace of mind, and appropriate confidence in Nature's preference to keep us alive and well. If we follow these parameters, the essence of naturopathy, we find inoculations to be irrelevant.

Now if you live on candy, hamburgers, shakes, and steaks, you'd best get inoculated. Just as overfed, undernourished laboratory rats get sick at any brush with disease, so do overfed, undernourished people. A weakened, polluted body is fertile ground for assorted microbes to multiply. To the extent that vaccines and drugs deal with microbes only, they are apparently effective.

That phrase was "apparently" effective. Like adding Drano to a polluted pond, the chemical intervention does produce some dead germs. But poison on top of poison fails to get at the root cause of all illness, which is "polluted body" or systemic toxemia. In fact, the added drugs and vaccines compound the body's problem, for they cause side effects and new troubles of their own. The person gets more vaccines and still more drugs, to try to cover all these new illnesses, and then even more illness results. The cycle can go on and on for a lifetime, never solving the real problem.

Body pollution from wrong diet and neglect of natural living principles is the cause of disease. How can inoculations be given for neglect? How can you vaccinate a body against abuse? How can you be immunized against bad diet and insufficient vitamins? It can't be done. The allopathic medical establishment is looking into test tubes for answers that are found at our dinner tables. Drug companies' chemicals and hospitals' equipment cannot eliminate disease because they do not bring health in its place. Only you, yourself, can live in such a way as to become and stay well. Then the underlying causes of illness, including those we're usually immunized against, are eliminated without vaccination.

This applies to children as well as adults. If children are fed vitamin-rich, raw and whole food diets, they will not require shots to stay healthy. They will be healthier without the vaccination. We would do well to remember the examples of the Hunza (in Pakistan) and other truly isolated "primitive" peoples who are so healthy they don't even have names for diseases that we're seeking immunizations for. They have no shots, no free clinics, and no filled-in vaccination charts—until they start eating "civilized man's" foods. When they start into a diet of processed foods, sugar, and white flour and rice, they promptly contract all the "infectious" diseases.

There is proof. Decades ago, Weston Price, a dentist, went around the world to observe primitive peoples and their diet. He found that a simple, natural diet of mostly raw and always whole foods was the common denominator among all healthy, disease-free primitive peoples. Once these peoples started developing a Western diet, however, cavities began to appear, along with tuberculosis, pneumonia, influenza, and other diseases.

There are alternatives to having one's children routinely vaccinated. There is the choice of simply not having shots. No one should order you to get shots for your kids or order you not to get them. A lot of people may try, however. I believe that the parents should decide. Many parents, including my wife and me, have chosen to decline vaccinations for their children after careful deliberation. In doing so, we sometimes run into not unexpected opposition for this decision. Among the arguments you're likely to hear against no-shots policies (all false) are:

1. You don't care about your kid's health. You're only thinking of your own ideologies.

2. Vaccination is legally required. You must have it done or your kids can't go to school.

3. Kids will get the diseases unless they're immunized against them.

4. You're taking a chance. Why not get the shots and be safe?

Let's consider each of these arguments in turn.

Argument 1: You Don't Care

The truth is, we really do care about our children and their health, and that is the number one reason why they are not getting inoculations. We don't want to inject unnecessary poisons into our children. We want our kids to be down deep, totally healthy. A well-nourished, near-vegetarian, no-drug, vitamin-supplemented child is a truly healthy child. We care for our children very, very much, as the vast majority of parents do.

281

Argument 2: It's the Law

Vaccination is not legally required. For entrance into public schools, yes, shots are normally required. For certain jobs, yes again. Naturally the military requires them. There are ways of getting around these individual regulations, though. The simplest way is to take religious exception to vaccination on personal, spiritual grounds. This is constitutionally valid; remember that the First Amendment guarantees freedom of religion. There are two religious avenues to consider, and we have used them both.

Church Membership

First, you can join a religious group that holds vaccinations in disfavor. If this is unacceptable or impractical, you can start a church organization that believes vaccinations are morally wrong. You can create a bona fide religious organization by first becoming a legally ordained minister through the mail for $25 or so from various churches. I do not assert that by-mail ordinations put you on a par with the Pope; I merely assert that they are legal. With such an ordination you can start your own religious group with your own set of doctrinal beliefs. These beliefs may certainly "forbid any serum, vaccine, foreign, unnatural, or chemical substance of any nature to be injected or ingested into a church member's body for any avowed medical purpose whatsoever."

Personal Religious Belief

Your second-approach option depends on your state's laws. Many states (such as New York, where I live) no longer require a designated church affiliation because to do so would probably be unconstitutional. Instead, parents or guardians must hold genuine and sincere religious beliefs that are contrary to vaccinations. This means that a simple affidavit stating those beliefs in one or two sentences may suffice. An affidavit is as simple as having both parents sign their two-sentence statement in the presence of a notary public. The notary will then stamp the paper, which instantly becomes a rather powerful document. Your bank or town clerk will likely notarize for little or no charge. What does such a vaccination exemption letter look like? Well, it might look a lot like the one my children used:

It is my sincerely held religious belief that immunization is detrimental to the health and purity of the body, mind, and spirit. Therefore, I respectfully request that my child (full name here), be allowed to attend school, namely (full name here) without being immunized.

Student's name: _____

Mother: _____ Father: _____

Sworn to before me this _____th day of _____, 20_____.

Notary Public: _____

Be sure to have both parents sign. That means, of course, that both parents agree. If they do not, you'd best stop there.

> "Andrew Saul, a natural-medicine specialist in Rochester, said parents in New York do not have to demonstrate they are a member of an organized religious group when submitting their letter. "The school district will almost always respond to this with a request for more information," said Saul, who advises parents on the topic on his website, www.DoctorYourself.com. "The parent does not have to provide any more information."
>
> (Klein M. Whooping cough outbreak. *The Journal News,* Westchester, NY, October 29, 2003. See www.doctoryourself.com/news/v3n25.html)

Changing Your Mind

It has always been relatively simple for well-informed, determined parents to have their children attend school without any shots if they choose a religious exemption. But what about parents of children who are already partially immunized, who change their mind? They have often been denied a religious exemption due to health department or school officials' claims that their religious beliefs are not "sincerely held" since they have already had vaccinations prior to their new request for religious exemption. In January 2002, however, U.S. District Court Judge Michael Telesca wrote an important precedent-setting decision: "This court may not pass on the wisdom of belief, nor on the manner upon which she came to hold that belief, provided that she maintains a sincere and genuine religious objection to immunization." In other words, once a person decides, for reasons of religious conscience, that she does not want any more shots, her decision is valid even if she previously had her child immunized. The case is also important because the family in question was devoutly Roman Catholic. The Vatican is not opposed to vaccination. This decision allows individual members of a mainstream church organization to hold personal spiritual beliefs that contradict their church's official doctrine.

283

VITAMIN C PREVENTS VACCINATION SIDE EFFECTS; INCREASES EFFECTIVENESS

by Thomas E Levy, M.D., J.D.

The routine administration of vaccinations continues to be a subject of controversy in the United States, as well as throughout the world. Parents who want the best for their babies and children continue to be faced with decisions that they fear could harm their children if made incorrectly. The controversy over the potential harm of vaccinating, or of not vaccinating, will not be resolved to the satisfaction of all parties anytime soon, if ever. This brief report aims to offer some practical information to pediatricians and parents alike who want the best long-term health for their patients and children, regardless of their sentiments on the topic of vaccination in general.

While there seems to be a great deal of controversy over how frequently a vaccination might result in a negative outcome, there is little controversy that at least some of the time vaccines do cause damage. The question that then emerges is whether something can be done to minimize, if not eliminate, the infliction of such damage, however infrequently it may occur.

CAUSES OF VACCINATION SIDE EFFECTS

When vaccines do have side effects and adverse reactions, these outcomes are often categorized as resulting from allergic reactions or the result of a negative interaction with compromised immune systems. While either of these types of reactions can be avoided subsequently when there is a history of a bad reaction having occurred at least once in the past as a result of a vaccination, it is vital to try to avoid encountering a negative outcome from occurring the first time vaccines are administered.

Due to the fact that all toxins, toxic effects, substantial allergic reactions, and induced immune compromise have the final common denominator of causing and/or resulting in the oxidation of vital biomolecules, the antioxidant vitamin C has proven to be the ultimate nonspecific antidote to whatever toxin or excess oxidative stress might be present. While there is also a great deal of dispute over the inherent toxicity of the antigens that many vaccines present to the immune systems of those vaccinated, there is no question, for example, that thimerosal, a mercury-containing preservative, is highly toxic when present in significant amounts. Rather than argue whether there is an infinitesimal, minimal, moderate, or significant amount of toxicity associated with the amounts of thimerosal or other potentially toxic components presently being used in vaccines, why not just neutralize whatever toxicity is present as completely and definitively as possible?

VITAMIN C IS A POTENT ANTITOXIN

In addition to its general antitoxin properties (Levy, 2004), vitamin C has been demonstrated to be highly effective in neutralizing the toxic nature of mercury in all of its chemical forms. In animal studies, vitamin C can prevent the death of animals given otherwise fatal doses of mercury chloride (Mokranjac and Petrovic, 1964). Having vitamin C onboard prior to mercury exposure was able to prevent the kidney damage the mercury otherwise typically caused (Carroll et al., 1965). Vitamin C also blocked the fatal effect of mercury cyanide (Vauthey, 1951). Even the very highly toxic organic forms of mercury have been shown to be effectively detoxified by vitamin C (Gage, 1975).

VITAMIN C IMPROVES VACCINE EFFECTIVENESS

By potential toxicity considerations alone, then, there would seem to be no good reason not to pre- and post-medicate an infant or child with some amount of vitamin C to minimize or block the toxicity that might significantly affect a few. However, there is another compelling reason to make vitamin C an integral part of any vaccination protocol: Vitamin C has been documented to augment the antibody response of the immune system (Prinz et al., 1977; Vallance, 1977; Prinz et al., 1980; Feigen et al., 1982; Li and Lovell, 1985; Amakye-Anim et al., 2000; Wu et al., 2000; Lauridsen and Jensen, 2005; Azad et al., 2007). As the goal of any vaccination is to stimulate a maximal antibody response to the antigens of the vaccine while causing minimal to no toxic damage to the most sensitive of vaccine recipients, there would appear to be no medically sound reason not to make vitamin C a part of all vaccination protocols. Except in individuals with established, significant renal insufficiency, vitamin C is arguably the safest of all nutrients that can be given, especially in the amounts discussed below. Unlike virtually all prescription drugs and some supplements, vitamin C has never been found to have any dosage level above which it can be expected to demonstrate any toxicity.

VITAMIN C REDUCES MORTALITY IN VACCINATED INFANTS AND CHILDREN

Kalokerinos (1974) demonstrated repeatedly and quite conclusively that Aboriginal infants and children, a group with an unusually high death rate after vaccinations, were almost completely protected from this outcome by dosing them with vitamin C before and after vaccinations. The reason articulated for the high death rate was the exceptionally poor and near-scurvy-inducing (vitamin C-depleted) diet that was common in the Aboriginal culture. This also demonstrates that with the better nutrition in the United States and elsewhere in the world, the suggested doses of vitamin C should give an absolute protection against death (essentially a toxin-induced acute scurvy) and almost absolute protection against lesser toxic outcomes from any vaccinations administered. Certainly, there appears to be no logical reason not to give a nontoxic substance known to neutralize toxicity and stimulate antibody production, which is the whole point of vaccine administration.

DOSAGE INFORMATION FOR PEDIATRICIANS AND PARENTS

Practically speaking, then, how should the pediatrician or parent proceed? For optimal antibody stimulation and toxin protection, it would be best to dose for three to five days before the shot(s) and to continue for at least two to three days following the shot. When dealing with infants and very young children, administering a 1,000 mg dose of liposome-encapsulated vitamin C would be both easiest and best, as the gel-like nature of this form of vitamin C allows a ready mixture into yogurt or any other palatable food, and the complete proximal absorption of the liposomes would avoid any possible loose stools or other possible undesirable bowel effects.

Vitamin C as sodium ascorbate powder will also work well. Infants under 10 pounds can take 500 mg daily in some fruit juice, while babies between 10 and 20 pounds could take anywhere from 500 mg to 1,000 mg total per day, in divided doses. Older children can take 1,000 mg daily per year of life (5,000 mg for a 5 year-old child, for example, in divided doses). If sodium must be avoided, calcium ascorbate is well-tolerated and, like sodium ascorbate, is nonacidic. Some, but not all, children's chewable vitamins are made with calcium ascorbate. Be sure to read the label. Giving vitamin C in divided doses, all through the day, improves absorption and improves tolerance. As children get older, they can more easily handle the ascorbic acid form of vitamin C, especially if given with meals. For any child showing significant bowel sensitivity, either use liposome-encapsulated vitamin C, or the amount of regular vitamin C can just be appropriately decreased to an easily tolerated amount.

Very similar considerations exist for older individuals receiving any of a number of vaccinations for preventing infection, such as the yearly flu shots. When there is really no urgency, and there rarely is, such individuals should supplement with vitamin C for several weeks before and several weeks after, if at all possible.

Even taking a one-time dose of vitamin C in the dosage range suggested above directly before the injections can still have a significant toxin-neutralizing and antibody-stimulating effect. It's just that an even better likelihood of having a positive outcome results from extending the pre- and post-dosing periods of time.

(Thomas Levy, M.D., J.D., is a board-certified cardiologist and admitted to the bar in Colorado and the District of Colombia.)

References

Amakye-Anim, J., T. Lin, P. Hester, et al. (2000) Ascorbic acid supplementation improved antibody response to infectious bursal disease vaccination in chickens. *Poultry Science* 79:680–688.

Azad, I., J. Dayal, M. Poornima, and S. Ali (2007) Supra dietary levels of vitamins C and E enhance antibody production and immune memory in juvenile milkfish, *Chanos chanos* (Forsskal) to formalin-killed *Vibrio vulnificus. Fish & Shellfish Immunology* 23:154–163.

285

Carroll, R., K. Kovacs, and E. Tapp (1965) Protection against mercuric chloride poisoning of the rat kidney. *Arzneimittelfor-schung* 15:1361–1363.

Feigen, G., B. Smith, C. Dix, et al. (1982) Enhancement of antibody production and protection against systemic anaphylaxis by large doses of vitamin C. *Research Communications in Chemical Pathology and Pharmacology* 38:313–333.

Gage, J. (1975) Mechanisms for the biodegradation of organic mercury compounds: the actions of ascorbate and of soluble proteins. *Toxicology and Applied Pharmacology* 32:225–238.

Kalokerinos, A. (1974) *Every Second Child*. New Canaan, CT: Keats Publishing, Inc.

Lauridsen, C. and S. Jensen (2005) Influence of supplementation of all-rac-alpha-tocopheryl acetate preweaning and vitamin C postweaning on alpha-tocopherol and immune responses in piglets. *Journal of Animal Science* 83:1274–1286 .

Levy, T. (2004) *Curing the Incurable. Vitamin C, Infectious Diseases, and Toxins*. Henderson, NV: MedFox Publishing.

Li, Y. and R. Lovell (1985) Elevated levels of dietary ascorbic acid increase immune responses in channel catfish. *The Journal of Nutrition* 115:123–131.

Mokranjac, M. and C. Petrovic (1964) Vitamin C as an antidote in poisoning by fatal doses of mercury. *Comptes Rendus Hebdomadaires des Seances de l'Academie des Sciences* 258:1341–1342.

Prinz, W., R. Bortz, B. Bregin, and M. Hersch (1977) The effect of ascorbic acid supplementation on some parameters of the human immunological defence system. *International Journal for Vitamin and Nutrition Research* 47:2248–257.

Prinz, W., J. Bloch, G., G. Gilich, and G. Mitchell (1980) A systematic study of the effect of vitamin C supplementation on the humoral immune response in ascorbate-dependent mammals. I. The antibody response to sheep red blood cells (a T-dependent antigen) in guinea pigs. *International Journal for Vitamin and Nutrition Research* 50:294–300.

Vallance, S. (1977) Relationships between ascorbic acid and serum proteins of the immune system. *British Medical Journal* 2:437–438.

Vauthey, M. (1951) Protective effect of vitamin C against poisons. *Praxis (Bern)* 40:284–286.

Wu, C., T. Dorairajan, and T. Lin (2000) Effect of ascorbic acid supplementation on the immune response of chickens vaccinated and challenged with infectious bursal disease virus. *Veterinary Immunology and Immunopathology* 74:145–152.

(Used with permission of the author.)

Required Proof

Now we need to take a closer look at the phrase, "sincere and genuine." Upon filing your religious objection, many school districts will contact you and demand that you come in and explain your religious beliefs, so they can verify that those beliefs are "sincere and genuine." This meeting will likely take on the appearance of a kangaroo court. You and your spouse may end up facing the principal, the school district's attorney, the assistant superintendent, the school physician, a school nurse or two, a few school board members, teachers, and who knows who else. Intimidating to say the least? Not at all. Remembering that this is America, here's all you have to do:

Their question: "Mrs. Smith, please explain your religious beliefs to us."

Your answer (reading from the document above): "It is my sincerely held religious belief that immunization is detrimental to the health and purity of the body, mind, and spirit."

Their inevitable follow-up question: "Yes, we saw that on the form you submitted. Please elaborate."

Your reply: "It is my sincerely held religious belief that immunization is detrimental to the health and purity of the body, mind, and spirit."

Their slightly irritated response: "Yes, Mrs. Smith. But we need to know more to make our determination."

Your answer: "Are you questioning my religion?"

Now, there is the fork in the road. And just as Yogi Berra said, "When you come to a fork in the road, take it." Why? Because you cannot lose.

They can either answer yes or no.

If they answer no, then you say: "Very well then. Thank you all for your time." And you leave. You won, and you are done.

If they answer yes, here is your reply: "Please put your request and your questions in writing."

They almost certainly will not. At this point, the school's attorney will lean over to the head inquisitor and start earnestly whispering, accompanied with a negative shaking of the lawyer's head. When that occurs, the school attorney just reminded them of the First Amendment, which specifically prohibits government from interfering in the practice of religion. A public school is a part of public government, and your personal beliefs are part of your religion. Private schools cannot violate your constitutional rights, either. If school officials demand details of your faith or any other spiritual information from you, they are breaking the law. The last thing they are going to do is put that request in writing. Among other things (such as inviting a lawsuit from you), they dislike a certain four-letter word: ACLU.

I was a teacher in both public and parochial schools, and two state prisons (no, not as an inmate). Do you really think I would have asked Jewish kids why they missed school on a High Holy Day? That I would have questioned late homework during Ramadan? All persons of all religions receive protection under the US Constitution. This includes you.

Medical Exemption

A completely different way to get around a vaccination requirement is to prove to a medical doctor that your children would suffer a great health risk by being vaccinated. A possible allergic reaction to the shot(s) would be an ideal reason, although great susceptibility to side effects or a pre-existing high-risk condition could also be given as reasons. This is hard to do; most physicians will side with orthodoxy and public health policy. And even if they did exempt you, it is very probable that they will be called on by authorities to defend why they think a child shouldn't be vaccinated. This approach, then, puts burden of proof on both you and the doctor, and will only be as strong as the weaker link. When faced with losing a medical license that the doctor worked twelve years to get, guess who the weaker link likely will be?

Alternative Education

Still another way to avoid shots for kids might be to enroll them in a private, cooperative, or alternative school that does not discriminate on medical grounds. It might be possible for a group of concerned parents to create such a school to ensure freedom of choice for family health decisions. However, most private and parochial schools are subject to, and in enthusiastic compliance with, the same public health regulations as public schools.

Home schooling is certainly an option. There are families in your community who teach their own children at home, and there are state education requirements that they must meet to do so. There are no inoculation requirements, however. You can keep the government happy and your kids' minds open at the same time by home schooling. Warning: it is labor intensive, to be sure.

Argument 3: Unvaccinated Kids Are Sitting Ducks

Kids don't automatically "get" all those so-called diseases of childhood. Just as insects eat weak crops, disease thrives in weak bodies. As I've said in this chapter, and as observations of primitive societies have shown, healthy lifestyles and diets are enough to prevent most of the diseases of modern life. Kids stay healthy not because of injections but because of correct eating and naturally strengthened immune systems.

The usual accompanying rejoinder to this is, "We need herd immunity. Everyone has to have shots for them to work." Wait a minute. This is saying that if you don't get your kids immunized, that choice threatens kids who have been immunized. How? They've *been* immunized. And immunization prevents the illness. Right?

Wrong. Vaccinations do not confer sufficient protection. New York in 2003, California in 2010, and Montana in 2012 experienced epidemics of whooping cough. Most of those that got it had been vaccinated against it.

I personally communicated with the reporter on the New York story[1] to get the facts: There were 25 whooping cough cases in Putnam County, and 29 whooping cough cases in Westchester County, for a total of 54. Ten of the 54 cases were in nonimmunized children. That means 44 of 54 cases of whooping cough were in vaccinated persons. That is 81 percent.

Seven years later, this turned out the same way in Marin County, California: 80 percent of children who developed whooping cough had been fully vaccinated.

Another interesting question would be, Exactly how many unimmunized children did *not* get whooping cough? I expect the number would be considerably higher. And, if you consider what I think amounts to an 80 percent vaccine failure rate, there should be a deafening chorus of millions of Americans, between the Atlantic and Pacific, whooping away with the "100 day cough" right this minute.

Whooping cough (pertussis) is caused by a bacteria. It is a pipe dream that we will ever kill every bacteria. And if we try to, they will mutate into resistant strains. Then, if we try to have a vaccination for every bacterial strain, we start an arms race that will make the Cold War look like a scouting jamboree, and make the pharmaceutical industry even richer. Vaccination does not work with influenza, which is viral. There are hundreds of flu viruses. Neither does it work with tuberculosis, which is bacterial like whooping cough.

The vaccines offered to your child have not been double-blind, placebo-tested. This is noteworthy. The medical profession is often sharply critical of natural-remedy or vitamin-therapy studies that are not sufficiently rigorous. I think vaccine evidence should be of the highest scientific standard. It is not. If you do not believe me, ask your doctor for the studies. Not just any studies, but double-blind placebo studies.

It looks to me as if shots are pretty much irrelevant in terms of effectiveness. Before you make your decision for your family, consider safety and effectiveness and alternatives. I choose to decline. Your decision should be your own.

Reference

Klein M. Whooping cough outbreak. *The Journal News,* Westchester, NY: October 29, 2003. http://www.doctoryourself.com/ news/ v3n25.html

Raging Contagion

When I registered my unvaccinated children for public school, the school nurse confirmed that my religious exemption was acceptable. I was further informed that, should there be an epidemic at the school, my children would have to stay home.

Wait a minute: if the other kids are vaccinated, what do they have to worry about? And if there *is* a worry, maybe those vaccinations aren't all they are cracked up to be. If their shots are so great, then why send my kids home? I would like to think that the school medical staff was actually saying that to protect my children from any outbreak. But that doesn't fit either, as contagious diseases are often contagious before observable symptoms erupt.

How come the nonvaccinated are not all sick all the time? Consider the Amish. They should, by the standards of school-district doctoring, all be dead, or paralyzed with polio, or crippled with lockjaw (tetanus), or at least plagued by a never-ending bevy of rampant life-threatening epidemics. Well, they aren't. If they were, you can be sure that our pharmaphilic (drug-lovin') news media would be quick to report that entire populations of "religious extremists" have been wiped out by their rejection of modern medicine.

That has not happened. And it's not because the Amish are isolated from the "germs" of others, either. The Amish maintain frequent contact with the rest of society. My parents lived right in the Amish epicenter: Lancaster, Pennsylvania. Everywhere they went, unvaccinated Amish people were there, too: horses, black buggies, and all. The Amish are not an isolated community and they are not a vaccinated community, yet they generally are a healthy community. Ever see a bunch of sickly farmers work horses in the field or raise a barn? No way. And they'd be an even healthier lifestyle model if they'd stop raising tobacco.

The practical answer for society in general? Natural immunity through optimum diet, and stand-by heavy-hitter therapy with huge doses of vitamin C. To think the needle is going to protect you is a fallacy.

WHOOPING COUGH VACCINATION IS INSUFFICIENTLY EFFECTIVE

New York Times: "Most of the people who contracted whooping cough during the current (2003) Westchester County outbreak of the disease had been immunized against it." (Kenny A. Whooping cough cases spread. *NY Times,* October 26, 2003)

Associated Press: " 'I was disturbed to find maybe we had a little more confidence in the vaccine than it might deserve,' lead researcher Dr. David Witt said. Witt is chief of infectious disease at the Kaiser Permanente Medical Center in San Rafael, Calif." (Whooping cough vaccination fades in 3 years. Associated Press, September 20, 2011.)

Considering these were major stories, controversial articles may nevertheless require a stiff Google search to find on the Internet. If you still have trouble, ask your public librarian for assistance. Librarians can find anything.

Argument 4: Just in Case, to Be Safe

Not getting vaccinations may actually be safer than getting them. Consider the checkered history of the DPT shot. Hundreds of millions of dollars have been paid out to parents of vaccine-disabled or vaccine-killed children. According to statistics compiled by the National Vaccine Information Center, between July 1990 and November 1993 "1,576 children died from adverse reactions to common vaccines" in the United States. Most deaths were from the pertussis (whooping cough) vaccine. In unimmunized Great Britain, in 1978 and 1979 there were 36 deaths attributed to whooping cough itself. Even allowing for wide variation in sample dates and population, it is impossible to dismiss the fact that *more American kids died from shots in a month than British kids died without shots in two years.*

Readers should also keep in mind that careful study of the medical profession's own statistics fails to verify the very common and highly emotional viewpoint that vaccination has been the major factor in the reduction of infectious diseases. Careful reviews of the medical literature show that the dramatic decline in typhoid, diphtheria, and whooping cough in this country occurred *before* vaccinations were available. Even polio fatalities decreased by nearly 90 percent from 1915 to 1955, before the polio vaccine became available. How can we truly say, then, that vaccination got rid of polio? There was a medical doctor in Canada who treated polio with iodine supplements in the 1950s. The method is called iodine prophylaxis, and the effectiveness of his treatments suggests that the popularization of iodized salt has had more to do with the elimination of polio in America than the polio vaccine!

Now I am not saying that there's no statistical significance to results with the Salk vaccine. But I do think that vitamin C, a vegetarian diet, and iodine will actually prevent polio more effectively. Much of the evidence supporting this theory can be found in papers written by Claus Jungeblut, M.D.. Dr. Jungeblut showed that vitamin C not only prevented polio, but actually killed polio viruses. For more on this, please turn to this book's section entitled "High-Dose Vitamin C Therapy for Major Diseases."

"No" Is Not Enough

It is not enough to say "no" to shots. You have to take active, alternative measures in their stead. There is a strong track record for preventing diseases through really good nutrition. That is why my children were raised virtually vegetarian and with daily vitamin supplementation. (Continues: When they were preschoolers, my children received 250–500 mg of vitamin C with each meal. As they got older, they got more C. In my opinion, a good prevention plan is to give kids half their age in grams of C per day. A gram being 1,000 milligrams, that means that an eight-year-old would get 4,000 mg/day and a twelve-year-old would get 6,000 mg/day, and so forth. (Always divide up the doses throughout day.) These are everyday health maintenance amounts. If you think they are too high, it is high time to read more on this subject in this book, and read more books on this subject. The bibliography is a good starting place for skeptics and their physicians.

It is vital (and also comforting) to remember that vitamin C is a proven antibiotic, antitoxin, and antiviral. (*The Healing Factor,* by Irwin Stone, discusses this in detail. Please also see my chapter on vitamin C therapy.) When my children had a fever or cough, they were put to bed with a temporarily all-fruit or vegetable-juice diet, saturation levels of vitamin C, and required to rest. They got better. And, although unvaccinated, they have never had whooping cough, polio, diphtheria, or measles. Was it just dumb luck, or was it smart eating?

Although I have offered my family's personal vaccination viewpoint to the reader, I do not pretend to tell anyone to get shots or not to get shots. Parents must make their own decisions based on all the facts they can gather. To assist in this search, I suggest reading the books by Robert Mendelsohn listed in the Recommended Reading, as well as *A Shot in the Dark* by Harris Coulter and Barbara Fisher, which focuses on the pertussis vaccine. I also recommend *Mothering* magazine's *Vaccinations: The Rest of the Story* and other well-written, well-referenced books by Neil Z. Miller.

Consent: Informed or Coerced?

When I asked my college students in health issues class to consider what so-called "informed consent" for vaccinations actually came down to, interesting discussions were sure to follow. As David Hume said, "Without freedom to refuse, there is no freedom of choice." Without full disclosure of risk, and time to think about it, there is no informed consent. So rather than shove a paper under Mrs. B.'s nose, with a needle in one hand and her baby in the other, genuine informed consent perhaps should go something like this:

Six weeks before Mrs. B.'s well-child visit for her infant, Dr. C.'s office telephones her.

"Hi, Mrs. B. This is Dr. C.'s office. We'd like to remind you that we think your child should receive immunizations in about six weeks, and that we are sending you a packet of abstracts, or summaries, of peer-reviewed research on both the advantages and the disadvantages of vaccination. Please carefully review these materials. If you have any difficulty in the reading, or have any questions, please call me, Mr. D., personally. I will answer, or look up the answer, to whatever concern you have, or I will connect you with Dr. C. if you prefer a direct discussion with her.

"You have the right to accept shots, or to refuse shots for your child, under the Bill of Rights of the U.S. Constitution. We earnestly believe that you should choose immunizations, but will also acquaint you with the simple legal options you have if you do not agree.

"Please call us back in about three weeks to schedule your appointment. Even if you decide to not immunize, we want you to know that we still want to have you and your child as our patients. You will be treated with friendliness and respect regardless of your position on vaccination."

Now *that's* informed consent.

FLU SHOTS FOR THE ELDERLY ARE INEFFECTIVE

Influenza vaccination has been widely touted even though evidence of effectiveness is lacking. One large scientific review looked at forty years' worth of influenza vaccine studies. It found that flu shots were ineffective for elderly persons living in the community, and flu shots were "non-significant against influenza" for elderly living in group homes.[2] The authors of another major review "found no correlation between vaccine coverage and influenza-like-illness attack rate."[3] Author Dr. Thomas Jefferson said, "The vaccine doesn't work very well at all. Vaccines are being used as an ideological weapon. What you see every year as the flu is caused by 200 or 300 different agents with a vaccine against two of them. That is simply nonsense."[4] Indeed, he commented, "What you see is that marketing rules the response to influenza, and scientific evidence comes fourth or fifth."[5]

As with all immunizations, flu shots can have harmful side effects. Vaccines may contain, among other things, ingredients such as mercury and aluminum, which are widely regarded as toxic. The elderly are more likely to be injured by, or even die from, flu vaccine side effects. Such incidents may remain unreported by hospitals or physicians.

The US Food and Drug Administration's Vaccine Adverse Effect Reporting System receives around 11,000 serious adverse reaction reports each year, mostly from doctors.[6] The FDA states that "VAERS tracks serious vaccine reactions, not common fevers and soreness from shots. Serious reactions include death, life-threatening illness, hospitalization, and disability resulting from a vaccine."[7] However, FDA admits that they probably receive reports for only about 10 percent of all adverse vaccine reactions.[8] The National Vaccine Information Center estimates the reporting percentage to be far lower, perhaps under 3 percent.[9]

The flu vaccine, notes the *New York Times*, has not been double-blind, placebo-control tested.[1] Faith in vaccination appears to be greater than the scientific evidence to justify vaccination.

References

1. Goodman B. Doubts grow over flu vaccine in elderly. www.nytimes.com/2008/09/02/health/02flu.html September 2, 2008.

2. Rivetti D, Jefferson T, Thomas R et al. Vaccines for preventing influenza in the elderly. Cochrane Database Syst Rev., 2006, 3:CD004876.

3. Jefferson T, Rivetti D, Rivetti A, et al. Efficacy and effectiveness of influenza vaccines in elderly people: a systematic review. *Lancet*, 2005, 366(9492):1165–74.

4. Gardner A. Flu vaccine only mildly effective in elderly. *HealthDay Reporter,* Sept 21, 2005.

5. Rosenthal E. Flu vaccination and treatment fall far short. *International Herald Tribune,* September 22, 2005.

6. National Technical Information Service, Springfield, VA 22161, 703–487–4650, 703–487–4600.

7. www.fda.gov/fdac/reprints/vaccine.html.

8. KM Severyn in the *Dayton Daily News*, May 28, 1993, cited at www.chiropracticresearch.org/NEWSVaccinations.htm .

9. "Investigative Report on the Vaccine Adverse Event Reporting System." National Vaccine Information Center (NVIC), 512 Maple Ave. W. #206, Vienna, VA 22180.

Recommended Websites

www.vaccinationnews.com

www.nccn.net/~wwithin/vaccine.htm

www.909shot.com

www.thinktwice.com

www.vaccines.bizland.com

www.vaccination.inoz.com

www.avn.org.au

Recommended Reading

Coulter HL and Fisher BL. *A Shot in the Dark.* Garden City Park, NY: Avery, 1991.

Hillemann HH. The illusion of American health and longevity. *Clinical Physiology* 2 (1960): 120–77.

Smith L, ed. *Clinical Guide to the Use of Vitamin C: The Clinical Experiences of Frederick R. Klenner, M.D.* Tacoma, WA: Life Sciences Press, 1988.

Mendelsohn RS. *Confessions of a Medical Heretic.* Chicago: Contemporary Books, 1979.

Mendelsohn RS. *How to Raise a Healthy Child in Spite of Your Doctor.* New York: Ballantine Books, 1985.

Miller NZ. *Vaccine Safety Manual for Concerned Families and Health Practitioners: Guide to Immunization Risks and Protection.* New Atlantean Press, 2008.

Miller NZ. *Vaccines: Are They Really Safe and Effective.* New Atlantean Press; Revised Updated Edition, 2008.

Mothering Magazine. *Vaccinations: The Rest of the Story.* Chicago: Mothering Books, 1993.

Price WA. *Nutrition and Physical Degeneration.* La Mesa, CA: Price-Pottenger Nutrition Foundation, 1945, revised 1970.

Tokasz J. Judge forces school to accept girl. Rochester, NY: *Democrat and Chronicle* (31 Jan 2002); B-1.

Williams RJ. *Physicians' Handbook of Nutritional Science.* Springfield, IL: Charles C. Thomas, 1975.

For More Information

Video questioning influenza vaccine: www.thinktwice.com/flu_show.htm.

A humorous look at flu vaccines: www.thinktwice.com/Flu_Farce.mov.

Varicose Veins

"When Ben Casey meets Kildare; that's a paradox."
—ALAN SHERMAN

What's black and white, and red all over? You remember the answer of course: a newspaper. So what is red and tan and purple all over? My father's legs, that's what. Pa loved to bake in the summer sun. His idea of an afternoon off was to take his Army surplus canvas cot into our backyard, unfold it, and wearing nothing but shorts, lie in the sun for hours. We kids were enjoined to leave him alone. Mom told us, and besides, we knew better. Well-rested parents are more likely to let you stay up on school nights and let you watch TV. Well, sometimes, anyway.

Still, unavoidably, Pa's legs were on neighborhoodwide display while he slept in the sun. The result of such community scrutiny could only have been the verdict that they were not an especially lovely sight. Pa had prominent varicose veins, from knees to the feet.

My dad also had an inordinate love of wearing Bermuda shorts, and, unfortunately, not just at home. As a teenager, this embarrassed me, as did his cavalier taste when it came to clothing in general. For a consummate artist who could discern two dozen different shades of blue, Pa had incredibly bad taste in wardrobe. Oh, he could put on a dark suit and do the Kodak patent-office thing okay; it's what he wore when he was not at work that was enough to give Calvin Klein a coronary. He would wear plaids with checks, bright red pants with bright blue jackets, and brazenly loud bow ties with anything.

The most outrageous outfits my dad ever wore, in my opinion, were his homemade pajamas. My mother liked to sew. She was not particularly good at sewing, but made up for it with sheer inventiveness. Inventions are not always successful, my father the patent draftsman would tell you, but that does not stop inventors. Neither did such constraints as good taste stop my parents. When my mother made my dad terrycloth pajamas, she must have been critically low on material. The pajamas turned out Bermuda-shorts' length, with conspicuous assorted off-color double-stitching and wild, patterned, chartreuse pockets cut from an entirely different fabric. Perhaps those pockets were not quite big enough to hold Volume One of the *Encyclopedia Britannica,* but it would have been a near thing. The worst part of it was that Pa absolutely loved them, and to prove it, wore the pajama pants in public. No, that was not quite the worst part; this was: he took me with him. When I was in ninth grade. To the neighborhood public library. Where my friends were.

I knew what was coming but was powerless to prevent it. The man whose best-known family phrase was, "Don't talk while I'm interrupting" was not to be dissuaded by the likes of me. Off we went to the Charlotte Branch of the Rochester Public Library, me hunching way, way down into the foam front seat of our sea-green 1960 Chevy. When we got to the library parking lot, I deliberately dragged behind, as far as humanly possible. It was looking good: I was thirty feet back now as we approached the front double doors. Up the steps he strode; back on the sidewalk I slowly slunk. He opened the door, and in full view of the world, called back to me in his never-soft voice, "C'mon, Andrew!"

Oh good grief. I followed him in and yes, right at the first lobby table were several of my friends. My memory blanks after that. I understand that is what post-traumatic stress can do.

But I digress. And isn't that why this book is so much fun to read? Huh? Huh?

Many years later, when he started taking vitamin E for his angina (as detailed in the Angina chapter), something unexpected happened: his varicose veins changed color. From a dark indigo, they became more of reddish-purple. A couple of years later, they were hardly purple at all, just a dark red. Next year, they were red-pink. A year or two later, pink. Then they were virtually all gone. Sure, it took time. But it is very uncommon for varicose veins to go away, ever. Especially in the retirement years. Well, my father's did. His angina went away with 1,600 IU of vitamin E daily. Side effects? None. Side benefits? Nicer legs. It took about six or seven years. But it worked.

Is this news to you, as it was to me when I saw it? Oddly enough, it is not new news at all. Back in 1950, vitamin E had already been shown to be effective treatment for varicose veins by Drs. Wilfrid and Evan Shute. (Reference: Shute E. *The Vitamin E Story*)

Over sixty years ago. In all that time, how many more people could vitamin E have helped?

And by the way, the varicose veins that I started developing as a young man are gone. Yep. Just checked again. I accessed my calves and they look simply lovely. I am nearly sixty. I take 800 IU of vitamin E a day and have for decades.

Now where are my Bermuda shorts?

"How can I get thinner? Give up lunch and dinner."

—ALAN SHERMAN

Some diets are nothing but quackery.

Sitting through high school chemistry class one gorgeous spring day, an equally bored friend of mine and I came up with a sure-fire diet program based entirely on the thermal properties of water.

Let me run it by you. In eleventh-grade chemistry, we were taught that water has a high specific heat. That is, it takes a lot of heat to raise the temperature of water even a little. A watched pot never boils, or so it seems, because even a gas stove's flames or the red-hot coil of an electric range must work extremely hard to bring that pot up to 212 degrees F. Why? It takes one unit of heat, called a calorie (small "c"), to raise one gram of water (which is one milliliter) by one degree Celsius (1.8 degrees F). Sorry about the math anxiety this may be arousing in you, but I'm going somewhere with this.

Your body temperature is surprisingly hot: 98.6 degrees F, to be exact. "Cold" tap water is perhaps 50 degrees F or less. Ice is 32 degrees F, and "ice water" might be in the high 30s. If ice water were 38.6 degrees, that is fully 60 degrees lower than your body temperature.

Now a dietetic Calorie (with the large C) is more properly termed a kilocalorie, equal to 1,000 small-c calories. It takes 1,000 little one-ml-of-water-one-degree heat calories to make one "food" Calorie.

Hmm. A small-c calorie of heat can only raise one ml of water 1.8 degrees F. A liter of water is 1,000 ml. One food big-C Calorie is 1,000 little calories. So you have to burn one Calorie to raise the temperature of one liter of water 1.8 degrees.

Uh huh. But that means that to raise the temperature of a liter of ice water sixty degrees, to body temperature, takes 33 Calories. Two liters would burn 67 Calories.

We know from dietitians that just 10 extra food Calories per day, for 10 years, will gain you 10 pounds. In other words, if you eat only 10 superfluous Calories each day, you will gain a pound a year. That is admittedly not much. On the other hand, you would have real trouble cutting me a 10-Calorie piece of chocolate cake. On a dessert plate, 10 Calories looks almost insignificant.

If, however, you drink two liters of ice water a day, you will burn 67 Calories each day just heating that water to your normal body temperature. That is almost seven pounds per year weight loss. In ten years, that's 67 pounds of weight lost.

Two liters is just over eight eight-ounce glasses, no more than many a physician would advise you to drink anyway. Make that water cold, and you burn calories watching TV. A pound or so every two months, on ice water. Up it to three liters a day and it's almost a pound a month. No exercise factored in; no dietary changes considered. Just add water. *Cold* water.

But wait, there's more. Many a person drinking more liquids will eat fewer solids. Even water is filling if you drink enough of it. Reduced food means reduced Calories. Take a daily multivitamin tablet to cover the nutrient losses inevitable in any diet. Americans consume more soft drinks than all other beverages put together (yes, that includes milk, tea, coffee, juices, sports drinks, bottled water, liquor, wine, and beer). Drink water instead of pop, and you will be consuming much less sugar (and fewer Calories) or, in the case of diet pop, far less of those questionable artificial sweeteners. You'll also avoid the carbonic acid found in all carbonated beverages, and the phosphoric acid added to colas. Dentists etch teeth with phosphoric acid, and carbonic acid isn't much easier on the enamel.

Can you get too much water? Not easily; your body is naturally mostly water. Your blood is mostly water. Your food is mostly water. Your bowels and kidneys require water for excretion of wastes. Why, you were conceived in an aquatic environment. Too little water is associated with kidney stones, urinary tract infections, febrile illness, dehydration, and worse. So drink yourself slim. Unless your doctor tells you otherwise, two to three liters per day is a reasonable plan.

Just warming up. Vegetable juicing is next.

Comedian Dick Gregory came to our college campus to speak against the Vietnam war. The year was 1970, and the controversy was running high. Draft cards were burned and demonstrations shut down classes. I personally saw the student body president, from an overhead stairway, dump the contents of a fifty-pound sack of flour on two Marines at their recruiting table. My hair was a whole lot shorter than the student president's, but a good deal longer than the Marines'. At the time I was on the student activities lecture committee, and we knew full well we were bringing in a speaker who would be as inflammatory as he was funny. Anything else I knew of Mr. Gregory's politics came from reading *Dick Gregory from the Back of the Bus* a few years earlier.

I was to be surprised. Gregory had pledged not to eat until the war was over. He started his fast at 308 pounds and was down to 135. To save his life, his promise was amended to not eat any solids until the war was over. Vietnam went on for years, so this was no wimp-out. He lived on nothing but juice, fresh vegetable juice. In his lengthy speaking contract were written specifications about which and how many organically grown vegetables we were to provide for him. So our lecture committee went shopping for Mr. Gregory and presented him with two large brown paper bags of fresh food. He carried them right into the Student Union's now very-crowded press conference room, put the overflowing bags on the big walnut table, and casually sat down.

I was four feet away from the man. The room was ablaze with the dazzlingly bright portable white lights of TV reporters. Cameras whirred and clicked and the questions flew. As he quietly answered, Mr. Gregory calmly commenced juicing. I don't quite remember where the juicer came from, but there it was. Cup after cup of orange or green drinks went into the man. The questions from the press stayed on his antiwar views. I don't recall any questions about his diet. It was weird to watch. I thought Mr. Gregory was off his rocker.

Years later, I learned of people weighing 600, 800, even 1,000 pounds losing weight with vegetable juicing when all else had failed. Guess who was behind it? Dick Gregory. He had been called in to get the morbidly obese into vegetable juicing, and did it. He got them doing exactly what he had done, and they lost hundreds of pounds. Plus, they got healthier in the process. Forget his politics; Gregory's enduring contribution will be saved lives.

I myself tried a half-hearted, perhaps one-third vegetable juice diet and lost over twenty pounds in three months. It was easy. Getting someone to try it is the only obstacle.

To summarize: there are four "noble truths" of weight loss.

1. *Fat is real.* And really unhealthy. Half of Americans are overweight, one in four is obese, and over four million are morbidly obese. If you are overweight, admit it now before you die early and miss seeing your grandchildren grow up. Obesity kills 250,000 Americans each year.

2. *Fat has a reason.* If you are overweight, you are either eating too many Calories or burning too few. It's about behaviors, not genetics. If you have heavy parents and you have heavy children, look for what I call dinner table heredity. You are not doomed by your DNA. It is far more likely that you have merely adopted your family's eating habits.

3. *There is a way out.* Behave differently. Eat fewer Calories, or burn more, preferably both. Both are within any human being's power, and don't try to tell me otherwise. Anyone, even a paraplegic, can exercise. Even in a wheelchair or bed you can lift small weights to start. And one of the few genuinely free choices everyone has is what they will or will not put into their mouths.

4. *It's not how much, but what.* Water and vegetable juices are low-calorie and very, very low-fat. There is almost no limit to how much water you can drink, or the amount of vegetables you can eat. Juicing vegetables is even better. Vegetable juicing increases both the quantity of vegetables that you will eat, and increases your absorption of those vegetables. Nutrient deficiency, a common obstacle with dieting, is therefore a nonissue. See my chapters "Saul's Jumpstart to Health" and "Juicing Hints" for more information on juicing.

You cannot live on water alone; Mahatma Gandhi and entirely too many others have approached death after weeks and months of total fasting. But, like Dick Gregory, you can live for a surprisingly long time on vegetable juices exclusively and be the better—and lighter—for it.

Just try it and see. Maria in New York did, and here is her story:

In 2003 I weighed 166 pounds at 5'6," wore a size 14, had a heart arrhythmia, chronic ITP (platelets between 10–20,000, the dangerous range), full-blown ulcerative colitis, rhinitis, rashes, and anemia. I was 35, grouchy, and generally irritable and fatigued, was on several prescriptions, and felt like I had no more energy for any activities. Whenever I saw my doctors I was told that surgery, avoiding certain strenuous activities, and lifelong medication were in my future. Men rarely gave me a glance, unsurprisingly, and I dressed to conceal.

In 2008 at age 41, I weigh 131 (size 6), just finished a half marathon, look like 33 on a bad day, work out six times a week because I am bursting with energy, am an active member of a gym and a running club, and have a generally outgoing disposition. Lunch most days is a large salad with sprouts and other nutrient-dense vegetables. Now I use my pharmacy only to buy toothpaste, because all my illnesses are gone, including the heart arrhythmia, and my platelets have been at 125–135,000 (normal) for almost a year now. I take no medication, feel like 25, and astound people whom I tell I am 41. I am brimming with interests, friends, hobbies, and activities in addition to my full-time job. I have become so accustomed to admiring looks from men that I hardly register them anymore. I shop for clothes wherever I want now, usually fashionable boutiques for younger women.

One funny effect of this change in health habits is that people initially thought I had resorted to some exotic treatment or procedure because of the dramatic change in my appearance and energy levels. When I told them what I was doing (not counting calories, not doing Atkins, not doing Weight Watchers, just cutting out certain foods, taking vitamins, and building my health) I encountered disbelief.

There are also some funny moments, such as on the lunch line when I order my organic salad toppings and always order two portions of sprouts and twice the vegetables the others order, or when I encounter overweight colleagues in the elevator when I am carrying my five-pound healthy lunch upstairs, or on a business trip when I start peeling a tangerine I keep in my hand- bag, and the business guys turn to see where the smell is coming from. On another business trip, when I had just run a 15 km race before jumping on an airplane, it turned out that I was the same age as an overweight, fatigued, graying, depressed businessperson in our group, who the next day skipped lunch with us and ate a granola bar instead.

Another funny effect is that people who did not know me in the bad old days find it hard to believe that I was ever overweight or unwell and think I must be exaggerating or even lying about having been those things. To lighten things up on business trips, when I take out my pumpkin seeds or piece of fruit or four glasses of water in a conference room, I say I am a "recovering fat person" and people are genuinely amazed when I tell them I lost almost 40 pounds.

Or in the pharmacy, of which I was once a frequent customer handing over three or four prescriptions at a time (for nasal sprays, prednisone, cortisone inserts for colitis, pain medi- cation, antibiotics, synthroid, asthma medication) when I hand over the toothpaste and they say expectantly, "anything else?" and I say, "Nope!" and bound out to enjoy the day.

Truly, there is no hidden "trick" to losing weight. It is simply a matter of deciding to, know- ing how, and following through. I've worked with people so overweight that they had difficulty squeezing into an armchair. I have seen them lose up to 65 pounds by following even some of the ideas mentioned above. The side benefits are tremendous: more energy, better self-image, and a longer, healthier life.

If they can do it, I believe that you can do it.

A reader from Oregon says:

I am seventy years of age and morbidly obese. Diagnosed with congestive heart failure four years ago, I have a prostate, diverticulosis (itis?), chronic esophagitis, and GERD, to name some of what my doc says. I do not have high blood pressure, but have a chronic arrhythmia that occurs when exposed to any significant amount of caffeine. I abused coffee when I was younger. And I am a pensioner with no resource except my Social Security and two other tiny pensions. I didn't mention the joint problems with two knees and the lumbar spinal region.

A mess? Surely, but a little over three weeks ago I started on your eating plan. I bake my own 100 percent whole-wheat bread, gobble frozen veggies and brown rice, and have become a juice drinker (100 percent juice with no additives, of course). I haven't had any kind of a soda since I started. I make bean soup to enjoy even in the hot weather. I feel good and will start supplements when I have a few more bucks to spend. I feel better now (three weeks, mind you) than I have in a very long time. I am losing weight slowly, but steadily. Does your plan of nutrition work? Absolutely! Thanks.

For Further, Slightly Humorous Reading

Put on your helmet for my infamous "Crash Course in Vegetarian Cooking," ready to delight your senses later in this book. But we will also have to face a fact: my beloved Mother was a lousy cook. That story will also be coming up as well. So on to Part Two!

Part Two

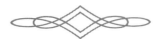

Natural Healing Tools and Techniques

Saul's Super Remedy

"The physician should not treat the disease but the patient who is suffering from it."
—MAIMONIDES

"Why, it's good for what ails you." That's how my great-uncle described the virtues of any food or edible plant he knew to be healthy. Quite a few made his list, and as a result, I disliked nearly everything he put on the dinner table when we came to visit. But I always remembered this saying of his, along with his standard greeting when he met us at his front door: "Come in, and make your miserable lives happy!"

Recently, a lady wrote to me wanting a cure for eczema. I get a lot of letters like that, all of which I answer with a suggestion to do some reading. Not everybody likes a response like that. I mentioned that she could do a site search at DoctorYourself.com, using the keyword "skin" as a starting point. That will bring up seventy-four matches. She replied that that was too general to really help her, for she wanted a specific cure for eczema.

And therein lies the problem.

Most folks want to know how to treat a particular disease condition, but are not interested in how to treat their whole body. Yet you cannot remove the first from the second. It sounds like a truism, but the way to get rid of a skin disease is to have healthy skin. Treating symptoms is allopathy (drug medicine). Natural healing is about treating the person with the symptoms. The quote at the beginning of this chapter is a good reminder for all of us. "Holistic" is more than a philosophy or catchy title. It is a way of life that is "good for what ails you." You can exclude illness by actively creating a healthy body every day.

As you've probably already noticed, I advocate megadoses of vitamins (generally in conjunction with exercise, good diet, and stress reduction) for a wide array of different health conditions. Is this because I'm a simpleton obsessed with vitamins? No, it's because what we call diseases are usually just different manifestations of the same problem: the huge vitamin deficiencies most of us silently and chronically endure. Get rid of the deficiency, and the disease disappears.

> The quantity of a nutritional supplement that cures an illness indicates the patient's degree of deficiency. It is therefore not a megadose of the vitamin, but rather a megadeficiency of the nutrient that we are dealing with.

Doctors would like you to believe that your health is very complicated, with thousands of diseases out there requiring thousands of patented drugs and trained experts to figure out what to use to keep you upright. But the truth is, health is pretty simple. The body evolved to last a long lifetime on only about two dozen naturally occurring nutrients. None of the basic building blocks of life are pharmaceutical drugs, not one. All living things in creation owe their lives to nature, not to technology. Emulate nature and medical intervention should play only a tiny role in your life.

In that spirit, I offer you my special do-it-yourself super remedy. If you do not feel well—and

I would go so far to say for almost any reason—try this deceptively simple game plan. Go out of your way to promptly get to saturation of the following four key nutrients: niacin, vitamin C, water, and carotene. Then cut the junk out of your diet. This plan is uncomplicated, fast-acting, and very effective on a wide variety of illnesses. Elsewhere in the book I offer megadosing routines customized to a particular condition, but often I just refer you back to this one, because so many diseases are caused by a need for these four nutrients. If in doubt, this is the place to start.

1. **Get to niacin saturation**, which is indicated by a mild, warm, pink-eared facial vasodilation known as a "flush." (Inside Windsor Castle it is doubtless known as a "royal flush.") If you are feeling stressed, anxious, depressed, worried, or just plain ticked off, try this while you are pouring that double shot of bourbon and counting to ten: immediately take 50 to 100 mg of niacin (not niacinamide) every ten minutes until you feel nice and toasty. . . and happy. Then continue to take enough niacin throughout the day so that each dose makes you feel just a tad warm. If you think this will not work, it's because you have not tried it. I refer to the niacin, not the bourbon.

While we're at it, some Fearless Flush Facts: If I had a dime for every person worried about the flushing they experienced when taking large doses of niacin, I'd be a rich man. Niacin flushes are harmless. Some people (including me) enjoy them, especially in winter, as they are accompanied by some welcome warmth. Dr. Abram Hoffer says that the more niacin you take now, the less you will flush later. (See my chapter "Niacin Saturation" for more information.)

Time needed to see improvement: less than an hour.

2. **Get to vitamin C saturation**, which is indicated by bowel tolerance. That means take a few thousand milligrams of vitamin C every ten minutes until you get, or feel like you are about to get, diarrhea. When you feel a rumbling in the bowel, you are close to bowel tolerance and can slightly reduce the amount of C that you've been taking. As you get well, you will find that the amount of C your body can hold automatically goes down. Follow my "take enough C to be symptom free" rule. This will both clean you out and jump-start your immune system. Vitamin C in quantity is the best broad-spectrum antitoxin, antibiotic, and antiviral there is. Cheapest, too. See my chapter "Vitamin C Megadose Therapy" for more information.

Time needed to see improvement: less than a day.

3. **Get to carotene (and water) saturation**. These can be simultaneously achieved by twice daily juicing a big stack of green or orange vegetables, such as carrots. Yes, green as well as orange veggies are absolutely loaded with carotene. Yes, you really do have to drink it. What are you afraid of? When's the last time a person died of vegetable overdose?

Saturation of carotene is reached when your skin turns a partial pumpkin color. Called "hypercarotenosis," it is harmless. Looks cool, too, much like a suntan.

Abundant water intake is guaranteed by abundant juicing. When your tummy is full of juice, you will need to urinate a lot. That is all I mean by water saturation. Inside your skin, you are an aquatic animal. Water is good. Veggie juice is better. If you are worried about getting enough trace minerals, relax: most are amply found in the vegetables. See my chapter "Juicing" for more information.

Time needed to see improvement: less than a week.

4. **Stop eating meat, sugar, and chemical food additives**. Be a near-vegetarian, or at least come as close as you can. There is nothing to it; just eat the other, good natural foods that you really

like anyway—salads, nuts, your favorite vegetables, brown rice and other whole grains, fruits, and beans. Buy fresh or read every label. No chemicals, no sugar. Just do it!

Time needed to see improvement: less than two weeks.

If you think I've lost what's left of my marbles, think again. I have never been more serious. When I work with very sick people, the first "homework" I give them is to go flush, reach bowel tolerance, hydrate, turn orange, and save a cow. Sounds preposterous, doesn't it? But people who do so feel better immediately. Their tests improve immediately. And they learn something of lasting practical value.

Many readers have written to say that when they try to talk to their physician about using nutritional medicine, the subject is promptly dismissed. Furthermore, such dismissal is often accompanied with doctor statements such as, "I have not seen any good research showing that vitamins work therapeutically."

That your doctor has not seen the research is probably true. However, the research has been there all along. The problem is that many health practitioners are often too busy, and sometimes too complacent, to look for it.

It is time to change that. Orthomolecular (nutritional) medicine is well-established as safe and effective. If your doctor still believes that somehow it is not, s/he is behind the times.

And speaking of doctors, another request readers frequently write in with is, "Can you help me find an orthomolecular nutrition doctor near where I live?" For that, you search the Internet.

Niacin Saturation

"You can fix your brain. You can fix your brain with nutrition."

—MARGOT KIDDER

Niacin is vitamin B₃, one of the water-soluble B-complex vitamins. One of niacin's unique properties is its ability to help you naturally relax and get to sleep more rapidly at night. And it is well established that niacin helps reduce harmful cholesterol levels in the bloodstream. Abram Hoffer, M.D., explains: "Niacin is one of the best substances for elevating high density lipoprotein cholesterol (the 'good' cholesterol) and so decreases the ratio of the total cholesterol over high density cholesterol."

Another niacin feature is its ability to greatly reduce anxiety and depression. Yet another feature of niacin is that it dilates blood vessels and creates a sensation of warmth, called a "niacin flush." This is often accompanied with a blushing of the skin. It is this "flush" or sensation of heat that indicates a temporary saturation of niacin, and that is our topic here.

When you flush, you can literally see and feel that you've taken enough niacin. The idea is to initially take just enough niacin to have a slight flush. This means a pinkness about the cheeks, ears, neck, forearms, and perhaps elsewhere. A slight niacin flush should end in about ten minutes or so. If you take too much niacin, the flush may be more pronounced and longer lasting. If you flush beet red for half an hour and feel weird, well, you took too much. As large doses of niacin on an empty stomach are certain to cause profound flushing, take your niacin right after a meal. With each additional dose, the intensity of the flush decreases. Most patients stop being bothered by the flush.

I have found that the best way for me to accurately control the flushing sensation is to start with very small amounts of niacin and gradually increase until the first flush is noticed. One method is to start with a mere 25 milligrams three times a day, say with each meal. The next day, try 50 mg at breakfast, 25 mg at lunch and 25 mg at supper. The following day, try 50 mg at breakfast, 50 mg at lunch, and 25 mg at supper. And, the next day, 50 mg at each of the three meals. The next day, 75, 50, and 50, and so on. Continue to increase the dosage by 25 mg per day until the flush occurs.

It is difficult to predict a saturation level for niacin because each person is different. As a general rule, the more you hold, the more you need. If you flush early, you don't need much niacin. If flushing doesn't happen until a high level, then your body is obviously using the higher amount of the vitamin.

Now that you've had your first flush, what next? Since a flush indicates saturation of niacin, it is desirable to continue to repeat the flushing, just very slightly, to continue the saturation. This could be done three or more times a day. To get to sleep sooner at night, niacin can be taken to saturation at bedtime, too. You might be asleep before you even notice the flush.

An important point here is that niacin is a vitamin, not a drug. It is not habit forming. Niacin does not require a prescription because it is that safe. It is a nutrient that everyone needs each day.

Says Dr. Hoffer, "A person's upper limit is that amount which causes nausea, and, if not reduced, vomiting. The dose should never be allowed to remain at this upper limit. The usual dose range is 1,500 to 6,000 mg daily divided into three doses, but occasionally some patients may need more. The toxic dose for dogs is about 5,000 mg per kilogram body weight. We do not know the toxic dose for humans since niacin has never killed anyone."

Inevitable physician skepticism and questions about niacin's proven safety and effectiveness are best answered in *Niacin: The Real Story* (2012) by Abram Hoffer, Harold Foster and myself. This therapeutic handbook provides details on niacin therapy. *People with a history of heavy alcohol use, liver disorders, diabetes, or who are pregnant will especially want to have their physician monitor their use of niacin in quantity.* Monitoring long-term use of niacin is a good idea for anyone. It consists of having your doctor check your liver function with a simple blood test. Personally, I have this done every few years. According to William B. Parsons Jr., M.D., the Mayo Clinic niacin expert, elevations in liver function tests are of no concern unless they are substantial. Proper interpretation of your test results is important, and most physicians do not know this. Do yourself and your doctor a favor and take a copy of Dr. Parson's book, *Cholesterol Control Without Diet* (Lilac Press, 2000) with you.

Niacin can be purchased in tablets at any pharmacy or health-food store. Tablets typically are available in 100 mg, 250 mg, and 500 mg doses. The tablets are usually scored down the middle so you can break them in half easily. You can break the halves in half, too, to get the exact amount you want.

If niacin is taken right after a meal, the flush may be delayed. In fact, the flush may occur long enough afterward that you forgot about it! Don't let the flush surprise you. Remember that niacin does that, and you can monitor it easily. If you want a flush right away, you can powder the niacin tablet. This is easily done by crushing it between two spoons. Powdered niacin on an empty stomach can result in a flush within minutes.

Sustained-release niacin is often advertised as not causing a flush at all. This may not be completely true; sometimes the flush is just postponed. It would probably be difficult to determine your saturation level with a time-released product like this. It is also more costly. But the biggest reason to avoid sustained-release niacin is that most reports of side effects stem from use of that form.

There is nothing wrong with niacinamide, by the way. That form of vitamin B_3 is frequently found in multivitamins and B-complex preparations. Niacinamide does not cause a flush at all. In my opinion, however, it is less effective in inducing relaxation and calming effects. Niacinamide also does not significantly lower serum cholesterol. This is an important distinction to make when purchasing.

It is a good idea to take all the other B-complex vitamins in a separate supplement in addition to the niacin. The B vitamins, like basketball players, work best as a team. Still, the body seems to need proportionally more niacin than the other B vitamins. Even the RDA for niacin is much more than for any other B vitamin. Many physicians consider the current RDA for niacin of only 20 mg to be way too low for optimum health. While the government continues to discuss this, you can decide for yourself based on the success of doctors that use niacin for their patients every day.

Recommended Reading

Hawkins DR and Pauling L. *Orthomolecular Psychiatry*. San Francisco: Freeman, 1973.

Hoffer A. *Vitamin B_3 and Schizophrenia: Discovery, Recovery, Controversy*. Kingston, Ontario Canada: Quarry Press, 1998.

Hoffer A and Saul AW. *Orthomolecular Medicine for Everyone: Megavitamin Therapeutics for Families and Physicians*. Laguna Beach, CA: Basic Health Publications, 2008.

Hoffer A, Saul AW, and Foster HD. *Niacin: The Real Story*. Laguna Beach, CA: Basic Health Publications, 2012.

Vitamin C Megadose Therapy

"Vitamin C should be given to the patient while the doctors ponder the diagnosis."
—FREDERICK R. KLENNER, M.D.

Vitamin C has varying activity in the body at varying levels of intake. At low levels of consumption, vitamin C is like a trace nutrient: you need very little of it to stay alive, but without any at all you die. Even a few mg a day will suffice to preserve life. At moderate levels of consumption—say 500 to 1,500 mg per day for an adult—the vitamin works to build health. Fewer colds will be reported; incidence, severity, and duration of influenza will be less. But it is at high levels—8,000 to 40,000 mg per day—that we begin to obtain therapeutic properties for the vitamin.

At this high level, vitamin C has antihistamine, antitoxin, and antibiotic properties. The pharmacological effects of a vitamin at high concentration do not disqualify our continuing to call it, and think of it, as a vitamin. Money still buys things even if you have a lot of it; its nature has not changed, but its power has. If it takes 100 gallons of gas to drive from New York City to Los Angeles, you simply are not going to make it on 10 gallons, no matter how you try. Likewise, if your body wants 70,000 mg of vitamin C to fight an infection, 7,000 mg won't do. The key is to take enough C, take it often enough, and take it long enough.

The safety of vitamin C is extraordinary, even in enormously high doses. Compared to commonly used prescription drugs, side effects are virtually nonexistent. I do not know of a single case of vitamin C toxicity anywhere in the world's medical literature. The major side effect of vitamin C overload is an unmistakable, urgent diarrhea. This indicates absolute saturation, and the daily dose is then promptly dropped to the highest amount that will not bring about diarrhea. That is a *therapeutic* level. Robert Cathcart, M.D., routinely employs high–ascorbic acid therapy with his patients with success. Frederick Klenner, M.D., has seen cures of diphtheria, staph and strep infections, herpes, mumps, spinal meningitis, mononucleosis, shock, viral hepatitis, arthritis, and polio using high doses of vitamin C. Dr. Klenner says, "Ascorbic acid is the safest and the most valuable substance available to the physician."

How much vitamin C is an effective therapeutic dose? Bowel tolerance. Physicians have administered as much as 200,000 mg per day. Generally, a therapeutic dose will be in the neighborhood of 350–700 mg per kilogram body weight per day. That is a lot of vitamin C. But then again, the goal is success, not political correctness. Physicians experienced with vitamin C all emphasize that small amounts do not work.

Perhaps the biggest misconception about vitamin C therapy is the assumption that one size fits all. It most certainly doesn't. Sicker bodies hold vastly more vitamin C than do healthy bodies.

Some people need to buffer their vitamin C if they have a sensitive tummy. You can take your C with a calcium-magnesium supplement, or use an already-buffered form of vitamin C such as calcium ascorbate or a neutral form such as sodium ascorbate.

VITAMIN C AND ACIDITY

WHAT FORM IS BEST?

Vitamin C is commonly taken in large quantities to improve health and prevent asthma, allergies, viral infection, and heart disease.[1,2] It is nontoxic and nonimmunogenic, and does not irritate the stomach as drugs like aspirin can. Yet vitamin C (L-ascorbic acid) is acidic. So, a common question is, what are the effects from taking large quantities?

Ascorbic acid is a weak acid (pKa= 4.2),[3] only slightly stronger than vinegar. When dissolved in water, vitamin C is sour but less so than citric acid found in lemons and limes. Can large quantities of a weak acid such as ascorbate cause problems in the body? The answer is, sometimes, in some situations. However, with some simple precautions they can be avoided.

ACID IN THE MOUTH

First of all, any acid can etch the surfaces of your teeth. This is the reason the dentist cleans your teeth and warns about plaque, for acid generated by bacteria in the mouth can etch your teeth to cause cavities. Cola soft drinks contain phosphoric acid, actually used by dentists to etch teeth before tooth sealants are applied. Like soft drinks, ascorbic acid will not cause etching of teeth if only briefly present. Often, vitamin C tablets are coated with a tableting ingredient such as magnesium stearate, which prevents the ascorbate from dissolving immediately. Swallowing a vitamin C tablet without chewing it prevents its acid from harming tooth enamel.

CHEWABLE VITAMIN C TABLETS

Chewables are popular because they taste sweet and so are good for encouraging children to take their vitamin C.[4] However, some chewable vitamin C tablets can contain sugar and ascorbic acid, which, when chewed, is likely to stick in the crevices of your teeth. So, after chewing a vitamin C tablet, a good bit of advice is to rinse with water or brush your teeth. But the best way is to specifically select nonacidic vitamin C chewables, readily available in stores. Read the label to verify that the chewable is made entirely with nonacidic vitamin C.

STOMACH ACIDITY

People with sensitive stomachs may report discomfort when large doses of vitamin C are taken at levels to prevent an acute viral infection (1,000–3,000 milligrams or more every 20 minutes).[1,5] In this case the ascorbic acid in the stomach can build up enough acidity to cause heartburn or a similar reaction. On the other hand, many people report no problems with acidity even when taking 20,000 mg in an hour. The acid normally present in the stomach, hydrochloric acid (HCl), is very strong: dozens of times more acidic than vitamin C. When one has swallowed a huge amount of ascorbate, the digestive tract is sucking it up into the bloodstream as fast as it can, but it may still take a while to do so. Some people report that they seem to sense ascorbic acid tablets "sitting" at the bottom of the stomach as they take time to dissolve. It is fairly easy to fix the problem by using buffered ascorbate, or taking ascorbic acid with food or liquids in a meal or snack. When the amount of vitamin C ingested is more than the gut can absorb, the ascorbate attracts water into the intestines creating a laxative effect. This saturation intake is called bowel tolerance. One should reduce the amount (by 20 to 50 percent) when this occurs.[1]

ACID BALANCE IN THE BODY

Does taking large quantities of an acid, even a weak acid like ascorbate, tip the body's acid balance (pH) causing health problems? No, because the body actively and constantly controls the pH of the bloodstream. The kidneys regulate the acid in the body over a long time period, hours to days, by selectively excreting either acid or basic components in urine. Over a shorter time period, minutes to hours, if the blood is too acid, the autonomic nervous system increases the rate of breathing, thereby removing more carbon dioxide from the blood, reducing its acidity. Some foods can indirectly cause acidity. For example, when more protein is eaten than necessary for maintenance and growth, it is metabolized into acid, which must be removed by the kidneys, generally as uric acid. In this case, calcium and/or magnesium are excreted along with the acid in the urine which can deplete our supplies of calcium and magnesium[6]. However, because ascorbic acid is a weak acid, we can tolerate a lot before it will much affect the body's acidity. Although there have been allegations about vitamin C supposedly causing kidney stones, there is no evidence for this, and its acidity and diuretic tendency actually tends to reduce kidney stones in most people who are prone to them.[1,7] Ascorbic acid dissolves calcium phosphate stones and dissolves struvite stones. Additionally, while vitamin C does increase oxalate excretion, vitamin C simultaneously inhibits the union of calcium and oxalate.[1,2]

FORMS OF VITAMIN C

Ascorbate comes in many forms, each with a particular advantage. Ascorbic acid is the least expensive and can be purchased as tablets, timed-release tablets, or powder. The larger tablets (1,000–1,500 mg) are convenient and relatively inexpensive. Timed-release tablets contain a long-chain carbohydrate which delays the stomach in dissolving the ascorbate, which is then released over a period of hours. This may have an advantage for maintaining a high level in the bloodstream. Ascorbic acid powder or crystals can be purchased in bulk relatively inexpensively. Pure powder is more quickly dissolved than tablets and therefore can be absorbed somewhat faster by the body. Linus Pauling favored taking pure ascorbic acid, as it is entirely free of tableting excipients.

Buffered Ascorbate

A fraction of a teaspoon of sodium bicarbonate (baking soda) has long been used as a safe and effective antacid which immediately lowers stomach acidity. When sodium bicarbonate is added to ascorbic acid, the bicarbonate fizzes (emitting carbon dioxide), which then releases the sodium to neutralize the acidity of the ascorbate.

Calcium ascorbate can be purchased as a powder and readily dissolves in water or juice. In this buffered form ascorbate is completely safe for the mouth and sensitive stomach and can be applied directly to the gums to help heal infections.[8] It is a little more expensive than the equivalent ascorbic acid and bicarbonate but more convenient. Calcium ascorbate has the advantage of being nonacidic. It has a slightly metallic taste and is astringent but not sour like ascorbic acid. 1,000 mg of calcium ascorbate contains about 110 mg of calcium.

Other forms of buffered ascorbate include sodium ascorbate and magnesium ascorbate.[9] Most adults need 800–1,200 mg of calcium and 400–600 mg of magnesium daily.[6] The label on the bottle of all these buffered ascorbates details how much "elemental" mineral is contained in a teaspoonful. They cost a little more than ascorbic acid.

Buffered forms of ascorbate are often better tolerated at higher doses than ascorbic acid, but they appear not to be as effective for preventing the acute symptoms of a cold. This may be because after they are absorbed they require absorbing an electron from the body to become effective as native ascorbate.[1] Some types of vitamin C are proprietary formulas that claim benefits over standard vitamin C.[9]

Liposomal Vitamin C

Recently a revolutionary form of ascorbate has become available. This form of vitamin C is packaged inside nano-scale phospholipid spheres ("liposomes"), much like a cell membrane protects its contents. The lipid spheres protect the vitamin C from degradation by the environment and are absorbed more quickly into the bloodstream. Liposomes are also known to facilitate intracellular uptake of their contents, which can cause an added clinical impact when delivering something such as vitamin C. This form is supposed to be five- to tenfold more absorbable than straight ascorbic acid. It is more expensive than ascorbic acid tablets or powder.

Ascorbyl Palmitate

Ascorbyl palmitate is composed of an ascorbate molecule bound to a palmitic acid molecule. It is amphipathic, meaning that it can dissolve in either water or fat, like the fatty acids in cell membranes. It is widely used as an antioxidant in processed foods, and used in topical creams where it is thought to be more stable than vitamin C. However, when ingested, the ascorbate component of ascorbyl palmitate is thought to be decomposed into the ascorbate and palmitic acid molecules so its special amphipathic quality is lost. It is also more expensive than ascorbic acid.

Natural Ascorbate

Natural forms of ascorbate derived from plants are available. Acerola, the "Barbados cherry," contains a large amount of vitamin C, depending on its ripeness, and was traditionally used to fight off colds. Tablets of vitamin C purified from acerola or rose hips are available but are generally low-dose and considerably more expensive than ascorbic acid. Although some people strongly advocate this type, Pauling and many others have stated that such naturally derived vitamin C is no better than pure commercial ascorbate.[2,9] Bioflavonoids are antioxidants found in citrus fruits or rose hips and are thought to improve uptake and utilization of vitamin C. Generally, supplement tablets that contain bioflavonoids do not have enough to make much difference. For consumers on a budget, the best policy may be to buy vitamin C inexpensively, whether or not it also contains bioflavonoids. Citrus fruits, peppers, and a number of other fruits and vegetables contain large quantities of bioflavinoids. This is one more reason to eat right as well as supplement.

References

1. Hickey S, Saul AW. (2008). *Vitamin C: The Real Story, the Remarkable and Controversial Healing Factor.* Laguna Beach, CA: Basic Health Publications.

2. Pauling L. (1986; 2006, revised version). *How to Live Longer and Feel Better.* Corvallis, OR: Oregon State University Press.

3. *Handbook of Chemistry and Physics.* (2004). Boca Raton, FL: CRC Press.

4. www.doctoryourself.com/megakid.html (for ideas on how to get children to take vitamin C).

5. Cathcart RF. (1981). Vitamin C, titrating to bowel tolerance, anascorbemia, and acute induced scurvy. *Med Hypotheses.* 7:1359–1376.

6. Dean, C. (2006). *The Magnesium Miracle.* New York: Ballantine Books.

7. www.doctoryourself.com/kidney.html.

8. www.doctoryourself.com/gums.html (healing gums with buffered ascorbate). See also: Riordan HD, Jackson, JA. (1991). Topical ascorbate stops prolonged bleeding from tooth extraction. *J Orthomolecular Med* 6:3–4. www.orthomolecular.org/library/jom/1991/pdf/1991-v06n03&04-p202.pdf or www.doctoryourself.com/news/v3n18.txt.

9. http://lpi.oregonstate.edu/infocenter/vitamins/vitaminC/vitCform.html (for information about different forms of vitamin C).

10. www.doctoryourself.com/bioflavinoids.html.

The safety and effectiveness of high vitamin C doses have been well established by medical physicians and decades of practice. Before accepting scare stories about ascorbic acid, you should investigate for yourself. If you haven't yet read the books listed below, you don't know what you're missing. Additionally, you and your doctor may well wish to read papers by William McCormick, M.D., Linus Pauling, Ph.D., Abram Hoffer, M.D., and Robert Cathcart III, M.D. *The Journal of Orthomolecular Medicine* is especially recommended.

DID YOU SAY ACID?

Vitamin C is most frequently supplemented as ascorbic acid. Ascorbic acid is a weak acid, having about the same pH as an orange. Ascorbic acid is weaker than vinegar or even Coca-Cola. I do not see any great amount of published periodontal panic over people routinely consuming these items. However, not everybody likes the taste of ascorbic acid crystals, even in juice. And if you do take vitamin C crystals in a liquid, it is a good policy to rinse your mouth afterwards. Acidity is not good for tooth enamel. Don't want to go through all that? Here is an easy alternative: you can buy ascorbic acid in capsule form. Capsules are easy to swallow, fast-dissolving, tasteless, and fairly cheap. Taking ascorbic acid vitamin C this way does not require mouth rinsing, because there is nothing in the mouth to rinse.

How to Get to a Therapeutic Level of Vitamin C

As I always say, "Take enough C to be symptom-free, whatever the amount might be." It's corny, but it works. The effective therapeutic level is also known as "saturation" or "bowel tolerance." Gradually increase your daily vitamin C dose until you have, or are on the verge of having, diarrhea. Vitamin C diarrhea is frequent, watery, and explosive. You may find that you do not have to get quite to that point to reach saturation. Try this: when you feel (or hear) a rumbling or gurgling in the bowel, back off the amount of C that got you there. You are now probably close to bowel tolerance.

Again you ask, why so much? Simply put, this is the quantity that gets results. At saturation levels, vitamin C has strong antibiotic, antihistamine, antiviral, and antipyretic effects. That means that a saturation level kills bacteria, reduces congestion, inactivates viruses, and lowers fevers.

It cannot be overemphasized that very large quantities of vitamin C are required if you want it to work against real illnesses. You don't take the amount of vitamin C you *think* you should need; you take the amount that does the job!

If you are taking large doses of vitamin C, and decide for any reason to stop doing so, I think it is important to *gradually* decrease the daily dose. This is best done over a week or two. An abrupt halt leaves the body in a lurch. A pilot gradually reduces the airspeed of a jet as the runway approaches; abrupt landings are not appreciated by the passengers. Avoiding sudden drops in your vitamin C level prevents a rebound effect where temporary vitamin C deficiency symptoms occur.

"Do I have to stay at saturation forever?" is another common question. The answer is, yes, yes, and no. Yes, in that you need to stay at or just below bowel tolerance as long as you are ill. The second "yes" is that bowel tolerance is self-adjusting. As a person gets better, he gets to saturation sooner and the dose comes down. A sick body holds an enormous amount of vitamin C. A healthy body holds much less. So the 70,000 mg of C that barely caused a fart when you had influenza would be a toilet-shattering catastrophe when you are in good health. So the real answer is, in effect, "no." As you get better, your saturation dose automatically decreases.

Isn't this neat? And you can monitor the entire process on your own.

Quantity and Frequency Are the Keys to Ascorbate Therapy

So what is it about a little left-handed molecule of six carbons, six oxygens, and eight hydrogens that ticks off so many in the medical community? Maybe it's cases like the one I described near the beginning of this book in the Antibiotic Alternatives chapter. Remember the health-professional couple who, out of desperation, decided to try something they previously had been taught to not try? Ray and his wife gave their very sick baby vitamin C about every fifteen minutes. As a result, the baby was noticeably improved in a matter of hours, and slept through the night. With frequent doses continuing, the child was completely well by the end of the next day. Ray calculated that the child had received just over 2,000 mg vitamin C per kilogram body weight per day. This is even more than what vitamin C expert Dr. Frederick Klenner customarily ordered for sick patients. Remarkably, at 20,000 milligrams of vitamin C/day, that baby never had bowel-tolerance loose stools.[1]

With such a little body, you have to marvel at where all that ascorbate was going. Of course, it is the opinion of those who promulgate the US RDA and related nutritional mythology that almost all of that baby's vitamin C went uselessly into the toilet. Ray and his wife would tell you differently. They would say that their sick child soaked it up like a sponge, and then promptly got better. You choose the answer that works for you.

Quantity of Dose

Dr. Frederick Robert Klenner earned his M.D. from Duke University School of Medicine and was subsequently board certified in diseases of the chest.[2] A working summation of Dr. Klenner's therapeutic use of vitamin C is 350 milligrams vitamin C per kilogram body weight per day (350 mg/kg/day), in divided doses.[3] Since a kilogram is about 2.2 pounds, this translates to:

VITAMIN C (MG)	BODY WEIGHT	NUMBER OF DOSES	AMOUNT PER DOSE
35,000 mg	220 lb	17–18	2,000 mg
18,000 mg	110 lb	18	1,000 mg
9,000 mg	55 lb	18	500 mg
4,500 mg	28 lb	9	500 mg
2,300 mg	14–15 lb	9	250 mg
1,200 mg	7–8 lb	9	130–135 mg

Although these quantities may seem high, *Dr. Klenner actually used as much as four times as much for serious viral illness,* administered by injection. The oral doses listed above are, for the doctor, comparatively moderate.

Frequency of Dose

For those unable to obtain intravenous vitamin C, it is essential to pay special attention to one of the most important aspects of vitamin C therapy: dividing the dosage improves absorption and retention of vitamin C. High oral doses of vitamin C yield higher blood levels of the

310

vitamin, and dividing the oral doses maintains those higher levels. Although initially seeming almost too obvious to mention, these are not self-evident concepts. Many a medical website and government-based dietary recommendation hinge on ignoring them. Hilary Roberts, Ph.D., writes: "Stressed and even mildly ill people can tolerate 1,000 times more vitamin C, implying a change in biochemistry that was ignored in creating the RDA. In setting the RDA, unsubstantiated risks of taking too much vitamin C have been accorded great importance, whereas the risks of not taking enough have been ignored. Real scientists understand that 'no scientific proof' is a fancy way of saying 'we don't like this idea.'"[4]

And there is ample proof to not like. Vitamin C, in very high doses, has been used to successfully treat several dozen illness,[5] with published, peer-reviewed literature spanning the last sixty years. Therefore, the effectiveness and safety of megadose vitamin C therapy should, by now, be yesterday's news. Yet I never cease to be amazed at the number of persons who remain unaware that vitamin C is the best broad-spectrum antibiotic, antihistamine, antitoxic, and antiviral substance there is. Equally surprising is the ease with which some people, most of the medical profession, and virtually all of the media have been convinced that, somehow, vitamin C is not only ineffective but is also downright dangerous.

Bias Against Ascorbate Therapy

When you pick up a health or nutrition book and need to know really fast if it is any good or not, just check the index for "Klenner" and three other key names: Cathcart, Stone, and Pauling. Robert F. Cathcart, an orthopedic surgeon, administered huge doses of vitamin C to tens of thousands of patients for decades,[6] without generating a single kidney stone. Irwin Stone, the biochemist who first put Linus Pauling onto vitamin C, is the author of *The Healing Factor: Vitamin C against Disease.*[7] Pauling cites Stone thirteen times in his landmark book *How to Live Longer and Feel Better,*[8] a recommendation if there ever was one. The importance of vitamin C's power against infectious and chronic disease is extraordinary. To me, omitting it is tantamount to deleting Shakespeare from an English Lit course.

Because of such bias, the primary way patients (and through them, their physicians) have been exposed to Dr. Klenner's work has been through Dr. Lendon Smith's sixty-eight-page *Clinical Guide to the Use of Vitamin C: The Clinical Experiences of Frederick R. Klenner, M.D.*[9] Upon discovering this book, one of my undergraduates submitted a paper to another class discussing a substantial number of medical references she had found on vitamin C as a cure for polio. That course's instructor told me privately that the student's work was absurd, and he literally described her as a "dial tone." I recall a nutritional presentation I made to a hospital staff. All was going well until I mentioned using vitamin C as an antibiotic, as Dr. Klenner did. The mood changed quickly. And how many of us have heard this old saw: "If vitamin C was so good, every doctor would be prescribing it!"

Cardiologist Thomas Levy, M.D., explains: "I could find no mainstream medical researcher who has performed any clinical studies on any infectious disease with vitamin C doses that approached those used by Klenner. Using a small enough dose of any therapeutic agent will demonstrate little or no effect on an infection or disease process."[10]

Preventive Doses

Dr. Klenner recommended daily preventive doses of 10,000 to 15,000 mg/day. He advised parents to give their children their age in vitamin C grams (1 g = 1,000 mg). That would be 2,000 mg/day for a two year old, 9,000 mg/day for a nine-year-old, and for older children, a level-ing-off at about 10,000 mg/day. As for me, I simply say, "Take enough C to be symptom free, whatever that amount may be." It worked for my family. I raised my children all the way into college and they never had a dose of any antibiotic. Not once.

It is high time for medical professionals to welcome vitamin C megadoses and their power to cure the sick. Cure is by far the best word there is in medicine. It would seem that you cannot spell *cure* without *C*. I do not think Dr. Klenner would dispute that.

References:

1. Bowel tolerance as an indicator of vitamin C saturation is discussed by Dr. R. F. Cathcart at www.doctoryourself.com/ titration. html and www.doctoryourself.com/cathcart_thirdface.html.

2. For more about Dr. Klenner's life and work: www.doctoryourself.com/klennerbio.html.

3. Klenner, FR. The significance of high daily intake of ascorbic acid in preventive medicine in *A Physician's Handbook on Orthomolecular Medicine,* Third Edition, Roger Williams, PhD, ed. Chicago, IL: Keats Publishing, 1979, 51–59.

4. Hickey, S and Roberts, H. Ascorbate: *The Science of Vitamin C.* Morrisville, NC: Lulu, 2004.

5. www.doctoryourself.com/vitaminc.html.

6. www.doctoryourself.com/biblio_cathcart.html.

7. The complete text of Irwin Stone's book *The Healing Factor* is posted for free reading at http://vitamincfoundation.org/stone/.

8. Pauling L. *How to Live Longer and Feel Better,* revised edition, 2006. Reviewed at www.doctoryourself.com/livelonger.html.

9. The full text of Dr. Frederick R. Klenner's *Clinical Guide to the Use of Vitamin C* is posted for free reading at www.seanet.com/~-alexs/ascorbate/198x/smith-lh-clinical_guide_1988.htm.

10. Levy, TE. *Vitamin C, Infectious Diseases, and Toxins: Curing the Incurable.* West Greenwich, RI: Livon Books/MedFox Publishing, 2002.

Objections to Vitamin C Megadoses

Many people wonder, in the face of strong evidence for vitamin C's efficacy, why the medical profession has not embraced vitamin C therapy with open and grateful arms. The reason is this: many studies that claim to "test" vitamin effectiveness are designed to disprove it.

You can set up any experiment to fail. One way to ensure failure is to make a meaningless test. A meaningless test is assured if you make the choice to use inappropriate administration of insufficient quantities of the substance to be investigated.

If I were to give every homeless person I met on the street 25 cents, I could easily prove that money will not help poverty. If a nutrition study uses less than 20,000 or 30,000 mg of vitamin C, it is unlikely to show any antihistamine, antibiotic, or antiviral benefit whatsoever. You have to give enough to get the job done. As long as such research as is done uses piddling little doses of vitamins, doses that are invariably too small to work, megavitamin therapy will be touted as "unproven."

Probably the main roadblock to studies of megavitamin therapy is the widespread belief that there must be unknown dangers to tens of thousands of milligrams of ascorbic acid. Yet, since the time such therapy was introduced in the 1940s by Frederick Klenner, M.D., and up to the present, there has been a surprisingly safe and effective track record to follow. One death from vitamin overdose occurs about every ten years in the United States. According to Lucian Leape, in a 1994 *JAMA* article, "Error in Medicine," there are more than 100,000 pharmaceutical drug deaths annually in America. By this yardstick, vitamins are literally one million times safer than medicines.

On top of this, several reported side effects of vitamin C have been found to be completely mythical. According to a NIH report published in *JAMA* in April 1999, none of the following problems are caused by taking too much vitamin C: Hypoglycemia, rebound scurvy, infertility, and destruction of vitamin B_{12}.

Safety and effectiveness should always be the benchmark for any therapeutic program. When one considers that even the AMA admits to more than 100,000 deaths annually from routine administration of prescription drugs, I think we need to consider anew the merits of truly large doses of vitamin C.

Over 1.5 million Americans are injured every year by drug errors in hospitals, doctors' offices, and nursing homes. If in a hospital, a patient can expect at least one medication error every single day (Associated Press, July 20, 2006).

Bioflavonoids and Vitamin C

So what exactly is a rose hip, anyway? Any biologist knows that roses don't have hips because they are not vertebrates. Ha! Actually, rose hips are the fruit of a rose bush. All flowers give rise to fruits, and the rose is no exception. When I hike, I look for wild or feral rosebushes and munch on the hips as soon as they are ready (usually early autumn). They are often found on the bushes throughout the entire winter, just waiting for you to come along. Eaten fresh or dried, they are good sources of vitamin C.

Rose hips are also a rich source of bioflavonoids, plant compounds that improve uptake and utilization of vitamin C. Albert Szent-Gyorgyi won the Nobel prize for his research with vitamin C and related factors back in the 1930s. He actually proposed the term "vitamin P" for the "protective" phytochemicals in bioflavonoids. In a rather adorable, unplanned bit of research, Szent-Gyorgyi was feeding pure vitamin C to his lab mice when one evening some of them snuck out of their cage and ate his dinner when he wasn't looking. The meal consisted of stuffed green peppers. Szent-Gyorgyi observed that the animals that ate the peppers seemed to require considerably less ascorbic acid than the other critters. Peppers, along with many fruits and vegetables, are high in bioflavonoids.

This bioflavonoid–vitamin C connection is why you often see "rose hip" vitamin C tablets offered for sale. Here is the kicker, though: there is so very little rose hips powder in most such tablets that it is a waste of money to pay extra for what amounts to zilch. I (in agreement with Linus Pauling) recommend that people buy the cheapest vitamin C they can find, and take a lot of it. In addition, people need to eat right—lots of fruits and veggies. Fruits and veggies are a mediocre source of vitamin C but an excellent source of bioflavonoids. Vitamin C tablets are a lousy source of bioflavonoids, but a good source of C. Good match.

Recommended Reading

Townsend Letter for Doctors, April, 1992.

Drug Abuse Warning Network (DAWN) Statistical Series I, Number 9, Annual Data 1989.

Leape L. Error in medicine. *Journal of the American Medical Association,* 272 (1994): 1851.

Levy T. *Vitamin C, Infectious Diseases, and Toxins: Curing the Incurable.* Philadelphia, PA: Xlibris, 2002.

Hickey S and Saul AW. *Vitamin C: The Real Story.* Laguna Beach, CA: Basic Health Publications, 2008.

Hughes RE and Jones PR. Natural and synthetic sources of vitamin C. *J Sci Food Agric* 22 (1971): 551–52.

313

Jones E and Hughes RE. The influence of bioflavonoids on the absorption of vitamin C. *IRCS Med Sci* 12 (1984): 320.

Vinson JA and Bose P. Comparative bioavailability of synthetic and natural vitamin C in Guinea pigs. *Nutr Rep Intl* 27 (1983): 875.

Vinson JA and Bose P. Comparative bioavailability to humans of ascorbic acid alone or in a citrus extract. *Am J Clin Nutr* 48 (1988): 6014.

Cathcart RF, III The method of determining proper doses of vitamin C for the treatment of disease by titrating to bowel tolerance. *Journal of Orthomolecular Psychiatry* 10 (1981a):125–32.

Cheraskin E, et al. *The Vitamin C Connection.* New York: Harper and Row, 1983.

McCormick WJ. Lithogenesis and hypovitaminosis. *Medical Record* 159 (1946): 410–13.

Pauling L. (1986; revised ed. 2006). *How to Live Longer and Feel Better.* Corvallis, OR: Oregon State University Press.

Pauling L. *Vitamin C, the Common Cold, and the Flu.* San Francisco: W. H. Freeman, 1976.

Smith LH, ed. *Clinical Guide to the Use of Vitamin C.* [This is a summary of Dr. Frederick Klenner's published papers.] Tacoma, WA: Life Sciences Press, 1988.

Stone I. *The Healing Factor: Vitamin C Against Disease.* New York: Putnam, 1972.

Juicing

"When you are sick of sickness, you are no longer sick."
—ANCIENT CHINESE SAYING

Infomercials do nothing for me personally, but the ones for juicers are in the main correct: juicing makes you healthier and makes you feel better. The first is a long-term observation, the second you can see for yourself in a few days.

Why not just eat all those vegetables raw? Because you won't, that's why. I often juice five pounds or more of carrots, plus six to eight apples, just for breakfast. I'd never find the time to eat all that without the shortcut of a juicer. Also, your body's absorption of fresh, raw juice is simply outstanding. A juicer is essentially a powerful motor with teeth. It breaks cell walls and releases all the plant's nutrients into a solution that your body sucks up like a sponge. Having taught cell biology for so long, I've become familiar with what that good stuff is: plant RNA and DNA (no, this will not grow leaves on your nose), cytoplasm, mitochondria, ribosomes, enzymes and coenzymes, vitamins and minerals, plus the usual proteins, lipids, and carbohydrates. Juicing gives you the lot, and all uncooked, which is important since cooking destroys many beneficial enzymes in raw foods.

I've been juicing for decades now, and have seen it change many lives besides mine. I have also heard two frequent complaints:

1. *"The juicer and the vegetables cost too much!"* Simple answer: A brake job on your car is three hundred dollars. That will get you a really good juicer—which will serve just as important a role in protecting your health. But if you just have to get that brake job first, you can go cheap to start with. I've picked up cheap juicers, new, for as little as $20. Garage sales are a resource for used ones. (Concerned about sanitation? Common household bleach will clean and disinfect plastic and metal juicer parts to a surgical-nurse's satisfaction.) The cost of the produce is no more than you'd spend on other foods that aren't even good for you. I've seen people at the supermarket check out two ritzy cuts of meat and not blink an eye at the $50 it cost them. You couldn't even fit fifty bucks worth of carrots in a grocery cart. Garden, and the price plummets further.

2. *"Juicing takes too much time!"* Simple answer: No, it doesn't. It takes no more time than fixing a regular meal, and probably less. How much time do you spend in doctors' waiting rooms? In line at the checkout? Watching TV? C'mon, everybody has a little time for their health.

The carotene in one cup of carrot juice is probably the equivalent of nearly 20,000 IU of vitamin A. So there's one nutrient you surely do not need to buy as a supplement. It's also worth noting that carotene in high doses has been shown to strengthen the immune system by helping the body to build more helper T cells.

Excess carotene causes the skin to turn slightly orange, once succinctly described in a newspaper as resembling an artificial suntan. This is harmless. Vitamin A toxicity is possible from the preformed, oil type of vitamin A, but not from carotene. In short, it is singularly difficult to kill yourself with carrots. Or juice.

Hints

I'm no Heloise, but by this point I've become a middling-fair juicing expert. Here are some tips for making your juicing experience a rewarding one.

To get more juice, reduce clogging, and simplify cleanup, add some peeled zucchini along with your carrots. My Carrottini (trademark!) juice tastes better than it sounds.

If there is a "head" of frothy foam on the top of your glass of juice, you can either enjoy the taste and milkshake-like texture of it (at least I do), or avoid it by drinking through a straw.

If the leftover vegetable pulp produced by your juicer seems damp or wet, you may be pushing vegetables through too fast. Take your time and let the machine do its job. Use only a subtle pressure, with the plunger supplied by the manufacturer, to send the produce through your juicer. Taking your time juicing can yield as much as a third more juice. It will also reduce the heat from pressing vegetables too hard against the juicer's blade assembly. Reduced friction means cooler juice, which is to be preferred. To this end, I frost up a couple of large drinking glasses, and the glass pitcher I collect the juice in, by sticking them in the freezer each night. Next morning, I begin. Naturally, refrigerating (but NOT freezing!) your fresh produce also keeps everything cooler.

Twice a year, juice a couple of pounds of grapes with seeds to clean the innards of the juicer. I like to use concord grapes, and afterwards let the juice sit for, oh, about five days. And *then* I drink it. Oh yeah!

JUICE EXCUSE

"There is no scientific reason to juice vegetables!"

Really? Anyone intoning that old saw had better check PubMed. Research has shown that drinking vegetable juice has specific medical value.

- Vegetable juice provides huge amounts of bioavailable antioxidants, which fight heart disease, cancer, and many other illnesses: Potter AS, Foroudi S, Stamatikos A, Patil BS, Deyhim F. Drinking carrot juice increases total antioxidant status and decreases lipid peroxidation in adults. *Nutr J.* 2011 Sep 24;10:96.

- More juice means less pancreatic cancer: Jansen RJ, Robinson DP, Stolzenberg-Solomon RZ, Bamlet WR et al. Fruit and vegetable consumption is inversely associated with having pancreatic cancer. *Cancer Causes Control.* 2011 Sep 14.

- Carrot juice is an effective treatment for leukemia: *J Med Food.* 2011 Aug 24. Zaini R, Clench MR, Le Maitre CL. Bioactive Chemicals from Carrot (Daucus carota) Juice Extracts for the Treatment of Leukemia.

This last one is particularly interesting, as I know a leukemia patient who greatly improved when glasses and glasses of vegetable juices were added to his daily diet. Here is what the study authors had to say:

"Overwhelming evidence indicates that consumption of fruits and vegetables with anti-oxidant properties correlates with reduced risk for cancers, including leukemia. Carrots contain beneficial agents, such as β-carotene and polyacetylenes, which could be effective in the treatment of leukemia. This study investigated the effect of carrot juice extracts on myeloid and lymphoid leukemia cell lines together with normal hematopoietic stem cells.

Leukemia cell lines and nontumor control cells were treated with carrot juice extracts for up to 72 hours in vitro. . . . Treatment of leukemia cell lines with carrot juice extract induced apoptosis (cell death) and inhibited progression through the cell cycle. Lymphoid cell lines were affected to a greater extent than were myeloid cell lines, and normal hematopoietic stem cells were less sensitive than most cell lines. This study has shown that extracts from carrots can induce apoptosis and cause cell cycle arrest in leukemia cell lines. The findings suggest that carrots may be an excellent source of bioactive chemicals for the treatment of leukemia."

Add a tablespoon or two of frozen natural juice concentrates (especially lemonade, grape, or pineapple) to kill the taste of any juice you do not like. Try it with cucumber or cabbage. Another way is to have a chaser ready. Pick your very favorite sweet juice and have a full glass ready as your reward for first drinking the good-for-you vegetable juice.

If your family runs for cover at first sight of your intent to liquefy everything in the fridge, then snag your dog. Our dog's ears perk up at the sound of a Champion revving up, for she knows that the vegetable pulp is all for her. We mix it with her dog food to greatly increase its vegetable, vitamin, and fiber content. It is also low-calorie and filling, so it keeps her thin. No dog? Then put the pulp in your compost pile. No compost pile? Well, why not? Okay, okay, one more option: carrot pulp is just the ticket for carrot cake. And that might even get your family back into the kitchen again.

Clean the clogs as you go. Carrots and other veggies can be very fibrous at certain times of the year. If you are really going at it, stop juicing every five pounds or so, unplug the juicer, and (carefully) rinse the blade assembly under running cold tap water. No soap needed.

Recommended Reading

Alexander M, et al. (1985). Oral beta-carotene can increase the number of OKT4 cells in human blood. *Immunology Letters* 9: 221–24.

Tang AM, et al. (1993). Dietary micronutrient intake and risk of progression to acquired immunodeficiency syndrome (AIDS) in human immunodeficiency virus type 1 (HIV-1)-infected homosexual men. *Am J Epidemiol* 138(11):937–51.

317

Breakfast Blast

"The test to which all methods of treatment are finally brought is whether they are lucrative to doctors or not."
—GEORGE BERNARD SHAW

I like to start the day with, oh, a quart and a half of carrot juice. It is carrot-and-zucchini in summer and carrot-and-apple in autumn. Off season, however, I am more likely to get my start with a breakfast concoction I lovingly call "slurry." Here's the recipe:

One pint fruit juice (Orange juice from frozen concentrate works fine and is frequently on sale. Pineapple juice is great, too. Buy unsweetened, bearing in mind that it is naturally, intensely sweet. And that's just as well, given what you're going to put into it.)

Three (or more) rounded tablespoons lecithin granules

One teaspoon vitamin C crystals (approximately 4,500 mg)

Mix together in a spacious stein, and chug-a-lug!

I also take the following supplements everyday, whether it's with the veggie juice or with the "slurry":

600 international units (IU) vitamin E (as natural mixed tocopherols, containing 80 percent d-alpha-tocopherol).

A few hundred milligrams (mg) niacin (more if I don't "flush"; less if I do). This is in addition to my multivitamin.

3 calcium-magnesium tablets (each supplying about 200 mg calcium and 100 mg magnesium. This also helps buffer the vitamin C).

5 multiple digestive enzyme tablets (to help your tummy more easily handle the lecithin. Pancreatin will do, although it is not vegetarian. Vegetarian enzyme sources, which usually include papaya and other fruits, cost more.).

1 high-potency multivitamin, providing:

> 400 IU vitamin D
>
> 25 mg thiamin (vitamin B_1)
>
> 25 mg riboflavin (vitamin B_2)
>
> 100 mg niacinamide (vitamin B_3)
>
> 25 mg pyridoxine (vitamin B_6)
>
> 400 micrograms (mcg) folic acid
>
> 25 mcg vitamin B_{12}
>
> 200 mcg biotin
>
> 25 mg pantothenic acid
>
> 15 mg zinc
>
> 25 mcg selenium
>
> 4 mg manganese
>
> 25 mcg chromium

The multivitamin also contains moderate additional amounts of vitamins A, C, and E. If the multivitamin's mineral quantities seem on the low side, bear in mind that I take this multivitamin again at lunch, and again at dinner, for total of three a day. I also take an additional 60 mg of zinc and 200 mcg of chromium at lunchtime. If you can make this a part of your routine, whether daily or weekly, I think you'll notice benefit.

After I scarf all this down, I enjoy a "chaser" cup of undoctored fruit juice. I am now good for six hours or more without any food or any hunger.

I must express a debt of gratitude to Dr. Jacobus Rinse, whose famous Rinse Formula is the inspiration for my modification presented above.

Vitamin B₁₂ Supplementation

"The standard is not perfection; the standard is the alternative."
—CALIFORNIA LAW ENFORCEMENT OFFICIAL

Let's set the matter straight from the start: If you do not like getting shots of B_{12}, you should be aware that intranasal absorption (discussed below) is the next best thing. Oral administration of B_{12} supplements is less effective. This goes for so-called sublingual B_{12} tablets as well.

Vitamin B_{12}, unlike other B vitamins, is stored in muscle and other organs of the body. A little B_{12} goes a long way, what is stored lasts a long time, and it may take years to deplete your body's reserves. But sooner or later, usually later (after age forty), not only do poor eating habits catch up with us, but we also lose the ability to efficiently absorb what B_{12} we do get from food.

Cobalamin is the proper name for vitamin B_{12}. It is a really huge molecule ($C_{63}H_{90}O_{14}PCo$). The "Co" is for the one cobalt atom at its core. B_{12} is obtained mostly, but not exclusively, by eating animal products such as dairy and meat. Grass-and-grain-eating cattle get their B_{12} from synthesis by microorganisms in their gastrointestinal tract. Yes, B_{12} is also synthesized in the human GI tract, but not enough. It can be enhanced by a good vegetarian diet that favors an internal population of beneficial, B_{12}-making bacteria, but we still need more than that. Nutritional yeast, fermented soy foods such as tempeh, and sprouts (according to some sources) are vegetarian sources of dietary B_{12}.

Absorption of dietary B_{12} takes place in the very last part of the small intestine, right before the colon. Absorption requires a biochemical helper molecule called "intrinsic factor," which is a glycoprotein normally secreted by cells lining your stomach. Strong stomach hydrochloric acid is also required to split up this huge molecule. (That's why a weak acid like vitamin C (ascorbic acid) is harmless to B_{12}, persistent myths to the contrary). Even sublingual (under-the-tongue) B_{12} supplements are probably ineffective because the cobalamin molecule is too large to diffuse through the mucosa of the mouth. And if your body no longer makes intrinsic factor like it should, you cannot absorb oral B_{12} supplements very well, either.

The end result can be pernicious anemia, which is more than the classic inability to make enough hemoglobin for your red blood cells. Pernicious anemia also results in a sore mouth and tongue, assorted burning and tingling sensations, and eventually neurological damage. I think Ménière's syndrome and dementia symptoms mistaken for Alzheimer's disease might be a manifestation of this as well.

While there is a urine test for B_{12} deficiency, to get accurate B_{12} readings it is necessary to measure the cerebrospinal fluid. If you are not a spinal tap fan, consider a simple, noninvasive therapeutic trial of B_{12}. This is so inexpensive and safe that it would be difficult to deny it to anyone. I would suggest your doctor try a 1,000 mcg injection at least once a week. Compared to the RDA of only about 3 mcg, that dose may appear hefty. But given the miserable nature of unappreciated B_{12}-deficiency diseases, erring on the high side may be preferable to unnecessarily delaying recovery. And I know of no side effects whatsoever with B_{12} overdose.

Intranasal (that is, by way of the nose) administration sounds pretty weird, but it is an efficient delivery method for large-sized molecules whether you like the sound of it or not. Your nose has two choices:

1. You can obtain ready-to-use B_{12} gel from a pharmacy. This will probably require a prescription, will not be covered by insurance, and can therefore be expected to be pricey.

2. Make your own B_{12} intranasal supplement. It is cheap, easy, and best done behind closed doors. Obtain your doctor's okay before trying this procedure. Take any B_{12} tablet (between 100 to 1,000 mcg) and grind it into a powder between two tablespoons. Add water, just a few drops at a time, to make a soft paste. With a "Q-Tip," its generic equivalent, or your clean pinkie finger, gently swab the paste inside your nose up to a comfortable level. Do not push; use no force whatsoever. The excipients (tableting ingredients) are more likely to bother your schnoz than the B_{12} is. If it irritates you, try using less, or a different brand of tablet. I'd try this two times a week for a month.

Feel free to quit at any time and get B_{12} shots instead. Once in a great while doctors will even teach you how to give yourself B_{12} shots, but that remains a singularly rare event. Hence this nose news.

A reader says:

"I have used nasal B_{12} ever since the FDA took it off the market to make a prescription drug. I now make my own, taking about six 2,500 mcg oral supplement tablets, putting them into about a 1-oz. nose dropper bottle, filling it $^3/_4$ full with water, shaking it up, and storing it in the refrigerator. I find it is good for any respiratory disease. I put a half dropper full in each nostril, and between 4 to 24 hours it works. It has never failed me or my friends."

Stress Reduction

"Learn and live. If you don't, you won't."
—WWII U.S. ARMY-TRAINING FILM

Frequently in this book I've suggested stress reduction as one key to alleviating many health problems. You already know some things you should be doing, or not doing, in order to relieve stress. Here is my three-step plan for even better results.

Step One: Experience Relaxation

It does no good to tell somebody to relax. They need to be shown how to relax, immediately and reliably. For me, the end of tension began with a book. That particular book was *Relief without Drugs,* by Australian psychiatrist Ainslie Meares. Shortly thereafter, I began to do a technique known as progressive relaxation. It is time-honored, easy, and works surprisingly well. Here's the version I learned while a visiting student in the psychiatric wing of Canberra Hospital:

While sitting with your eyes closed, pay attention to your toes. Yes, *those* toes. Relax your toes. Really relax them, too. If you do not know what this means, tense them up and *then* relax them. Then, without tensing, relax them some more. Next, relax the soles of your feet in the same way. Then your ankles. Then your calves. Then thighs, hips, abdomen, and so forth. Relax each region of your body as you progress upward, ending with your head. Relaxing each part of the face is especially effective. Keeping your eyes closed, feel how relaxed you are. Feel your whole body relaxed. Feel your mind relaxed. Now just sit and enjoy it for a few minutes. Then slowly open your eyes, take a deep breath or two, and off you go.

Step Two: Regular Practice Brings Progress

State University of New York emeritus professor of biology John Mosher (whom we will hear from later) has provided the following six suggestions for a breath-based method of stress reduction, which you may find even more profoundly settling than Step One was. Because this practice is very settling and relaxing, it is best done before eating, in the morning and evening.

1. Choose a quiet comfortable place. It is best to do the meditation sitting up with your back comfortably straight.

2. With eyes closed, be aware of your breathing. Be sure you are breathing from the diaphragm ("belly breathing") and not the chest. Your lower abdominal area should easily rise and fall as you inhale and exhale.

3. Try some "alternating breathing." The alternating breathing simply consists of breathing through one nostril at a time. Use your thumb to gently close your right nostril, and inhale through the left nostril. Then, release the right, close the left nostril with your fingers, and now exhale through the right nostril. Then, in through the right nostril, close the right with your thumb, and exhale through the left. Now in with the left, close, and out through the right. Continue this alternating breathing for about five minutes, with the eyes closed.

4. Now discontinue the alternating breathing technique and continue to sit quietly with eyes closed, bringing your attention to your normal breath. Continue to breathe from the diaphragm.

5. Be mindful of inhaling and exhaling. Continue this "mindful" breathing for fifteen or twenty minutes. If during the breathing your mind wanders and gets off on thoughts, as soon as you realize your attention is not on the breathing, very gently turn your attention from the thought to the breathing. Do not try to control your thoughts! Do not dwell on thoughts.

6. At the end of fifteen or twenty minutes of the "mindful" breathing, lie down and relax with eyes closed for ten minutes. At the end of your rest, come back into activity very gradually and easily.

Step Three: Centering Prayer

Contemplatives and scholars alike have pointed out that many religious and secular traditions share interest in stress reduction that may be gained from meditation or prayer. One widely practiced faith-based technique is known as Centering Prayer, or Prayer of the Heart. The following books discuss and describe this method:

Bacovcin H, trans. *The Way of a Pilgrim and the Pilgrim Continues His Way: A New Translation.* New York: Image Books, 1978.

Johnston W, ed. *The Cloud of Unknowing and the Book of Privy Counseling.* New York: Image Books, 1996.

Peers E, trans. Teresa of Avila. *Interior Castle.* New York: Image Books, 1972.

Pennington M. *Daily We Touch Him: Practical Religious Experiences.* Chicago: Sheed and Ward, 1997.

More than Just an "Out-There" Hippie Idea

Therapeutic meditation is an especially well-researched area of medicine. A free PubMed search (www.nlm.nih.gov) for "meditation" will yield over 2,400 scientific papers on the subject. And "stress reduction" will get you almost 39,000 matches. Complete text of many of these articles will be found in *Scientific Research on the Transcendental Meditation Program: Collected Papers, Volumes 1–6.* Fairfield, IA: Maharishi University of Management, 1990.

Evading Exercise

"I hate exercise, but I like the results."

—JACK LALANNE

Organized nudity is responsible for it.

When I was a little kid, we boys all swam naked at the YMCA. The one exception was when moms and sisters were invited for special events. I still remember the one kid who forgot it was Family Swim Night and innocently strolled out of the showers and into the pool room in his birthday suit. He did the fastest about-face I've ever seen, and we never let him live it down.

What's more, we were still swimming nude in boy's gym class when I graduated from Charlotte High School in 1970. Back dives were especially revealing. I know this sounds a bit hard to believe, but it was true: nude swimming was the rule all the way through grade twelve in the Rochester, New York, public schools. I am reliably informed that the girls got to wear swimsuits in their gym classes.

But not us.

Of course we all showered together as well. In a scene reminiscent of a juvenile prison movie, after gym class we were compelled to shower. In the scant three minutes given to us for the purpose, enough teen trauma was accumulated to last a lifetime. I mean, how do you cope with such a situation? Everybody had to do it, so evidently we managed. And we learned valuable skills in the process. For example, one of my acquaintances taught me how to get dressed without drying first.

It did not help that my high-school gym teacher took a special dislike to me. I was about 6' 1" and weighed, maybe, 100 pounds. This guy, an obese ex-Marine, was also the wrestling coach. He combined the only two marketable skills he possessed into a brilliant method of selecting sparring teams: he'd line us up by height and have us count off by twos. This meant, of course, that I inevitably ended up with a 6' 1", 220-pound varsity football lineman as my wrestling "partner." I therefore developed the fastest sit-out in wrestling history.

Under such circumstances, it is no surprise that I developed an enduring dislike of all things related to sport. It's not that I haven't tried. Like all the neighborhood boys, I played ball all summer. I mean, that's what boys *did*. My teams never got even remotely close to being in the playoffs, but my brothers did. Which figures.

For the first fifteen years of his life, my older brother was a round-shouldered, horn-rimmed, skinny little twerp. The he started working out in our basement. Like a mushroom planted in the dark and forgotten, he thrived. Weightlifting utterly transformed him. Good diet, natural maturation, and contact lenses didn't hurt, either, but that Sears and Roebuck weight kit did wonders.

The secret, of course, is that he spent the time using it.

And that brings me to my real point.

You either talk about doing it, or you do it. I do not like to exercise. But I like even less having a pudgy belly, skinny arms, no chest, and health conditions. The health benefits of exercise are vast and well-known. So are the purely physical benefits. That is why I exercise. Of course you and I know it is good to exercise, in the same way that smokers know it is good not to smoke, but knowledge is not enough. You have to do it.

My exercise hints? Thought you'd never ask.

Exercise for a really honest reason: vanity.

Exercise with a friend (or relative, if you are desperate) who has the same goals you do. This is very important for staying on the wagon.

Exercise to music. I recommend the Who, the Rolling Stones, good blues, early Beatles, and maybe a little Badfinger for the rest of you eclectic ex-hippies.

Start small and work up. I began, at my son's insistence, with crunches. When I started, I thought thirty was a lot. After six years, I now do 2,100 crunches in under 50 minutes.

Invest as little money as possible. A cheap exercise bike and a pair of dumbbells is a good start. Maybe add a weight set and a bench. Check garage sales, for a lot of people purchase this stuff, and that act constitutes their entire exercise program: the buying of equipment. Consequently, you can outfit your garage, attic, or basement for very little cash.

Better yet, keep it all in your living room. If you see it, you will use it. Still better, keep all your gear within a remote's distance of your TV. You can watch the tube while you bike. You can kill an hour of brainless network programming and bike miles in the process.

BODY BUILDING

A reader writes, "I'm a body builder and wonder how much protein supplementation I should do to increase muscle mass."

None. No protein supplementation. Yes, you heard that right. The average meat-eating American consumes over 100 grams of protein daily, and only needs about 45 grams to maybe, possibly, 65 grams—if they are a real weight-training beast. A good near-vegetarian diet can provide this amount. You can get protein from foods other than meat, milk, and eggs. If you check the food composition tables in any nutrition textbook you will see that beans (not just soybeans), whole grain breads, sprouts, nuts, and even vegetables have significant amounts of protein. I raised my kids ovolacto-vegetarian and they are now tall, healthy adults. Elephants never even eat eggs or dairy. They are even bigger. It is not about how much protein you shovel in. It is about how much you work out.

325

Keep a record. My brother told me that you need to simply beat your own record to be a winner. That's a pretty profound point. I would never have gotten to 2,100 crunches unless I'd wanted to beat 2,000, or 1,000, or 30.

Vary your program. Although I am a crunch-meister, I also use dumbbells for my arms and chest. I happen to already have strong legs from childhood paper routes, chasing my brothers so I'd not be left behind, biking everywhere as a teenager, and living at the top of a hill in Vermont as a car-less young man. So I don't use the bike as much as you might want to. I also walk home with my groceries, and try for a four-mile walk along the nearby Erie Canal on alternate days to my crunching. Again, take a friend, or a dog, for safety, companionship, and mutual encouragement.

Watch the cable exercise channels, especially if you are a beginner. Seeing all those supple, writhing bodies exercising with one great smile is stimulating. Use Richard Simmons exercise tapes, Jane Fonda workout tapes, any workout tapes that appeal to you. Personally, I think the porno industry should come up for air for a minute, and make totally nude workout tapes.

And that brings us full circle: it really *is* all about nudity. Especially how you, with your clothes off, look in the mirror. You will be pleased, your friends will be jealous, and your family will be thrilled to know how much longer they will have you around. Well, they will if you first put your clothes back on.

Removing Pesticides from Food

*"If you drink much from a bottle marked "poison" it is almost certain
to disagree with you sooner or later."*

—ALICE IN WONDERLAND

Real-world people shop at supermarkets, and real-world affordable fruits and vegetables contain pesticide residues. Not everybody can buy organic; not everybody is a gardener. Here are easy and effective ways to reduce your chemical consumption.

Rule number one: wash your fruits like you wash your hands: use soap! Mom was right: just running your mitts under tap water does little to remove oily grime. Agricultural pesticides do not come off in water, either. If they did, farmers would have to apply them after each rain or even a heavy dew. That would be both labor-intensive and expensive. So companies make pesticides with chemical "stickers" that are insoluble in water. They stay on the fruit, rain or shine.

Soap, or detergent, is more effective in removing pesticide residues than you think. You can prove this for yourself. Take a big bunch of red or green grapes, and place them, with a squirt of dishwashing detergent, in a large bowl of water. Mix the detergent in thoroughly, and swish the grapes around for a minute. Carefully watch the water. You will see evidence that detergent works. If you do not think that that stuff is pesticide residue, try another bowl of grapes in water without detergent, and try another bowl of organically grown grapes in water with detergent. Seeing is believing.

It is necessary to rinse detergent-washed fruits before eating, of course, but that is hardly a burden. Rinse until the water is clear. When you handle the detergent-washed fruit, you will also notice that it feels different, too. We are so used to fruit with chemical coatings that when we touch truly clean fruit, it's a new tactile experience. Go ahead, try it. Nobody's looking.

Even if you do not believe that pesticides pose the slightest health risk, there is no down side to not eating them. Whatever benefits they may confer on the tree, pesticides do you no good in your gut. Children may consume disproportionately large amounts of pesticides because kids eat a lot of fruit relative to their body weight. For parents, there is a measure of comfort in knowing that their kid's chemical intake has been minimized.

Newly detergent-washed fruit does not keep as well. The former petrochemical coating probably served as a moisture barrier and even an oxidation barrier (as does the wax coating on many fruits and vegetables). No worries; you only wash before you eat.

In case you think I am taking too easygoing a view of chemical farming, I would like to point out that I am an avid organic gardener. I also advocate purchasing organically grown foods whenever possible. It costs more to buy organic, but it is probably money well spent. Home gardening is an incredibly cheap alternative. All those stories that you hear about a thirty-dollar investment in seed and fertilizer yielding seven hundred dollars' worth of fresh food are true. If you think I'm more full of fertilizer than my garden is, I recommend that you try it and see. For starters, try leaf lettuce, zucchini, cucumbers, bush green beans, and a dozen tomato plants. You will soon be supplying half the neighborhood. None of the veggies require any pesticides to grow well.

A cheapskate hint: save those potatoes that are no good because they've sprouted eyes. The eyes are actually sprouts, each of which will grow into an entire potato plant bearing several spuds. Cut the tater up and plant each piece that has a sprout on it. No pesticides needed here, either.

Many fruits and vegetables are not merely sprayed, but are waxed as well. So-called "food grade" waxes improve shelf life and appearance, but also coat over and lock in any previously applied pesticides. This poses a problem, for waxes do not readily dissolve in detergent solution. You might find a product or two on the market that is certified to remove waxes from fruits, but I am skeptical. In order to dissolve food wax, the product should be able to dissolve a birthday candle. I had lots of solvents in my biochemistry lab that would do that pronto, but I have not seen any *safe* products that can. The easiest alternative is simply to peel them. Frequently waxed produce includes apples, pears, eggplants, cucumbers, squash, and even tomatoes. The lack of a high gloss is not proof positive that a fruit is not waxed: many waxes, like many types of floor polyurethane or spray varnish, are not at all shiny. One way to tell if a fruit or vegetable is waxed is to run your fingernail over it and see if you can scrape anything off. Another way is to read the label and see if the produce is waxed. This may require a trip in back to the warehouse to see the carton that the produce came in. Lotsa luck on that.

A peeler costs about a buck and effectively removes wax. A squirt of dish detergent costs a few cents. Lots more information on pesticides is free and readily available on the Internet and from your public library.

327

Free Food. No, Really

"Good health makes a lot of sense, but it does not make a lot of dollars."
—SOURCE: MODESTY PREVENTS ME. OK, *I* SAID IT, IN THE MOVIE *FOODMATTERS*

Free food. For once in your life, this statement is literally true, with no catch, and no one trying to sign you up or sell you anything.

Free Potatoes

Save all old, "spoiled" potatoes that have sprouted "eyes." Get anyone crazy enough to save theirs to give them to you, and it's free. Plant them. You will get a potato bush (vine) from each one, which will yield several to many potatoes each when you dig.

Free Carrots

When you juice fresh carrots, save the tops. Not, not the box tops or package tops. No, not the big fern-like carrot tops. Save the top inch of each carrot. Some will be sprouting light green shoots while in the bag, even fresh from the store. They will sprout further if you plant them. With carrots, a growing top means a growing bottom. The orange root below ground is storage for food their green chlorophyll factories make above ground in the sun. The new green tops will generate white flowers that look exactly like Queen Anne's Lace, the wild carrot. These will then seed. Save the seeds or let them fall, and you get free carrots next year.

You might think this is an expendable, optional, even trivial pursuit. It is not. A lack of potatoes nearly wiped out Ireland. A lack of carrots causes 100,000 cases of preventable blindness in children worldwide every year. More wars have been lost for lack of food than by battlefield defeat. More sickness has been caused by malnutrition than by any microbe.

Free Onions

The first botanical experiment I recall ever doing is sticking an onion in a half-filled glass of water. It sprouted. Try this at home, then plant the results. You will get onion plants, then onion flowers (really), and then onion seed. Save the seed for the next season.

Free Garlic

Same as onions. When the garlic cloves you did not use start to sprout, plant them.

Free Tibet

While you are at it, don't forget that growing your own food makes you independent from what General and President Dwight David Eisenhower called the "military-industrial complex." Every person on earth could grow enough food for themselves and their family if they had just two or three acres of arable land.

Sure, my kitchen looks like the set of *Invasion of the Body Snatchers.* But what is a kitchen for, anyway?

And my garden is, well, casual. At the end of the season I leave some broccoli and lettuce to go to seed . . . and collect the seeds. Same with lupin flowers. I also let some green beans, squash, and other fruits (yes, botanically they are) get overripe, dried on the vine, and gathered and saved for next year. I further dry the seed in the barn in open containers, with some live-catch mousetraps strategically placed nearby. By the way: be sure you store your seed in paper, not plastic. It will keep the air circulating and there is less chance of mold or rot.

A Crash Course in Vegetarian Cooking

"Hey, I won't say I'm a bad cook, but all the flies chipped in to fix the screen door."
—AFTER RODNEY DANGERFIELD

Put on your helmet: It's time for my infamous "Crash Course in Vegetarian Cooking." When I was a kid, eating was a necessary evil. Mom, a former history teacher, did not exactly have a passion for cooking. Her casual disregard of any advances ever made in culinary science approached the legendary. Years ago, my daughter based an essay for English class on the time in my boyhood when my mother mixed a box of lime Jell-O with a box of cherry Jell-O and got gray Jell-O. Yes, we had to eat it. You didn't waste food in our home.

"Well done," at least in my experience, is the ultimate oxymoron. Mom could have burned ice cream. She overcooked everything, justifying it with the ever-ready apology, "Your father likes it this way." After years and years of eating overdone, dry, tooth-stressing meals, I finally asked Pop why he liked everything overcooked. He said, "That's the way your mother makes it." O. Henry would have been pleased.

By the way, Mom also mixed partly open boxes of breakfast cereal "to save space." I was raised on Cheerios, Corn Flakes, Wheaties, Puffed Rice, Shredded Wheat, and Grape Nuts . . . all in the same bowl at the same time.

But in fairness, Mom also gave each of us a multivitamin every day. The moment Dad walked into the house after work, he had a glass of orange juice stuck into his hand and a Eastman Kodak penny-a-piece vitamin pill plunked in his mouth before he could say, "What's for dinner?" And since "What's for dinner?" was such a fruitless question anyway, everything being uniformly charred to a tasteless slab, the pill no doubt did him good.

Mom also drank the water the canned spinach was packed in. She saved fresh vegetable cooking water and made soup from it. I now know that such behaviors result in increased consumption of vitamins and minerals. Back then, I simply thought she was a little nuts. Obviously, it is hereditary.

Perhaps it was this palate-punishing perversion of what should have been home cooking that sent me running in the other direction as an adult. Whatever it was, I've been cooking with whole, natural, vegetarian foods for thirty years now. Here are my ten best kitchen tips. (Remember, however, that you are getting these suggestions from a guy who, as a college graduate, still thought allspice was a mixture of all the spices together in one convenient jar.)

1. If there is one secret of vegetarian cooking, it is salt. OK, that was also Marge Simpson's secret ingredient for pork chops. But still. Grains and legumes (peas, beans, and lentils) especially need it for good taste. Now don't go worrying that you are getting too much sodium. Homemade foods have less salt than most store-bought processed foods, and certainly are less salty than restaurant foods. Use (just) enough salt to make people want to eat what you serve, and you have won half the battle. If you overdo it, too much salt can be removed from food by cooking a halved raw potato into your mistake and then removing the potato before serving. Adding more water, or more of all the other ingredients, will also reduce the salt concentration.

2. Taste your cooking as you go. If you like it, others probably will. Learning from mistakes is less costly if you own a nice, hungry, tolerant doggie. Such animals are readily available from your local pound or humane society. Believe me, anything you were previously thinking of tossing out is far better than the stuff that goes into most commercial pet foods.

3. Consult easy vegetarian cookbooks. I especially like *The Deaf Smith Country Cookbook* and *Laurel's Kitchen*. Health food stores tend to have a good selection of cookbooks, and often have free recipes for the asking.

4. When in doubt, leave it out. If you are not sure whether to use an ingredient, don't. I've made bread with just whole wheat flour, water, and salt. Period. It yields a flatbread or Johnny-cake, but it tastes great. I never add shortening or oil to my raised breads; you really don't miss it. Extra-sneaky hint: get and use a bread machine. Easy!

5. Over the years, you will save a fortune cooking vegetarian. (Just don't make your fortune cooking vegetarians, which is illegal in most states.) Maybe you didn't get that raise, and we know that taxes never go down. We have here a way to make money getting healthy. This is not a trivial benefit. Back when he was age seventeen, my son conservatively estimated that our family's simple eating for his entire lifetime to date had saved us nearly the purchase price of our house. I checked both his math and the mortgage: he was right.

The best foods in the supermarket are often the cheapest; the worst foods cost the most. Yes, fruit is mind-numbingly expensive. But so is meat. And especially so are convenience foods. We buy fruit (among other good things) and still spend only about one third as much on food as our neighbors do. We have here a way to make money getting healthy. And every buck you save is effectively tax-free cash in your pocket. Can you beat that?

6. Start small, but when you get experienced try to cook in quantity. A big pot of soup will feed you all week. Keep it in meal-sized containers in your refrigerator. Open one of those instead of a can of something. Just as convenient, but cheaper and healthier, too.

7. Be sure to cook beans and dry legumes thoroughly. They taste dreadful if you don't. After checking to remove any little stowaway stones, soak your legumes tonight to reduce cooking time tomorrow. Change the soaking water twice before cooking to remove dirt or soap residues.

8. If you are not used to baking with whole wheat flour, work it in gradually. Start with $2/3$ white (unbleached) flour and $1/3$ whole wheat. Then try half and half. Over time, you can increase the fraction of whole wheat so subtly that no one will notice. Baking with all whole wheat (or any other whole grain) generally requires more leavening and more cooking time. Pull up a chair by the oven and check from time to time. Baking with honey requires less liquid, because honey is one. Honey tastes sweeter than sugar, so two-thirds to one-half as much honey is enough.

9. To stimulate your cooking habit, keep *less* food in the house. The more convenience crutches we have, the less we work at self-reliance. Stock up on grains and legumes. Being dry, they keep a long time in glass jars or plastic bags. With salt, oil, some herbs and spices, and of course fruits and vegetables, you are set. Butter and yogurt are part of our menu, but need not be for some. Tofu, tempeh, sprouts or seed for sprouting, honey, molasses, and fruit juice fill out our cheap diet. We are most creative in the kitchen when the pickings are slim.

331

The above statement is more subversive than it looks. Food stamps and other well-meant programs encourage supermarket spending. That may be good for the economy, but it is not always good for the body.

My First Law of Nutrition: The best foods in the supermarket are often the cheapest; the worst foods cost the most. Take along a copy of the *Supermarket Handbook* (N. and D. Goldbeck, Signet, 1976) to help you shop, and always eat first.

10. Do not fret if you succumb to a Big Mac Attack or wolf down the occasional box of chocolates. To me, it is not a matter of life or death if you have turkey at the holidays (though it is to the turkey). What matters is not what you do on any one day but what you do on the other 364. In total, are you doing it right? Check your debts; check your medicine cabinet use; check the bathroom scales: if they are all going down, you are doing fine.

Your spouse or children may not necessarily go for all of this. The rest of the world should be so lucky, but they are not. You know, the reason the Chinese eat lots of grains, legumes, and vegetables is not because they are seeking health. It is because they can't afford to eat any other way. Their lower rates of heart disease, cancer, and osteoporosis are a by-product of frugality.

Natural Versus Synthetic Vitamins

Nobody really likes what I have to say on this subject. Vitamin salespeople think it's too medical, and medical people think it's too quacky. But facts are facts, and here are mine:

1. Most vitamin products sold in health-food stores contain synthetic vitamin powders. There are only a few manufacturers of vitamin powders, and they are generally large pharmaceutical companies. This is not an inherently bad thing, however, because laboratory-made vitamins are far cheaper than whole food concentrates, synthetic vitamins *usually* work quite well, and labs can get a significant potency into a small tablet.

One of the biggest differences in "health-food store" versus "drug store" brands is what is *not* in the tablet. For example, most natural brands leave out artificial chemical colors, which is a good thing to do. Just about all brands contain tablet fillers and excipients, needed to physically hold the pill together. Since these will vary, the only way to find out exactly who uses what is to write to the company and find out. Some tableting ingredients are pretty standard: calcium-phosphate compounds, maltodextrin, silica or silicon dioxide, cellulose, and the stearates or stearic acid are common and widely accepted as harmless.

2. Vitamins can be called "natural" even if made in a laboratory. Vitamin C, for example, is factory-made from starch, which is a natural product. Is this starch-based vitamin C identical to orange-juice-based vitamin C? Most biochemists say yes. But the real test is effectiveness. High doses of factory-made ascorbic acid vitamin C work against viral and bacterial illness, and in numerous other illnesses. It is possible that food-concentrate vitamin C may be somewhat more efficient, but because it would be so much more expensive, it isn't worth it.

CHEAP VITAMIN C

Milligram for milligram, vitamin C supplementation is cheaper than trying to get vitamin C from food. A single large orange costs at least 50 cents and may easily cost one dollar. It provides less than 100 milligrams (mg) of vitamin C. A bottle of 100 tablets of ascorbic acid vitamin C, 500 mg each, costs about five dollars. The supplement gives you 10,000 mg per dollar. In terms of vitamin C, the supplement is 50 to 100 times cheaper, costing about one or two cents for the amount of vitamin C in an orange.

3. In some cases, however, the natural form of a vitamin *is* clearly superior to the synthetic form. The best example is vitamin E, discussed in the next chapter.

It is remarkable how many natural-looking brown bottles, with naturally decorated labels and natural-sounding brand names, contain the synthetic form. I once bought just such an innocent-looking package, only to discover that the pills inside were a dazzling, nearly radioactive pink color. Strange, but true. I still have them, and I like to trot them out during lectures as proof.

333

Supplements: The Real Story—Foods or Tablets?

It's a nutritional "Catch 22": The public is told, confusingly: "Vitamins are good, but vitamin supplements are not. Only vitamins from food will help you. So just eat a good diet. Do not take supplements! But by the way, there is no difference between natural and synthetic vitamins."

Wait a minute. What's the real story here?

A recent health study reported that the risk of heart failure decreased with increasing blood levels of vitamin C[1]. The benefit of vitamin C (ascorbate) was highly significant. Persons with the lowest plasma levels of ascorbate had the highest risk of heart failure, and *persons with the highest levels of vitamin C had the lowest risk of heart failure.* This finding confirms the knowledge derived over the last fifty years that vitamin C is a major essential factor in cardiovascular health.[2,3] The study raises several important questions about diet and vitamin supplements.

Was It Food or Supplements?

The report discussed vitamin C as if it were simply an indicator of how many fruits and vegetables were consumed by the participants. Yet, ironically, the study's results show little improvement in the risk for heart failure from consuming fruits and vegetables. This implies that the real factor in reducing the risk was indeed the amount of vitamin C consumed. Moreover, the study appears to utterly ignore the widespread use of vitamin C supplements to improve cardiovascular health. In fact, out of four quartile groups, the quartile *with the highest plasma vitamin C had six to ten times the rate of vitamin C supplementation* of the lowest quartile, but this fact was not emphasized. This type of selective attention to food sources of vitamin C, while dismissing supplements as an important source, appears to be an attempt to marginalize the importance of vitamin supplements.

Many medical and nutritional reports have maintained that there is little difference between natural and synthetic vitamins. This is known to be true for some essential nutrients. The ascorbate found in widely available vitamin C tablets is identical to the ascorbate found in fruits and vegetables.[3] Linus Pauling emphasized this fact, and explained how ordinary vitamin C, inexpensively manufactured from glucose, could improve health in many important ways.[4] Indeed, the above-mentioned study specifically measured the plasma level of ascorbate, which was shown to be an important factor associated with lower risk of heart failure.[1, 2] The study did not measure blood plasma levels of the components of fruits and vegetables. It measured vitamin C.

A known rationale for this dramatic finding is that vitamin C helps to prevent inflammation in the arteries by several mechanisms. It is a necessary co-factor for the synthesis of collagen, which is a major component of arteries. Vitamin C is also an important antioxidant throughout the body that can help to recycle other antioxidants like vitamin E and glutathione in the artery walls.[2,3] This was underscored by a report that *high plasma levels of vitamin C are associated with a 50% reduction in risk for stroke.*[5]

Yes, Synthetic Vitamin C Is Clinically Effective

I can almost hear my books being incinerated as I state it, but here it is: synthetic vitamin C works, in real people with real illnesses. Ascorbate's efficacy has little direct relation to food intake. A dramatic case of this was a dairy farmer in New Zealand who was on life support with lung whiteout, kidney failure, leukemia, and swine flu.[6] He was given 100,000 mg of vitamin C daily and his life was saved. We have nothing against oranges or other vitamin C-containing foods. Fruits and vegetables are good for you for many, many reasons. However, you'll need to get out your calculator to figure out how many oranges it would take to get t 100,000 mg, and then also figure how to get a sick person to eat them all.

It is established that liver function improves with vitamin C supplementation, and it is equally well known that adequate levels of vitamin C are essential for the proper functioning of the immune system. Vitamin C improves the ability of the white blood cells to fight bacteria and viruses. The Orthomolecular News Service (OMNS) has more articles expanding on this topic, available for free access, at http://orthomolecular.org/resources/omns/index.shtml.

Deficiency of vitamin C is very common. According to US Department of Agriculture (USDA) data,[7] *nearly half of Americans do not get even the US RDA of vitamin C,* which is a mere 90 mg.

Synthetic Vitamin E Is Less Effective

For some other nutrients, there is a significant difference in efficacy between synthetic and natural forms. Vitamin E is a crucial antioxidant, but also has other functions in the body, not all well understood. It comprises eight different biochemical forms—alpha-, beta-, delta-, and gamma-tocopherols, and alpha-, beta-, delta-, and gamma-tocotrienols. All of these forms of vitamin E are important for the body. Current knowledge about the function of vitamin E is rapidly expanding, and each of the eight forms of natural vitamin E is thought to have a slightly different function in the body. For example, gamma-tocotrienol actually kills prostate cancer stem cells better than chemotherapy does. (Orthomolecular Medicine News Service, Oct 14, 2011. http://orthomolecular.org/resources/omns/v07n11.shtml).

Synthetic vitamin E is widely available and inexpensive. It is "DL-alpha-tocopherol." Yes, it has the same antioxidant properties in test tube experiments as does the natural "D-alpha-tocopherol" form. However, the DL-form has only 50 percent of the biological efficacy, because the body utilizes only the natural D isomer, which makes up half of the synthetic mix.[8] Therefore, studies utilizing DL-alpha-tocopherol that do not take this fact into account are starting with an already-halved dose that will naturally lead to a reduction in the observed efficacy.

Then there are the esterified forms of vitamin E such as acetate or succinate. These esterified forms, either natural or synthetic, have a greater shelf life because the ester protects the vitamin E from being oxidized and neutralized. When acid in the stomach cleaves the acetate or succinate component from the original natural vitamin E molecule, the gut can then absorb a good fraction and the body receives its antioxidant benefit. But when esterified vitamin E acetate is applied to the skin to prevent inflammation, it is ineffective because there is no acid present to remove the acetate ester.

Based on USDA data[9] an astonishing *90 percent of Americans do not get the RDA of vitamin E,* which is, believe it or not, under 23 IU (15mg) per day.

Well, Which? Natural or Synthetic?

While the natural form of vitamin E (mixed natural tocopherols and tocotrienols) is at least twice as effective as the synthetic form, this is not true of vitamin C. The ascorbate that the body gets from fruits and vegetables is the same as the ascorbate in vitamin C tablets. On first thought, this may sound confusing, because there are many so-called "natural" forms of vitamin C widely available. But *virtually every study that demonstrated that supplemental vitamin C fights illness used plain, cheap, synthetic ascorbic acid.* Other forms of ascorbate—for instance, the sodium or magnesium salt of ascorbic acid—are digested slightly differently by the gut, but once the ascorbate molecule is absorbed from these forms, it has identical efficacy. The advantage of these ascorbate salts is that they are non-acidic and can be ingested or topically applied to any part of the body without concern about irritation from acidity.

Further, it is known that essential nutrients are symbiotic—that is, they are more effective when taken as a group in proper doses. For example, vitamin E is more effective when taken along with vitamin C and selenium, because each of these essential nutrients can improve the efficacy of the others. Similarly, the B vitamins are more effective when taken together. Readers with dosage questions will want to consult their healthcare provider and also look at freely available information archived at http://orthomolecular.org/resources/omns/index.shtml.

Food Factors

Natural food factors are also important. Bioflavonoids and other vitamin C-friendly components in fresh fruits and vegetables (sometimes called "vitamin C complex") do indeed have health benefits. These natural components are easily obtained from a healthy, unprocessed whole foods diet. However, eating even a very good diet does not supply nearly enough vitamin C to be effective against illness. A really good diet might provide several hundred milligrams of vitamin C daily. An extreme raw food diet might provide two or three thousand milligrams of vitamin C, but this is not practical for most people. Supplementation, with a good diet, is.

The principle that "natural" vitamins are better than synthetic vitamins is a widely quoted justification for actually avoiding vitamin supplements. The argument goes, because vitamins and minerals are available from food in their natural form, that somehow one might suppose that we are best off by ignoring supplements. Apparently this is what the authors of the above-mentioned study had in mind, because the report hardly mentions vitamin supplements.

The Bottom Lines

In the real world of today's processed food, most of us don't get all the nutrients we need in adequate doses. *Most people are deficient in* several *of the essential nutrients.* These deficiencies are responsible for much suffering, including heart disease, cancer, premature aging, dementia, diabetes, and other diseases such as eye disease, multiple sclerosis, and asthma. The above-mentioned study showing the efficacy of vitamin C in reducing heart failure is but one of the many studies showing the value of vitamins. Others are discussed and available at http://orthomolecular.org/resources/omns/index.shtml.

For vitamin E, the natural form, taken in adequate doses along with a nutritious diet, is the best medicine. However, for most vitamins, including vitamin C, the manufactured form is identical to the natural one. Both are biologically active and both work clinically. It all comes down to dose. Supplements enable optimum intake; foods alone do not.

Don't be fooled: nutrient deficiency is the rule, not the exception. That's why we need supplements. When ill, we need them even more.

References

1. Pfister R, Sharp SJ, Luben R, Wareham NJ, and Khaw KT. (2011) Plasma vitamin C predicts incident heart failure in men and women in European Prospective Investigation into Cancer and Nutrition-Norfolk prospective study. *Am Heart J.* 162:246–253. See also: http://orthomolecular.org/resources/omns/v07n14.shtml

2. Levy TE. (2006). *Stop America's #1 Killer: Reversible Vitamin Deficiency Found to be Origin of All Coronary Heart Disease.* Henderson, NV: LivOn Books.

3. Hickey S, Saul AW. (2008). *Vitamin C: The Real Story—the Remarkable and Controversial Healing Factor.* Laguna Beach, CA: Basic Health Publications.

4. Pauling L. (2006). *How to Live Longer And Feel Better.* Corvallis, OR: Oregon State University Press.

5. Kurl S, Tuomainen TP, Laukkanen JA, Nyyssönen K, Lakka T, Sivenius J, and Salonen JT. (2002). Plasma vitamin C modifies the association between hypertension and risk of stroke. *Stroke* 33:1568–1573.

6. Watch the Channel 3 New Zealand news report at www.3news.co.nz/Living-Proof-Vitamin-C-Miracle-Cure/tabid/371/articleID/171328/Default.aspx or www.dailymotion.com/video/xh70sx_60-minutes-scoop-on-new-zealand-farmer-vit-c-miracle_tech [Note that each video is proceeded by a commercial, over which we have no control, and with which we have no financial connection whatsoever.]

7. Free, full text paper at www.ncbi.nlm.nih.gov/pmc/articles/PMC1405127/pdf/amjph00225-0021.pdf

8. Papas A. (1999) *The Vitamin E Factor: The Miraculous Antioxidant for the Prevention and Treatment of Heart Disease, Cancer, and Aging.* New York: HarperCollins.

9. http://lpi.oregonstate.edu/infocenter/vitamins/vitaminE/; scroll down to "Deficiency."

Vitamin E

"Let no one who has the slightest desire to live in peace and quietness be tempted, under any circumstances, to enter upon the chivalrous task of trying to correct a popular error."
—WILLIAM THOMS, DEPUTY LIBRARIAN FOR THE HOUSE OF LORDS, C. 1873

Vitamin E increases oxygen availability to the heart. One might expect vitamin E deficiency to cause heart trouble. Evidently it does, and "122 independent reports have been published in the world's medical journals in support of vitamin E" according to an uncredited article in *Popular Science Digest* . . . from 1953!

Wilfrid and Evan Shute, both medical doctors, with Dr. Arthur Vogelsang, traced a national vitamin E deficiency back to the turn of the century when the milling of flour and consumption of this and other refined foods increased greatly. They saw an increase of heart disease parallel the increase of refined foods. In *Coronet* there appeared an article by J. D. Ratcliff (1948) entitled "For Heart Disease: Vitamin E" that described this work: "The Shutes and Vogelsang note that heart disease is almost unknown among primitive peoples—until they start eating civilized man's food. Further, they emphasize that in 1910—before our national diet had become too refined—heart disease was the fourth cause of death instead of the first as it is today (1948); and that the rate of heart deaths is up 250 percent in this period" (p. 31).

The Shutes described this phenomenon in their books, particularly in *Vitamin E for Ailing and Healthy Hearts* (1969). The more refined, denatured foods eaten, the more heart disease. And what is refined out? Among other things, the vitamin E that helps keep the heart prospering, and you alive.

Since the 1940s, cardiovascular disease has continued to be our biggest killer disease. But also since then, certain doctors have treated tens of thousands of coronary patients with vitamin E. Drs. Wilfrid and Evan Shute have personally supervised vitamin E therapy for over 30,000 heart patients, making them the world's most experienced cardiologists. You would think that the medical profession would be most enthusiastic about their success with vitamin therapy.

That has not been the case. The Canadian, British, and American Medical Associations have not voiced serious support for vitamin E against heart disease. Why not? "The Fight Over Vitamin E" (Hutton, 1953) discusses the early stages of the controversy in detail. The article also expands on vitamin E's therapeutic uses:

> The Shutes' theory about vitamin E is this: it is not specifically a heart medication . . . The chief effect of vitamin E is to reduce the amount of oxygen which the cells and tissues of the body and its organs require for efficient, healthy functioning. Heart diseases happen to be the most dramatic example of the result of vitamin E deprivation, and vitamin E's effect, simply stated, is to condition the tissues involved so that they are able to function normally, or at any rate to survive, on the greatly reduced amount of oxygen available to them when a coronary clot cuts down the oxygen-bearing blood supply reaching them. The Shutes' and other investigators claim it is effective in a wide variety of other conditions: burns, wounds,

338

radiation damage, gangrene, ulceration, phlebitis . . . diabetes and its complications, nephritis, eye diseases, psychoses, post-surgical shock, plastic surgery and post-poliomyelitis (p. 4).

Much controversy comes out of the wide application that these scientists claim for vitamin E. However: A nutritional substance that cures many ills is a substance whose deficiency causes many ills. This is the case with any vitamin deficiency: the deficiency of one vitamin may show up as many different disease symptoms. One person lacking in vitamin E may develop arteriosclerosis; another may develop diabetic gangrene; another might just have poor skin; another might drop dead of a heart attack. This is because a vitamin is important for the entire organism, in all its organs and functions. No vitamin works just in or for the heart or any one sector. Each vitamin is essential to total body health, and all the vitamins collectively are needed for freedom from disease.

Safe, Effective, and Heart-Healthy

Heart disease is the number one killer in the United States, and the evidence supporting vitamin E's efficacy in preventing and reversing heart disease is strong.

Two landmark studies published in the *New England Journal of Medicine*[1,2] followed a total of 125,000 men and women healthcare professionals for a total of 839,000 person study-years. It was found that those who supplement with at least 100 IU of vitamin E daily reduced their risk of heart disease by 59 to 66 percent. The studies were adjusted for lifestyle differences (smoking, physical activity, dietary fiber intake, aspirin use) in order to determine the heart effect of vitamin E supplementation alone. Because a diet high in foods containing vitamin E as compared to the average diet further showed only a slight heart-protective effect, the authors emphasized the necessity of vitamin E supplementation.

Researchers at Cambridge University[3] in England reported that patients who had been diagnosed with coronary arteriosclerosis could lower their risk of having a heart attack by 77 percent by supplementing with 400 IU to 800 IU per day of the natural (d-alpha tocopherol) form of vitamin E.

Pioneer vitamin E researchers and clinicians Drs. Wilfrid and Evan Shute treated some 30,000 patients over several decades and found that people in average health received maximum benefit from 800 IU of the d-alpha tocopherol form of vitamin E. Vitamin E has been proven effective in the prevention and treatment of many heart conditions. "The complete or nearly complete prevention of angina attacks is the usual and expected result of treatment with alpha tocopherol," according to Wilfrid Shute, M.D., a cardiologist. Shute prescribed up to 1,600 IU of vitamin E daily and successfully treated patients for acute coronary thrombosis, acute rheumatic fever, chronic rheumatic heart disease, hypertensive heart disease, diabetes mellitus, acute and chronic nephritis, and even burns, plastic surgery, and mazoplasia.

339

A reader says:

"Back in 1970 my hubby had the killer kind of heart attack. He was alive but a sick man with serious heart troubles a year later. We learned about Dr. Shute's therapy with vitamin E. Dr. Wilfrid Shute called Coumadin "poison," took him off it, and within weeks (it seemed) had him heart healthy. My husband took only our current vitamins, plus he worked up to 1,600 IUs of vitamin E. This took him to age 90 without health problems."

How It Works

The reason one nutrient can cure so many different illnesses is because a deficiency of one nutrient can cause many different illnesses.

Vitamin E is a powerful antioxidant in the body's lipid (fat) phase. It can prevent LDL lipid peroxidation caused by free radical reactions. Its ability to protect cell membranes from oxidation is of crucial importance in preventing and reversing many degenerative diseases.

In addition, vitamin E inhibits blood clotting (platelet aggregation and adhesion) and prevents plaque enlargement and rupture.

Finally, it has anti-inflammatory properties, which may also prove to be very important in the prevention of heart disease.

Among other things, vitamin E supplementation:

* reduces the oxygen requirement of tissues[4]

* gradually melts fresh clots, and prevents embolism[5]

* improves collateral circulation[6]

* prevents scar contraction as wounds heal[7]

* decreases the insulin requirement in about one-forth of diabetics[8]

* stimulates muscle power[9]

* preserves capillary walls[10]

* reduces C-reactive protein and other markers of inflammation[11]

Epidemiological evidence also suggests that a daily supplement of vitamin E can reduce the risk of developing prostate cancer and Alzheimer's disease.[12, 13]

If all Americans daily supplemented with a good multivitamin-multimineral, plus extra vitamins C and E, thousands of lives a month could be saved.

References

1. Stampfer MJ, Hennekens CH, Manson JE, Colditz GA, Rosner B, and Willett WC. (1993). Vitamin E consumption and the risk of coronary disease in women. *N Engl J Med.* 328:1444–1449.

2. Rimm EB, Stampfer MJ, Ascherio A, Giovannucci E, Colditz GA, and Willett WC. (1993). Vitamin E consumption and the risk of coronary heart disease in men. *N Engl J Med.* 328:1450–1456.

3. Stephens NG, Parsons A, Schofield PM, Kelly F, Cheeseman K, and Mitchinson MJ.(1996). Randomised controlled trial of vitamin E in patients with coronary disease: Cambridge Heart Antioxidant Study (CHAOS). *Lancet* 347:781–86.

4. Hove EL, Hickman KCD, and Harris PL. (1945). *Arch. Biochem.* 8:395.

5. Shute EV, Vogelsang AB, Skelton FR, and Shute, WE. (1948). *Surg., Gyn. and Obst.* 86:1.

6. Enria G. and Fererro R. (1951). *Arch. per la Scienze Med.* 91:23.

7. Shute EV, Vogelsang AB, Skelton FR, and Shute WE. (1948). *Surg., Gyn. and Obst.* 86:1.

8. Butturini U. (1950). *Gior.di Clin. Med.* 31:1.

9. Percival L. (1951). *Summary* 3:55.

10. Ames BN, Baxter JG, and Griffith JZ. (1951). *International Review of Vitamin Research* 22:401.

11. RidkerPM, Hennekens CH, Buring JE. (2000). C-reactive protein and other markers of inflammation in the prediction of cardio-vascular disease in women. *New England Journal of Medicine* 342:836–843.

12. Ni J, Chen M, Zhang Y, Li R, Huang J and Yeh S. (2003). Vitamin E succinate inhibits human prostate cancer cell growth via modulating cell cycle regulatory machinery. *Biochem Biophys Res Commun-* 300(2):357–63.

13. Morris, MC, Evans DA, Bienias JL, Tangney CC, et al. (2002). Dietary intake of antioxidant nutrients and the risk of incident Alzheimer's disease in a biracial community study. *JAMA* 287(24):3230–3237.

Vitamin E Is Attacked Because It Works

The very first course I ever taught was called "Forgotten Research in Medicine."[1] Among other vitamins, it highlighted the clinical benefits of vitamin E. I taught that course thirty-six years ago. In fact, the battle over vitamin E has been going full-tilt for over sixty years.[2]

Well, you can say one thing for vitamin critics: at least they are consistent. Consistently wrong, but consistent.

A recent accusation against vitamin E is that somehow it increases risk of prostate cancer.[3] That is nonsense. If you take a close look at the numbers, you will see that "Compared with placebo, the absolute increase in risk of prostate cancer per 1,000 person-years was 1.6 for vitamin E, 0.8 for selenium, and 0.4 for the combination." That works out to be a claimed 0.63 percent increase in risk with vitamin E alone, 0.24 percent increase in risk with vitamin E and selenium, and 0.15 percent increase in risk for selenium alone.

Note the decimal points: these are very small figures. But more importantly, note that the combination of selenium with vitamin E resulted in a much smaller number of deaths. If vitamin E were really the problem, vitamin E with selenium would have been a worse problem. Selenium recharges vitamin E, recycling it and effectively rendering it more potent. Something is wrong here, and it isn't the vitamin E. Indeed, a higher dose of vitamin E might work as well as E with selenium, and be more protective.

And, in fact, this study did show that supplementation was beneficial. Vitamin E and selenium reduced risk of all-cause mortality by about 0.2 percent, and also reduced the risk of serious cardiovascular events by 0.3 percent. Vitamin E reduced risk of serious cardiovascular events by 0.7 percent. But what you were told, and just about all you were told, was "Vitamin E causes cancer!"

The oldest political trick in the book is to create doubt, then fear, and then conformity of action. The pharmaceutical industry knows this full well. One does not waste time and money attacking something that does not work. Vitamin E works, and the evidence is abundant.

Specifically in regards to prostate cancer, new research published in the *International Journal of Cancer* has shown that gamma-tocotrienol, a cofactor found in natural vitamin E preparations, actually kills prostate cancer stem cells.[4] As you would expect, these are the very cells from which prostate cancer develops. They are or quickly become chemotherapy-resistant. And yet natural vitamin E complex contains the very thing to kill them. Mice given gamma-tocotrienol orally had an astonishing 75 percent decrease in tumor formation. Gamma-tocotrienol also is effective against existing prostate tumors.[5,6]

Additionally:

- **Vitamin E reduces mortality by 24 percent in persons 71 or older**. Even persons who smoke live longer if they take vitamin E. Hemila H and Kaprio J. *Age Ageing,* 2011. 40(2): 215–220. January 17. http://ageing.oxfordjournals.org/content/40/2/215.short.

- **Taking 300 IU vitamin E per day reduces lung cancer by 61 percent**. (Mahabir S, et al. Dietary alpha-, beta-, gamma- and delta-tocopherols in lung cancer risk. *Int J Cancer.* 2008 Sep 1; 123(5):1173–80). www.ncbi.nlm.nih.gov/pubmed/18546288. For further information: Vitamin E prevents lung cancer. Orthomolecular Medicine News Service, Oct 29, 2008. http://orthomolecular.org/resources/omns/v04n18.shtml.

- **Vitamin E is an effective treatment for atherosclerosis**. Drs. Wilfrid and Evan Shute knew this half a century ago.[1] In 1995, *JAMA* published research that confirmed it, saying: "Subjects with supplementary vitamin E intake of 100 IU per day or greater demonstrated less coronary artery lesion progression than did subjects with supplementary vitamin E intake less than 100 IU per day." (Hodis HN, et al. Serial coronary angiographic evidence that antioxidant vitamin intake reduces progression of coronary artery atherosclerosis. *JAMA,* 1995, 273:1849–1854), http://jama.ama-assn.org/content/273/23/1849.short.

- **400 to 800 IU of vitamin E daily reduces risk of heart attack by 77 percent**. (Stephens NG, et al. Randomized controlled trial of vitamin E in patients with coronary artery disease: Cambridge Heart Antioxidant Study (CHAOS). *Lancet,* 1996, 347:781–786), www.ncbi.nlm.nih .gov/pubmed/8622332.

- **Increasing vitamin E with supplements prevents COPD** [Chronic obstructive pulmonary disease, emphysema, chronic bronchitis]. (Agler AH, et al. Randomized vitamin E supplementation and risk of chronic lung disease (CLD) in the Women's Health Study. American Thoracic Society 2010 International Conference, May 18, 2010). Summary at www.thoracic .org/newsroom/press-releases/conference/articles/2010/vitamine-e.pdf

- **800 IU vitamin E per day is a successful treatment for fatty liver disease**. (Sanyal AJ, Chalasani N, Kowdley KV. 2010. Pioglitazone, vitamin E, or placebo for nonalcoholic steatohepatitis. *N Engl J Med.* 362(18):1675–85), www.ncbi.nlm.nih.gov/pubmed/20427778.

- **Alzheimer's patients who take 2,000 IU of vitamin E per day live longer**. (Pavlik VN, Doody RS, Rountree SD, and Darby EJ. Vitamin E use is associated with improved survival in an Alzheimer's disease cohort. *Dement Geriatr Cogn Disord.* 2009, 28(6):536–40.) Summary at www. associatedcontent.com/article/719537/alzheimers_patients_who_take_vitamin.html ?cat=5.

  See also: Grundman M. Vitamin E and Alzheimer disease: the basis for additional clinical trials. *Am J Clin Nutr.* 2000, 71(2):630S–636S. Free access to full text at www.ajcn.org/cgi/content/full/71/2/630s).

- **Vitamin E supplements help prevent amyotrophic lateral sclerosis (ALS)**. This important finding is the result of a ten-year-plus Harvard study of over a million persons. (Wang H, O'Reilly EJ, Weisskopf MG, et al. Vitamin E intake and risk of amyotrophic lateral sclerosis: a pooled analysis of data from 5 prospective cohort studies. *Am. J. Epidemiol,* 2011, 173(6): 595–602) , http://aje.oxfordjournals.org/content/173/6/595.short.

- **Vitamin E is more effective than a prescription drug in treating chronic liver disease** (nonalcoholic steatohepatitis). Said the authors: "The good news is that this study showed that cheap and readily available vitamin E can help many of those with this condition." Sanyal AJ, Chalasani N, Kowdley KV, et al. Pioglitazone, vitamin E, or placebo for nonalcoholic steatohepatitis. *N Engl J Med.* 2010, 362(18):1675–85, www.nejm.org/doi/full/10.1056/NEJMoa0907929.

What Kind of Vitamin E?

Which work best: natural or synthetic vitamins? The general debate might not end anytime soon (more on that further below). However, with vitamin E, we already know. The best E is the most natural form, generally called "mixed natural tocopherols and tocotrienols."

This is very different from the synthetic form, DL-alpha tocopherol. There is considerable evidence that the natural form of vitamin E is more useful to the body than is the synthetic (*Am J Clin Nutr* 65; 785–89, 1997). The natural form is also more expensive. In choosing a vitamin E supplement, you should carefully read the label . . . the entire label. It is remarkable how many natural-looking brown bottles with natural-sounding brand names contain a synthetic vitamin. And no, I do not make brand recommendations. Furthermore, I have no financial connection with the health products industry, and no commercial affiliations period.

Follow the Money

Unfortunately, that's not the case with some authors of the negative vitamin E paper.[3] You will not see this in the abstract at the *JAMA* website, of course, but if you read the entire paper, and get to the very last page (1556), you'll find the "Conflict of Interest" section. Here you will discover that a number of the study authors have received money from pharmaceutical companies, including Merck, Pfizer, Sanofi-Aventis, AstraZeneca, Abbott, GlaxoSmithKline, Janssen, Amgen, Firmagon, and Novartis. In terms of cash, these are some of the largest corporations on the planet.

Well how about that: a "vitamins are dangerous" article, in one of the most popular medical journals, with lots of media hype . . . and the pharmaceutical industry's fingerprints all over it.

How Much Vitamin E?

More than the RDA, and that's for certain. A common dosage range for vitamin E is between 200 and 800 IU/day. Some orthomolecular physicians advocate substantially more than that. The studies cited above will give you a ballpark idea. However, this is an individual matter for you and your practitioner to work out. Your own reading and research, before you go to your doctor, will help you determine optimal intake. If your doctor quotes a negative vitamin study, then haul out the positive ones. You may start with this article. There are more links to more information at http://orthomolecular.org/resources/omns/v06n09.shtml and http://ortho molecular.org/resources/omns/v06n25.shtml.

Safety

And as for the old saw argument that supplement-users are supposedly dying like flies, consider this: Over 200 million Americans take vitamin supplements. So where are the bodies? Well, there aren't any. There has not been a single death from vitamins in twenty-seven years. Share that with your doctor as well. And with the news media.

References

1. At the Genesee Co-Op's Wholistic Health Education Center, Rochester, NY. http://orthomolecular.org/resources/omns/ v01n01. shtml.

2. Saul AW. Vitamin E: A cure in search of recognition. *J Orthomolecular Med*, 2003, 18(3,4):205–212. Free download at http:// orthomolecular.org/library/jom/2003/pdf/2003-v18n0304-p205.pdf or html at www.doctoryourself.com/evitamin.htm . See also: Saul AW. Review of the vitamin E story, by Evan Shute. *J Orthomolecular Med*, 2002, 17(3):179–181, www.doctoryourself .com/ estory.htm.

3. Klein EA, Thompson IM Jr, Tangen CM, et al. Vitamin E and the risk of prostate cancer: the Selenium and Vitamin E Cancer Preven-

343

tion Trial (SELECT). *JAMA,* 2011, 306(14):1549–1556, http://jama.ama-assn.org/content/306/14/1549. Also, as an example of many media spins: www.webmd.com/prostate-cancer/news/20111011/vitamin-e-supplements-may-raise-prostate-cancer-risk

4. Luk SU, Yap WN, Chiu YT, Lee DT, Ma S, Lee TK, Vasireddy RS, Wong YC, Ching YP, Nelson C, Yap YL, and Ling MT.Gamma-tocotrienol as an effective agent in targeting prostate cancer stem cell-like population. *International Journal of Cancer,* 2011, 128(9):2182–2191, http://onlinelibrary.wiley.com/doi/10.1002/ijc.25546/abstract.

5. Nesaretnam K, Teoh HK, Selvaduray KR, Bruno RS, and Ho E. Modulation of cell growth and apoptosis response in human prostate cancer cells supplemented with tocotrienols. *Eur. J. Lipid Sci. Technol.* 2008, 110:23–31, http://onlinelibrary.wiley.com/doi/10.1002/ejlt.200700068/abstract.

6. Conte C, Floridi A, and Aisa C. Gamma-tocotrienol metabolism and antiproliferative effect in prostate cancer cells. *Annals of the New York Academy of Sciences,* 2004, 1031: 391–4, www.ncbi.nlm.nih.gov/pubmed/15753178?dopt=AbstractPlus.

Also of Interest

Vitamin E research ignored by major news media. Orthomolecular Medicine News Service, May 25, 2010 (http://orthomolecular.org/resources/omns/v06n19.shtml).

Vitamin D

WHY YOU NEED MORE VITAMIN D. A LOT MORE.
by William B. Grant, Ph.D.

Vitamin D has emerged as the nutrient of the decade. Numerous studies have found benefits for nearly 100 types of health conditions. These health benefits include reduced risk of bone diseases, many types of cancer, cardiovascular disease (CVD), diabetes mellitus, bacterial and viral infectious diseases, and autoimmune diseases such as multiple sclerosis,[1] neurological conditions such as cognitive dysfunction,[2] and improved athletic and physical performance.[3]

Sunshine, Skin, Sunburn, and Sunscreen

The primary source of vitamin D for most people is solar ultraviolet-B (UVB) light. Skin pigmentation has adapted to where a population lives for a thousand years or more as those with skin too dark or light do not survive as well as those with the appropriate skin pigmentation.[4] Dark skin protects against the harmful effects of UV, but also blocks the UVB from penetrating deeply enough into the skin to produce vitamin D from 7-dehydrocholesterol. Those with lighter skin can produce vitamin D more rapidly, but are more prone to melanoma and other skin cancer. Sunscreens block UVB and thus limit vitamin D production. While sunscreens are useful in reducing risk of sunburning, they do not block the long wave UV (UVA) as well as UVB. UVA is linked to risk of melanoma. Wearing sunscreen when there is no danger of burning can actually increase the risk of melanoma.[5]

Understanding Vitamin D Research

Since vitamin D production is the primary source of vitamin D, ecological and observational studies have been very useful in teasing out the effects of vitamin D on health. There are two types of ecological studies, based on geographical and temporal (over time) variations. In geographical studies, populations are defined geographically and both health outcome and risk-modifying factors are averaged for each geographical unit. Statistical analyses are then used to determine the relative importance of each factor. The first paper linking UVB and vitamin D to reduced risk of colon cancer was published in 1980.[6] This link has now been extended to about 15 types of cancer in the United States with respect to average noontime solar UVB doses in July.[7] Solar UVB doses in July are highest in the Southwest and lowest in the Northeast.[8] Mortality rates are generally lowest in the Southwest and highest in the Northeast.[9] Similar results have been found in Australia, China, France, Japan, Russia, and Spain, and the entire world.[10]

In temporal studies, seasonal variations in health outcomes are sought. A good example of a seasonal effect linked to solar UVB doses and vitamin D is influenza, which peaks in winter.[11]

Observational studies are generally of three types: case-control, cohort, and cross-sectional. In case-control studies, those diagnosed with a disease have serum 25-hydroxyvitamin D [25(OH)D] level or oral vitamin D intake determined at that time and are compared statistically with others with similar characteristics but without that disease. In cohort studies, people are enrolled in the study and the vitamin D index determined at that time. The cohort is followed

345

for a number of years and those who develop a specific disease are compared statistically with matched controls who did not. The main problem with cohort studies is that the single value of the vitamin D index may not relate to the time in the individual's life when vitamin D had the most impact on the disease outcome. Cross-sectional studies are essentially snapshots of a population and look at various factors in relation to the prevalence of health conditions. As biochemistry can be affected by health status, such studies provide less reliable information on the role of UVB and vitamin D on health outcome.

The role of vitamin D in CVD and diabetes mellitus type 2 have largely been studied using cohort studies. Significantly reduced risk of CVD and diabetes mellitus incidence have been reported in a number of studies in the past three years.[12]

Health policy officials like to see randomized controlled trials (RCTs) reporting health benefits with limited adverse effects. RCTs are certainly appropriate for pharmaceutical drugs which, by definition, are artificial substances that the human body has no experience with. RCTs with vitamin D are problematic for a number of reasons. For one, many RCTs used only 400 IU/day vitamin D_3, which is much lower than the 10,000 IU/day that can be produced with whole-body exposure to the midday sun in summer, or 1500 IU/day from casual sunlight exposure in summer.[13] For another, there are both oral and UVB sources of vitamin D, so the amount taken in the study will compete with the other sources. There is considerable individual variation in serum 25(OH)D for a given oral vitamin D intake.[14] Unfortunately, serum 25(OH)D levels are generally not measured in oral vitamin D RCTs.

Nonetheless, there have been several vitamin D RCTs that found significant health benefits beyond preventing falls and fractures.[15] These include ones for cancer,[16,17] influenza and colds,[18] type A influenza,[19] and pneumonia.[20]

Important Benefits of Vitamin D

The evidence of beneficial roles of UVB and vitamin D for a large number of health conditions have recently been posted at the Vitamin D Council's website: www.vitamindcouncil .org/health-conditions/

In addition to an overview of the literature, the website also includes a feature to pull up a large number of titles on each condition from www.pubmed.gov.

Sufficient information is currently available from observational studies with support from ecological studies and RCTs to determine relationships between serum 25(OH)D levels and incidence rates for breast and colorectal cancer,[21] CVD,[22] and influenza.[23] Risk decreases rapidly for small increases in 25(OH)D for those with initial values below 10 ng/ml (25 nmol/L), then decrease at a slower rate to levels above 40 ng/ml (100 nmol/L). These relations have been used to estimate the change in mortality rates and life expectancy if population mean serum 25(OH)D levels were raised from current levels of 20–25 ng/ml (50–63 nmol/L) to 45 ng/ml (113 nmol/L). For the U.S., it was estimated that 400,000 deaths/year could be delayed,[24] which is about 15% of all deaths/year. For the entire world, it was estimated that the reduction in all-cause mortality rates would correspond to an increased life expectancy of two years.[22]

The mechanisms whereby vitamin D reduces the risk of disease are largely understood. For cancer, they include effects on cellular differentiation and proliferation, angiogenesis and metastasis.[25] For infectious diseases, they include induction of cathelicidin and defensins[26] and shifting cytokine production from proinflammatory T-helper 1 (Th1) cytokines to Th2 cyto-

346

kines.[27] For CVD, they may include reducing blood pressure and keeping calcium in the bones and teeth and out of the vascular tissues.[28] For diabetes mellitus type 2, they may include improving insulin sensitivity.[29]

Current Government-Sponsored Recommendations Are Too Low

In spite of the large and expanding body of scientific evidence that vitamin D has many health benefits, the US Institute of Medicine issued a report in November 2010 claiming that the evidence was strong only for effects on bones.[30,31] The reason given was lack of convincing randomized controlled trials on other health conditions. The one on cancer showing a 77% reduced risk of all-cancer incidence between the ends of the first and fourth years involved 1100 IU/day vitamin D plus 1450 mg/day calcium.[16] However, the IOM Committee relied on the findings from the start of the study, which was not statistically significant. In addition, the IOM Committee pointed to observational studies reporting a U-shaped serum 25(OH)D-disease incidence relation as a reason to be concerned about higher doses of vitamin D. However, these studies used a single serum 25(OH)D value from the time of enrollment followed by follow-up times as long as 17 years. Two studies reported that the sign of the correlation between disease outcome and serum 25(OH)D level changes from negative to positive after seven-to-15 years.[32,33] Thus, the U-shaped relations are not reliable and should not be used as the basis for policy decisions, especially since the committee refused to consider the largely beneficial findings from observational studies.

How Much Vitamin D Do We REALLY Need?

The IOM committee set the recommended vitamin D intake at 600 IU/day for those under the age of 70 years and 800 IU/day for those over 70, and stated that 20 ng/ml (50 nmol/L) was an adequate level. The scientific consensus is that oral intake should be 1,000–5,000 IU/day vitamin D with a goal of 30–40 ng/ml (75–100 nmol/L).[34] The vitamin D research community has responded to the IOM report on vitamin D with over 60 letters and articles in peer-reviewed journals pointing out the absurdity and illogic of the IOM report.[35] The Endocrine Society published a paper recommending 1,500–2,000 IU/day and 30 ng/ml.[36] Meanwhile, members of the IOM Committee have been publishing articles in mainstream journals promoting their report.

For More Information

For additional information on vitamin D, the reader is directed to PubMed at http://orthomolecular.org/resources/omns/ v07n07. shtmlwww.ncbi.nlm.nih.gov/pubmed or www.pubmed.gov to search "vitamin D" along with any keyword of interest. Some representative papers found there, with free access, are listed below. Papers published in the *Journal of Orthomolecular Medicine* are (still) not listed on PubMed. Reasons for this are presented at http://orthomolecular.org/resources/omns/v06n03.shtml and http://orthomolecular.org/resources/omns/v06n07.shtml . All *J Orthomolecular Med* papers may all be accessed at the Journal's free archive: http://orthomolecular.org/library/jom/index.shtml .

Adams JS, Hewison M. Update in vitamin D. J Clin Endocrinol Metab. 2010 Feb;95(2):471–8. Review. http://jcem.endojournals .org/content/95/2/471.full.pdf+html

Bikle DD. Vitamin D: newly discovered actions require reconsideration of physiologic requirements. Trends Endocrinol Metab. 2010 Jun;21(6):375–84. Epub 2010 Feb 10. Review. www.ncbi.nlm.nih.gov/pmc/articles/PMC2880203/pdf/nihms-170960.pdf

Herr C, Greulich T, Koczulla RA, Meyer S, Zakharkina T, Branscheidt M, Eschmann R, Bals R. The role of vitamin D in pulmonary disease: COPD, asthma, infection, and cancer. Respir Res. 2011 Mar 18;12:31. Review. http://respiratory-research.com/content/pdf/1465–9921–12–31.pdf

Hewison M. Vitamin D and the immune system: new perspectives on an old theme. Endocrinol Metab Clin North Am. 2010 Jun;39(2):365–79, table of contents. Review. www.ncbi.nlm.nih.gov/pmc/articles/PMC2879394/pdf/nihms180153.pdf

Raman M, Milestone AN, Walters JR, Hart AL, Ghosh S. Vitamin D and gastrointestinal diseases: inflammatory bowel disease and colorectal cancer. Therap Adv Gastroenterol. 2011 Jan;4(1):49–62. www.ncbi.nlm.nih.gov/pmc/articles/PMC3036961/pdf/10.1177_1756283X10377820.pdf

Zhang R, Naughton DP. Vitamin D in health and disease: current perspectives. Nutr J. 2010 Dec 8;9:65. Review. www.nutritionj.com/content/pdf/1475–2891–9-65.pdf

OFFICIAL RECOMMENDED INTAKE FOR VITAMIN D IS TOO LOW: 2,000 IU/DAY OR MORE NEEDED FOR OPTIMAL HEALTH

Vitamin D has been a natural part of man's experience forever, and 90% of vitamin D is derived from solar ultraviolet-B (UVB) irradiance. The health effects of vitamin D can be and have been determined from a variety of studies including ecological, observational (case-control and cohort), and cross-sectional studies.

Vitamin D helps both to prevent and to treat chronic diseases including many types of cancer, cardiovascular disease (coronary heart disease, stroke, etc.), congestive heart failure, diabetes mellitus (types 1 and 2), osteoporosis, falls, and fractures. It is also effective against infectious diseases including both bacteria and viral infections: bacterial vaginosis, pneumonia, dental caries, periodontal disease, tuberculosis, sepsis/septicemia, Epstein-Barr virus, and influenza type A such as A/H1N1 influenza. The autoimmune diseases include asthma, type 1 diabetes mellitus, multiple sclerosis, and perhaps rheumatoid arthritis.

Pregnancy outcomes are also adversely affected by low serum D levels. 40% of primary Cesarean-section deliveries in the United States are linked to low D levels (9% of births in the United States involve primary C-section), and preeclampsia is also linked to low serum levels of D. In regards to cancer, vitamin D helps cells fit into the organs properly or commit suicide (apoptosis), and also reduces angiogenesis (new blood vessel growth) around tumors and reduces metastasis. For metabolic diseases, the mechanisms include increased insulin sensitivity and insulin production. For infectious diseases, vitamin D induces production of cathelicidin and defensins, which have antimicrobial and antiendotoxin activities.

Due to current lifestyles in the United States, most people do not spend sufficient time in the sun to produce the higher serum D levels associated with optimal health. Black Americans are particularly vulnerable to low levels due to their darker skin, which reduces the amount of UVB that reaches the 7-dehydrocholesterol in the lower epidermis to produce previtamin D. Black Americans have a 25% higher mortality rate than White Americans, and this difference may be explained in terms of lower serum 25(OH)D levels. Solar UVB is an excellent source of vitamin D during about half of the year. The way to take advantage of the sun as a source of vitamin D is to expose as much of the body as possible without sunscreen near solar noon, the time when one's shadow is shorter than one's height, for 10–30 minutes depending on skin pigmentation, being careful not to turn pink or red or burn. (www.doctor yourself.com/holick.html)

Supplements represent an efficient way to obtain sufficient vitamin D. African-Americans should consider taking 3,000 international units (IU) per day while White Americans should consider taking 2,000 IU/day. The current dietary guideline, approximately 400 IU/day, was based on the amount of vitamin D in a spoonful of cod liver oil, which prevented rickets.

There are few adverse effects of vitamin D. With whole-body exposure to the sun, one can make at least 10,000 IU/day in a short time. Adverse effects such as hypercalcemia have been found in general only for 20,000–40,000 IU/day for very long periods. However, those with certain diseases such as adenoma of the parathyroid gland, granulomatous diseases, lymphoma, sarcoidosis, and tuberculosis, should limit their vitamin D intake or production due to the fact that the body's innate immune system produces too much 1,25-dihydroxyvitamin D in the serum, which can raise serum calcium levels too high.

Several studies have examined how much mortality rates and economic burdens of disease could be lowered if the population had more vitamin D. These studies were for Western Europe, Canada, the Netherlands, and the United States. They generally found that mortality rates could be reduced by about 15%.

During pregnancy and lactation, women should be taking about 6,000 IU/day. The current US "Adequate Intake" recommendation is a mere 200 IU/day. Bruce W. Hollis and Carol L. Wagner, Medical University of South Carolina, recently completed a randomized controlled trial vitamin D supplementation for pregnant and nursing women and found that even 2,000 IU/day was inadequate, and that there were no adverse effects with 6,000 IU/day.

For the text of a Vitamin D Scientists' Call to Action, please go to www.grassroots health. net.

(William Grant, PhD, is the director of the Sunlight, Nutrition, and Health Research Center [SUNARC] in San Francisco, California, www.sunarc.org.)

For Further Reading

[No authors listed]. Vitamin D—monograph. Altern Med Rev. 2008 Jun;13(2):153–64. www.thorne.com/altmedrev/.fulltext/13/2/153.pdf

Bodnar LM, Catov JM, Simhan HN, Holick MF, Powers RW, Roberts JM. Maternal vitamin D deficiency increases the risk of pre-eclampsia. J Clin Endocrinol Metab. 2007 Sep;92(9):3517–22. http://jcem.endojournals.org/cgi/reprint/92/9/3517

Cannell JJ, Hollis BW. Use of vitamin D in clinical practice. Altern Med Rev. 2008 Mar;13(1):6–20. www.thorne.com/ altmedrev/.fulltext/13/1/6.pdf

Dietrich T, Joshipura KJ, Dawson-Hughes B, Bischoff-Ferrari HA. Association between serum concentrations of 25-hydroxyvitamin D3 and periodontal disease in the US population. Am J Clin Nutr. 2004 Jul;80(1):108–13. www.ajcn.org/cgi/reprint/80/1/108

Dunning JM. The influence of latitude and distance from seacoast on dental disease. J Dent Res. 1953 Dec;32(6):811–29. http://jdr.sagepub.com/cgi/reprint/32/6/811

East BR. Mean annual hours of sunshine and the incidence of dental daries. Am J Public Health Nations Health. 1939 Jul;29(7):777–80. www.ajph.org/cgi/reprint/29/7/777

Garland CF, Garland FC, Gorham ED, Lipkin M, Newmark H, Mohr SB, Holick MF. The role of vitamin D in cancer prevention. Am J Public Health. 2006 Feb;96(2):252–61. www.ajph.org/cgi/reprint/96/2/252

Giovannucci E, Liu Y, Rimm EB, Hollis BW, Fuchs CS. Stampfer MJ, Willett WH. Prospective study of predictors of vitamin D status and cancer incidence and mortality in men. JNCI 2006; 98:451–9. http://jnci.oxfordjournals.org/cgi/reprint/98/7/451

Giovannucci E, Liu Y, Hollis BW, Rimm EB. 25-hydroxyvitamin D and risk of myocardial infarction in men: a prospective study. Arch Intern Med. 2008 Jun 9;168(11):1174–80. http://archinte.ama-assn.org/cgi/reprint/168/11/1174

Grant WB. How strong is the evidence that solar ultraviolet B and vitamin D reduce the risk of cancer? An examination using Hill's criteria for causality. Dermato-Endocrinology. 2009;1(1):17–24. www.landesbioscience.com/journals/dermatoendocrinology/article/7388/

Grant WB. In defense of the sun: An estimate of changes in mortality rates in the United States if mean serum 25-hydroxyvitamin D levels were raised to 45 ng/mL by solar ultraviolet-B irradiance. Dermato-Endocrinology, 2009;1(4):207–14. www.landesbioscience.com/journals/dermatoendocrinology/archive/volume/1/issue/4/

Grant WB, Cross HS, Garland CF, Gorham ED, Moan J, Peterlik M, Porojnicu AC, Reichrath J, Zittermann A. Estimated benefit of increased vitamin D status in reducing the economic burden of disease in Western Europe. Prog Biophys Mol Biol. Prog Biophys Mol Biol. 2009 Feb-Apr;99(2–3):104–13. (posted at www.sunarc.org)

Holick MF. Vitamin D deficiency. N Engl J Med. 2007 Jul 19;357(3):266–81. http://content.nejm.org/cgi/content/short/357/3/266

349

Hyppönen E, Power C. Hypovitaminosis D in British adults at age 45 y: nationwide cohort study of dietary and lifestyle predictors. Am J Clin Nutr. 2007 Mar;85(3):860–8. www.ajcn.org/cgi/reprint/85/3/860

Lappe JM, Travers-Gustafson D, Davies KM, Recker RR, Heaney RP. Vitamin D and calcium supplementation reduces cancer risk: results of a randomized trial. Am J Clin Nutr. 2007 Jun;85(6):1586–91. www.ajcn.org/cgi/reprint/85/6/1586

Looker AC, Pfeiffer CM, Lacher DA, Schleicher RL, Picciano MF, Yetley EA. Serum 25-hydroxyvitamin D status of the US population: 1988–1994 compared with 2000–2004. Am J Clin Nutr. 2008 Dec;88(6):1519–27. www.ajcn.org/cgi/reprint/88/6/1519

Martins D, Wolf M, Pan D, Zadshir A, Tareen N, Thadhani R, Felsenfeld A, Levine B, Mehrotra R, Norris K. Prevalence of cardio-vascular risk factors and the serum levels of 25-hydroxyvitamin D in the United States: data from the Third National Health and Nutrition Examination Survey. Arch Intern Med. 2007 Jun 11;167(11):1159–65. http://archinte.ama-assn.org/cgi/reprint/167/11/1159

Melamed ML, Michos ED, Post W, Astor B. 25-hydroxyvitamin D levels and the risk of mortality in the general population. Arch Intern Med. 2008 Aug 11;168(15):1629–37.http://archinte.ama-assn.org/cgi/reprint/168/15/1629

Merewood A, Mehta SD, Chen TC, Bauchner H, Holick MF. Association between vitamin D deficiency and primary cesarean section. J Clin Endocrinol Metab. 2009 Mar;94(3):940–5.

Papandreou D, Malindretos P, Karabouta Z, Rousso I. Possible Health Implications and Low Vitamin D Status during Childhood and Adolescence: An Updated Mini Review. Int J Endocrinol. 2010;2010:472173. www.ncbi.nlm.nih.gov/pmc/articles/ PMC2778445/ pdf/IJE2010–472173.pdf

Schwalfenberg G. Not enough vitamin D: health consequences for Canadians. Can Fam Physician, 2007;53(5):841–54. www.cfp.ca/cgi/reprint/53/5/841

Wang TJ, Pencina MJ, Booth SL, Jacques PF, Ingelsson E, Lanier K, Benjamin EJ, D'Agostino RB, Wolf M, Vasan RS. Vitamin D deficiency and risk of cardiovascular disease. Circulation. 2008 Jan 29;117(4):503–11. http://circ.ahajournals.org/cgi/content/full/117/4/503

Why You Need More Vitamin D. A Lot More

1. Holick MF. Vitamin D deficiency. N Engl J Med. 2007;357(3):266–81.

2. Llewellyn DJ, Lang IA, Langa KM, Melzer D. Vitamin D and cognitive impairment in the elderly U.S. population. J Gerontol A Biol Sci Med Sci. 2011;66(1):59–65.

3. Cannell JJ, Hollis BW, Sorenson MB, Taft TN, Anderson JJ. Athletic performance and vitamin D. Med Sci Sports Exerc. 2009;41(5):1102–10.

4. Jablonski NG, Chaplin G. Colloquium paper: human skin pigmentation as an adaptation to UV radiation. Proc Natl Acad Sci U.S.A. 2010;107 Suppl 2:8962–8.

5. Gorham ED, Mohr SB, Garland CF, Chaplin G, Garland FC. Do sunscreens increase risk of melanoma in populations residing at higher latitudes? Ann Epidemiol. 2007;17(12):956–63.

6. Garland CF, Garland FC. Do sunlight and vitamin D reduce the likelihood of colon cancer? Int J Epidemiol. 1980;9(3):227–31.

7. Grant WB, Garland CF. The association of solar ultraviolet B (UVB) with reducing risk of cancer: multifactorial ecologic analysis of geographic variation in age-adjusted cancer mortality rates. Anticancer Res. 2006;26(4A):2687–99.

8. Leffell DJ and Brash DE: Sunlight and skin cancer. Sci Am. 275(1): 52–53, 56–59, 1996. http://toms.gsfc.nasa.gov/ery_uv/ dna_exp.gif (accessed March 9, 2011).

9. Devesa SS, Grauman DJ, Blot WJ, Pennello GA, Hoover RN, Fraumeni JF Jr: Atlas of Cancer Mortality in the United States, 1950–1994. NIH Publication No. 99–4564, 1999. http://ratecalc.cancer.gov/ratecalc//

10. Grant WB, Mohr SB. Ecological studies of ultraviolet B, vitamin D and cancer since 2000. Ann Epidemiol. 2009;19(7):446–54.

11. Cannell JJ, Vieth R, Umhau JC, Holick MF, Grant WB, Madronich S, Garland CF, Giovannucci E. Epidemic influenza and vitamin D. Epidemiol Infect. 2006;134(6):1129–40.

12. Parker J, Hashmi O, Dutton D, Mavrodaris A, Stranges S, Kandala NB, Clarke A, Franco OH. Levels of vitamin D and cardiomet-abolic disorders: systematic review and meta-analysis. Maturitas. 2010;65(3):225–36.

13. Hyppönen E, Power C. Hypovitaminosis D in British adults at age 45 y: nationwide cohort study of dietary and lifestyle predictors. Am J Clin Nutr. 2007;85(3):860–8.

14. Garland CF, French CB, Baggerly LL, Heaney RP. Vitamin D supplement doses and serum 25-hydroxyvitamin D in the range associated with cancer prevention. Anticancer Res 2011:31:617–22.

15. Bischoff-Ferrari HA, Willett WC, Wong JB, Stuck AE, Staehelin HB, Orav EJ, Thoma A, Kiel DP, Henschkowski J. Prevention of nonvertebral fractures with oral vitamin D and dose dependency: a meta-analysis of randomized controlled trials. Arch Intern Med. 2009;169(6):551–61.

16. Lappe JM, Travers-Gustafson D, Davies KM, Recker RR, Heaney RP. Vitamin D and calcium supplementation reduces cancer risk: results of a randomized trial. Am J Clin Nutr. 2007;85(6):1586–91.

17. Bolland MJ, Grey A, Gamble GD, Reid IR. Calcium and vitamin D supplements and health outcomes: a reanalysis of the Women's Health Initiative (WHI) limited-access data set. Am J Clin Nutr. 2011 Aug 31. [Epub ahead of print]

18. Aloia JF, Li-Ng M. Re: epidemic influenza and vitamin D. Epidemiol Infect. 2007;135(7):1095–6; author reply 1097–8.

19. Urashima M, Segawa T, Okazaki M, Kurihara M, Wada Y, Ida H. Randomized trial of vitamin D supplementation to prevent seasonal influenza A in schoolchildren. Am J Clin Nutr. 2010;91(5):1255–60.

20. Manaseki-Holland S, Qader G, Isaq Masher M, Bruce J, Zulf Mughal M, Chandramohan D, Walraven G. Effects of vitamin D supplementation to children diagnosed with pneumonia in Kabul: a randomised controlled trial. Trop Med Int Health. 2010;15(10):1148–55.

21. Grant WB. Relation between prediagnostic serum 25-hydroxyvitamin D level and incidence of breast, colorectal, and other cancers. J Photochem Photobiol B, 2010;101:130–136.

22. Grant WB. An estimate of the global reduction in mortality rates through doubling vitamin D levels. Eur J Clin Nutr, 2011;65:1016–1026.

23. Sabetta JR, DePetrillo P, Cipriani RJ, Smardin J, Burns LA, Landry ML. Serum 25-hydroxyvitamin d and the incidence of acute viral respiratory tract infections in healthy adults. PLoS One. 2010;5(6):e11088.

24. Grant WB. In defense of the sun: An estimate of changes in mortality rates in the United States if mean serum 25-hydroxyvitamin D levels were raised to 45 ng/mL by solar ultraviolet-B irradiance. Dermato-Endocrinology, 2009;1(4):207–14.

25. Krishnan AV, Feldman D. Mechanisms of the anti-cancer and anti-inflammatory actions of vitamin D. Annu Rev Pharmacol Toxicol. 2011;51:311–36.

26. Liu PT, Stenger S, Tang DH, Modlin RL. Cutting edge: vitamin D-mediated human antimicrobial activity against Mycobacterium tuberculosis is dependent on the induction of cathelicidin. J Immunol. 2007;179(4):2060–3.

27. Cantorna MT, Mahon BD. Mounting evidence for vitamin D as an environmental factor affecting autoimmune disease prevalence. Exp Biol Med (Maywood). 2004;229(11):1136–42.

28. Zagura M, Serg M, Kampus P, Zilmer M, Eha J, Unt E, Lieberg J, Cockcroft JR, Kals J. Aortic stiffness and vitamin D are independent markers of aortic calcification in patients with peripheral arterial disease and in healthy subjects. Eur J Vasc Endovasc Surg. 2011 Aug 24. [Epub ahead of print]

29. Alvarez JA, Ashraf AP, Hunter GR, Gower BA. Serum 25-hydroxyvitamin D and parathyroid hormone are independent determinants of whole-body insulin sensitivity in women and may contribute to lower insulin sensitivity in African Americans. Am J Clin Nutr. 2010;92(6):1344–9.

30. Institute of Medicine (US) Committee to Review Dietary Reference Intakes for Vitamin D and Calcium; Ross AC, Taylor CL, Yaktine AL, Del Valle HB, editors. Dietary Reference Intakes for Calcium and Vitamin D. Washington (DC): National Academies Press (US); 2011.

31. Ross AC, Manson JE, Abrams SA, Aloia JF, Brannon PM, Clinton SK, Durazo-Arvizu RA, Gallagher JC, Gallo RL, Jones G, Kovacs CS, Mayne ST, Rosen CJ, Shapses SA. The 2011 report on dietary reference intakes for calcium and vitamin D from the Institute of Medicine: what clinicians need to know. J Clin Endocrinol Metab. 2011;96(1):53–8.

32. Lim U, Freedman DM, Hollis BW, Horst RL, Purdue MP, Chatterjee N, Weinstein SJ, Morton LM, Schatzkin A, Virtamo J, Linet MS, Hartge P, Albanes D. A prospective investigation of serum 25-hydroxyvitamin D and risk of lymphoid cancers. Int J Cancer. 2009;124(4):979–86.

33. Robien K, Cutler GJ, Lazovich D. Vitamin D intake and breast cancer risk in postmenopausal women: the Iowa Women's Health Study. Cancer Causes Control. 2007;18(7):775–82.

34. Souberbielle JC, Body JJ, Lappe JM, Plebani M, Shoenfeld Y, Wang TJ, Bischoff-Ferrari HA, Cavalier E, Ebeling PR, Fardellone P, Gandini S, Gruson D, Guérin AP, Heickendorff L, Hollis BW, Ish-Shalom S, Jean G, von Landenberg P, Largura A, Olsson T, Pierrot-Deseilligny C, Pilz S, Tincani A, Valcour A, Zittermann A. Vitamin D and musculoskeletal health, cardiovascular disease, autoimmunity and cancer: Recommendations for clinical practice. Autoimmun Rev 2010;9:709–15.

35. Heaney RP, Grant WB, Holick MF, Amling M. The IOM Report on Vitamin D misleads. J Clin Endocrinol Metab. eLetter. (4 March 2011). http://jcem.endojournals.org/cgi/eletters/96/1/53

36. Holick MF, Binkley NC, Bischoff-Ferrari HA, Gordon CM, Hanley DA, Heaney RP, Murad MH, Weaver CM. Evaluation, Treatment, and Prevention of Vitamin D Deficiency: an Endocrine Society Clinical Practice Guideline. J Clin Endocrinol Metab, 2011;96(7):1911–30.

Ten Ways to Spot Antivitamin Biases in a Scientific Study

*"It's not what we don't know that harms us,
but what we do know that ain't so."*

—MARK TWAIN

1. Where's the beef? How much of the original study is quoted in the media? Are you just getting factoids, or are data provided? Has the journalist writing about the subject read the original paper?

2. What exactly was studied, and how? Was it an *in vitro* (test tube) study or an *in vivo* (animal) study? Was there a *clinical study* on people, or is its application to real life a matter of conjecture?

3. Follow the money. Who paid for the study? Cash from food processors, pharmaceutical giants, and other deep pockets decides what gets studied, and how. It is very difficult, if not impossible, for researchers to present findings that embarrass their financial backers. Published research will often indicate sources of funding, possibly at the end of the paper in an acknowledgments paragraph. If not, correspondence addresses of principle authors are invariably provided. Write and ask.

4. Check the dosages. Any vitamin C study using less than 2,000 mg a day is a waste of time. Any vitamin E study employing less than 400 IU is a waste of time. Any niacin study using less than 1,000 mg a day is a waste of time.

5. Check the form of supplement used. Was the vitamin used in the study natural or synthetic? Any carotene study using the synthetic form of beta-carotene only is useless. Any vitamin E study using the synthetic DL-alpha-tocopherol form is useless.

6. Use the "Pauling Principle": read the entire study and interpret the data for yourself. Do not rely on the summary or conclusions of the authors. As Linus Pauling pointed out repeatedly, many researchers miss, or dismiss, the statistical significance of their own work. Such behavior may be human error, or it may be politically motivated. Beware of editorializing.

7. Beware of Pauling-bashers. If a media article is critical about Nobel prize–winning Linus Pauling, you can be sure it has been spin-doctored.

8. Watch for assumptions from the authors that we get all the vitamins we need from food, or that there is no scientific support for large vitamin doses.

9. Watch for ultra-cautious public recommendations at the end of the article such as "Just eat a balanced diet" or "If you must take vitamins, take no more than the RDA."

352

HOW TO MAKE PEOPLE BELIEVE ANY ANTI-VITAMIN SCARE

Media-trumpeted anti-vitamin news can be the product of pharmaceutical company payouts. No, this is not one of "those" conspiracy theories. Here's how it's done:

1. **Cash to study authors**. Many of the authors of a recent negative vitamin E paper[1] have received substantial income from the pharmaceutical industry. The names are available in the last page of the paper (1556) in the "Conflict of Interest" section. You will not see them in the brief summary at the *JAMA* website. A number of the study authors have received money from pharmaceutical companies, including Merck, Pfizer, Sanofi-Aventis, AstraZeneca, Abbott, GlaxoSmithKline, Janssen, Amgen, Firmagon, and Novartis.

2. **Advertising revenue**. Many popular magazines and almost all major medical journals receive income from the pharmaceutical industry. The only question is, how much? Pick up a copy of the publication and count the pharmaceutical ads. The more space sold, the more revenue for the publication. If you try to find their advertisement revenue, you'll see that they don't disclose it. So, just count the Pharma ads. Look in them all: *Readers Digest, JAMA, Newsweek, Time, AARP Today, NEJM, Archives of Pediatrics.* Even *Prevention* magazine. Practically any major periodical.

3. **Rigged trials**. Studies denying the health benefits of vitamins and essential nutrients appear to be rigged. This can be easily done by using low doses to guarantee a negative result, and by biasing the interpretation to show statistical increase in risk.

4. **Bias in what is published, or rejected for publication**. The largest and most popular medical journals receive very large income from pharmaceutical advertising. Peer-reviewed research indicates that this influences what they print, and even what study authors conclude from their data.[2]

5. **Censorship of what is indexed and available to doctors and the public**. Public tax money pays for censorship in the largest public medical library on the planet: the U.S. National Library of Medicine (MEDLINE/PubMed). You will not find certain medical journals indexed by MEDLINE, such as the *Journal of Orthomolecular Medicine* and the journal *Fluoride*. Both are peer-reviewed and both have been published for over forty years.

References

1. Klein EA, Thompson, IM Jr, Tangen CM, et al. Vitamin E and the risk of prostate cancer: the Selenium and Vitamin E Cancer Prevention Trial (SELECT). *JAMA*, 2011, 306(14):1549–1556. http://jama.ama-assn.org/content/306/14/1549.

2. Kemper KJ, and Hood KL. Does pharmaceutical advertising affect journal publication about dietary supplements? BMC Complement Altern Med., 2008, 8:11. Full text at www.biomedcentral.com/1472–6882/8/11 or www.pubmedcentral.nih.gov/articlerender.fcgi?tool=pubmed&pubmedid=18400092.

10. Use the media backwards. The more headlines about a particular study, the more politically charged the subject and the less likely that the reporting, or the original study, is objective. Positive new drug studies get headlines. So do vitamin scare stories. The more media hoopla, the worse the research. Truly valuable research does not scare people; it helps people get well.

High-Dose Vitamin C Therapy for Major Diseases

*"Have no respect for the authority of others,
for there are always contrary authorities to be found."*

—BERTRAND RUSSELL

We are going to hit this important topic very hard here, so brace yourself. **There is no longer doubt about it: vitamin C therapy works.** Decades of physicians' reports and controlled studies support the use of very large doses of ascorbate. Effective doses are high doses, often 1,000 times more than the US Recommended Dietary Allowance (RDA) or Daily Reference Intake (DRI). It is a cornerstone of medical science that dose affects treatment outcome. This premise is accepted with pharmaceutical drug therapy, but not with vitamin therapy. Most vitamin C research has used inadequate, low doses. Low doses do not get clinical results. Investigators using vitamin C in high doses have consistently reported excellent results. The medical literature has ignored nearly seventy-five years of laboratory and clinical studies on high-dose ascorbate therapy.

High doses were advocated immediately after ascorbic acid was isolated by Albert Szent-Gyorgyi, M.D., Ph.D. (1893–1986). Szent-Gyorgyi received the Nobel prize for ascorbate-related work in 1937.

The early pioneers of high-dose vitamin C therapy include:

Claus Washington Jungeblut
William J. McCormick
Frederick Robert Klenner
Modern pioneers of high-dose vitamin C therapy include:
Robert F. Cathcart, III
Hugh D. Riordan

CLAUS WASHINGTON JUNGEBLUT, M.D. (1898–1976)

Professor of Bacteriology, Columbia University College of Physicians and Surgeons (New York).

Jungeblut first published on ascorbate as prevention and treatment for polio in 1935. (Jungeblut CW. Inactivation of poliomyelitis virus by crystalline vitamin C (ascorbic acid). *J Exper Med* 62:317–321.)

Jungeblut's other polio papers, 1937–1939, include:

Jungeblut CW. (1937). Vitamin C therapy and prophylaxis in experimental poliomyelitis. *J Exp Med,* 65: 127–146.

Jungeblut CW. (1937). Further observations on vitamin C therapy in experimental poliomyelitis. *J Exper Med* 66: 459–477.

Jungeblut CW, Feiner RR. (1937).Vitamin C content of monkey tissues in experimental poliomyelitis. *J Exper Med* 66: 479–491.

Jungeblut CW. (1939). A further contribution to vitamin C therapy in experimental poliomyelitis. *J Exper Med* 70:315–332.

On September 18, 1939, *Time* magazine reported that Jungeblut, while studying the 1938 Australian polio epidemic, said that low vitamin C status was associated with the disease. Unlike oral polio vaccination, vitamin C has never caused polio. Few know that vitamin C has been known to prevent and cure poliomyelitis for nearly seventy-five years.

Whatever Happened to Vitamin C Therapy for Polio?

Jungeblut used fairly low doses. Albert Sabin used even lower doses, normally only one-third of Jungeblut's. Sabin's unsuccessful "replication" was taken as the standard, and is to this day. Even with relatively low doses of vitamin C, Jungeblut made the correct conclusion: "Vitamin C can truthfully be designated as the antitoxic and antiviral vitamin."

In 1935, Jungeblut showed that vitamin C inactivated diphtheria toxin. (Jungeblut CW, Zwemer RL. Inactivation of diphtheria toxin in vivo and in vitro by crystalline vitamin C (ascorbic acid). *Proc Soc Exper Biol Med* 1935, 32:1229–34.) By 1937, Jungeblut demonstrated that ascorbate inactivated tetanus toxin. (Jungeblut CW. Inactivation of tetanus toxin by crystalline vitamin C (l-ascorbic acid). *J Immunol* 1937; 33:203–214.)

Of Dr. Jungeblut's many research reports, twenty-two were published in the *Journal of Experimental Medicine.* Free online access at www.jem.org/contents-by-date.0.shtml

Jungeblut's biography and bibliography:

Saul AW. Taking the cure: Claus Washington Jungeblut, M.D.: Polio pioneer; ascorbate advocate. *J Orthomolecular Med,* 2006, 21(2):102–106.

www.doctoryourself.com/jungeblut.html and http://orthomolecular.org/library/jom

WILLIAM J. MCCORMICK, M.D. (1880–1968)

Practicing physician in Toronto, Canada

Over sixty years ago, McCormick saw vitamin C deficiency as the essential cause of, and effective cure for, numerous communicable illnesses. He was one of the very first to advocate injected, gram-sized doses of vitamin C as an antiviral and antibiotic. (McCormick WJ. The changing incidence and mortality of infectious disease in relation to changed trends in nutrition. *Medical Record,* 1947. September.)

Vitamin C does not cause kidney stones. Modern writers consistently pass by the fact that McCormick used vitamin C to prevent and cure kidney stones . . . in 1946. (McCormick WJ. Lithogenesis and hypovitaminosis. *Medical Record,* 1946. 159:7, July, pp. 410–413.)

Vitamin C is a specific antagonist of chemical and bacterial toxins.

—W. J. MCCORMICK.M.D.

McCormick also noted that four out of five coronary cases in hospital show vitamin C deficiency. (McCormick WJ. Coronary thrombosis: a new concept of mechanism and etiology. *Clinical Medicine,* 1957. 4:7, July.) Vitamin C is essential to strengthen the walls of blood vessels, small and large. A vitamin C deficient artery can literally "bleed" into itself. Blood clot forms; stroke may result.

Over fifty years ago, McCormick "found, in clinical and laboratory research, that the smoking of one cigarette neutralizes in the body approximately 25 mg of ascorbic acid." (McCormick WJ. Intervertebral-disc lesions: a new etiological concept. *Arch Pediatr.* 1954 Jan; 71(1):29–32.)

McCormick recognized that cigarette smoking, in causing vitamin C deficiency, causes artery damage and cardiovascular disease. Thirty years later, Linus Pauling and Matthias Rath would go on to demonstrate how vitamin C was a cure for cardiovascular disease.

Further Reading

Rath M, Pauling L. (1991). Solution to the puzzle of human cardiovascular disease: Its primary cause is ascorbate deficiency leading to the deposition of lipoprotein(a) and fibrinogen/fibrin in the vascular wall. *Journal of Orthomolecular Medicine,* 6: 125.

Rath M, Pauling L. (1992). A unified theory of human cardiovascular disease leading the way to the abolition of this diseases as a cause for human mortality. *Journal of Orthomolecular Medicine,* 7:5.

For a review of McCormick's work, with bibliography: Saul AW. (2003). Taking the cure: The pioneering work of William J. McCormick, M.D. *J Orthomolecular Med,*18(2):93–96. www.doctoryourself.com/mccormick.html and http://orthomolecular.org/library/jom.

FREDERICK ROBERT KLENNER, M.D. (1907–1984)

North Carolina, USA, Board-certified chest physician

For decades, Dr. Klenner treated patients with injections of vitamin C, ranging from 350 to 1,200 mg per kg body weight per day. Vitamin C at 350 mg/kg is about 20,000 to 35,000 mg/day for an adult. Vitamin C at 1,200 mg/kg is about 70,000 to 120,000 mg/day for an adult.

Klenner successfully treated polio, pneumonia, and other serious infectious diseases. (Klenner FR. Observations on the dose of administration of ascorbic acid when employed beyond the range of a vitamin in human pathology. *Journal of Applied Nutrition,* 1971. 23(3,4):61–68.), www.doctoryourself.com/klennerpaper.html.

Klenner treated an astounding variety of diseases with massive doses of vitamin C: bladder infections, arthritis, leukemia, atherosclerosis, ruptured intervertebral discs, high cholesterol, corneal ulcer, diabetes, glaucoma, burns and secondary infections, heat stroke, radiation burns, heavy metal poisoning, chronic fatigue, and complications resulting from surgery.

Additionally, Klenner arrested and reversed multiple sclerosis with very high doses of vitamin C and other vitamins. (Klenner FR. Response of peripheral and central nerve pathology to mega-doses of the vitamin B-complex and other metabolites. Parts 1 and 2. J *Applied Nutrition,* 1973, 25:16–40. Free download at www.townsendletter.com/Klenner/KlennerProtocol _forMS.pdf)

Klenner's specific treatment protocols are described in:

Smith, LH. Clinical guide to the use of vitamin C: The clinical experiences of Frederick R. Klenner, M.D. Portland, OR: Life Sciences Press, 1988. The full text of this book is posted at www.seanet.com/~alexs/ascorbate/198x/smith-lh-clinical_guide_1988.htm.

For a biography and bibliography: Saul AW. Hidden in plain sight: the pioneering work of Frederick Robert Klenner, M.D. *J Orthomolecular Med,* 2007, 22(1):31–38. www.doctor yourself.com/klennerbio.html and http://orthomolecular.org/library/jom.

ROBERT F. CATHCART III, M.D. (1932–2007)

California, USA, Board-certified orthopedic surgeon

From the 1960s onward, Dr. Cathcart successfully treated tens of thousands of patients with large doses of vitamin C. He found it highly effective against pneumonia, influenza, hepatitis, and most recently, the most severe symptoms of AIDS.

Further Reading

Cathcart RF. (1981). Vitamin C, titration to bowel tolerance, anascorbemia, and acute induced scurvy. *Medical Hypotheses,* 7:1359–1376, www.doctoryourself.com/titration.html.

———. (1984). Vitamin C in the treatment of Acquired Immune Deficiency Syndrome (AIDS) *Medical Hypotheses,* 14(4):423–433.

———. (1985). Vitamin C, the nontoxic, nonrate-limited antioxidant free radical scavenger. *Medical Hypotheses,* 18:61–77.

To read a full Cathcart bibliography: www.doctoryourself.com/biblio_cathcart.html.

HUGH D. RIORDAN, M.D. (1932–2005)

Kansas, USA, Board-certified psychiatrist

Dr. Riordan successfully used large doses of intravenous vitamin C against cancer, beginning in the 1970s. He and his colleagues published on this for many years. Their work has been largely ignored. A list of the team's published research can be found under References at the end of in this section. For an additional Riordan bibliography, please go to www.doctoryourself.com/biblio_riordan.html.

In 2008 the National Institutes of Health investigated high-doses of injected vitamin C as chemotherapy against cancer. (Chen Q, et al. [2008]. Pharmacologic doses of ascorbate act as a prooxidant and decrease growth of aggressive tumor xenografts in mice. *Proc Natl Acad Sci,* August 4.) The medical journals and popular mass media reported this as something new, somewhat promising, and definitely unproven. Yet, in 1954, fifty-four years ago, Dr. McCormick noted that persons with cancer typically have exceptionally low levels of vitamin C in their tissues, a deficiency of approximately 4,500 mg. (McCormick, WJ. [1954]. Cancer: The preconditioning factor in pathogenesis. *Archives of Pediatrics of New York* 71:313.)

We learn from history that we do not learn from history."

—GEORG WILHELM FRIEDRICH HEGEL, 1770–1831

The medical literature has ignored nearly seventy-five years of laboratory and clinical studies on high-dose ascorbate therapy. Doses of tens of thousands of milligrams of vitamin C is the most unacknowledged successful research in medicine.

For More Information

Free access to the online archive of the *Journal of Orthomolecular Medicine* can be found at http://orthomolecular.org/library/jom. To receive free, noncommercial news updates on nutritional (orthomolecular) medicine by email, visit http://orthomolecular.org /resources/omns/index.shtml.

References

Gonzalez MJ, Miranda-Massari, JR, Mora, EM, Jimenez, IZ, Matos, MI, Riordan HD, Casciari, JJ., Riordan NH, Rodriguez, M., Guzman, A. Orthomolecular Oncology: a Mechanistic View of Intravenous Ascorbate's Chemotherapeutic Activity. *Puerto Rico Health Sciences J,* March, 2002, 21:1.

Gonzalez MJ, Mora, E., Riordan NH, Riordan HD, Mojica, P. Rethinking Vitamin C and Cancer: An Update on Nutritional Oncology. *Cancer Prevention International,* 1998, 3: 215–224.

Gonzalez MJ, Mora, E.M., Miranda-Massari, JR., Matta, J., Riordan HD, Riordan NH. Inhibition of Human Breast Carcinoma Cell Proliferation by Ascorbate and Copper. *Puerto Rico Health Sciences J,* March 2002, 21:1.

Jackson JA, Riordan HD, Hunninghake, RE., Riordan NH. High Dose Intravenous Vitamin C and Long Term Survival of a Patient with Cancer of Head of the Pancreas. *J. Orthomolecular Med,* 1995, 10(2).

Padayatty, S.J., Sun, H., Wang, Y., Riordan HD, Hewitt, S.M., Katz, A., Wesley, R.A., Levine, M. Vitamin C Pharmacokinetics: Implications for Oral and Intravenous Use. *Annals of Internal Medicine,* April 6, 2004, 140(7): 533–537.

Riordan HD, et al. High-Dose Intravenous Vitamin C in the Treatment of a Patient with Renal Cell Carcinoma of the Kidney. *J. Orthomolecular Med,* 1998, 13:2.

Riordan HD, Hunninghake, RE, Riordan NH, Jackson, JA, Meng, XL, Taylor, P, Casciari, JJ, Gonzalez MJ, Miranda-Massari, JR, Mora, EM, Norberto, R, Rivera, A. Intravenous Ascorbic Acid: Protocol for its Application and Use. *Puerto Rico Health Sciences Journal,* September 2003, 22:3.

Riordan HD, Jackson JA, Schultz, M. Case Study: High-Dose Intravenous Vitamin C in the Treatment of a Patient With Adenocarcinoma of the Kidney. *J. Orthomolecular Med,* 1990, 5:1.

Riordan HD, Riordan NH, Jackson JA, Casciari, JJ, Hunninghake, R, Gonzalez MJ, Mora, EM, Miranda-Massari, JR, Rosario, N., Rivera, A.: Intravenous Vitamin C as a Chemotherapy Agent: a Report on Clinical Cases. *Puerto Rico Health Sciences J,* June 2004, 23(2): 115–118.

Riordan NH, Jackson JA, Riordan HD. Intravenous Vitamin C in a Terminal Cancer Patient. *J. Orthomolecular Med,* 1996, 11:2.

Riordan NH, Riordan HD, Meng, X., Li, Y., Jackson JA. Intravenous Ascorbate as a Tumor Cytotoxic Chemotherapeutic Agent. *Medical Hypotheses,* 1995, (44):207–213.

ABOUT "OBJECTIONS" TO VITAMIN C THERAPY

Many physicians refuse to employ vitamin C in the amounts suggested simply because it is counter to their fixed ideas of what is reasonable. There is no doubt that physicians are being brainwashed with the current journal advertising. I have never seen a patient that vitamin C would not benefit.

—FREDERICK ROBERT KLENNER, M.D.

In massive doses, vitamin C (ascorbic acid) stops a cold within hours, stops influenza in a day or two, and stops viral pneumonia (pain, fever, cough) in two or three days.[1] It is a highly effective antihistamine, antiviral, and antitoxin. It reduces inflammation and lowers fever. Administered intravenously, ascorbate kills cancer cells without harming healthy tissue. Many people therefore wonder, in the face of statements like these, why the medical professions have not embraced vitamin C therapy with open and grateful arms.

Probably the main roadblock to widespread examination and utilization of this all-too-simple technology is the equally widespread belief that there *must* be unknown dangers to tens of thousands of milligrams of ascorbic acid. Yet, since the time megascorbate therapy was introduced in the late 1940s by Fred R. Klenner, M.D.[2], there has been an especially safe, and extremely effective track record to follow.

Still, for some, questions remain. Here is a sample of what readers have asked OMNS about vitamin C:

Is 2,000 mg/day of vitamin C a megadose?

No. Decades ago, Linus Pauling and Irwin Stone showed that most animals make at least that much (or more) per human body weight per day.[3,4]

RDA FOR VITAMIN C IS TEN PERCENT OF USDA STANDARD FOR GUINEA PIGS

Are you healthier than a lab animal? The US RDA for vitamin C for humans is only 10 percent of the government's vitamin C standards for Guinea pigs.

Wait a minute; that cannot possibly be true. Can it?

The US Department of Agriculture states that "the Guinea pig's vitamin C requirement is 10 to 15 mg per day under normal conditions and 15 to 25 mg per day if pregnant, lactating, or growing."[1] Well, that sounds reasonable. But how much is that compared to humans?

An adult guinea pig weighs about one kilogram (2.2 pounds). Guinea pigs therefore need between 10 and 25 milligrams of C per kilogram. In the US, an average human weighs (at least) 82 kg (180 lbs).[2] That means the USDA's standards, if fairly applied to us, would set our vitamin C requirement somewhere between 820 mg and 2,000 mg vitamin C per day.

The US RDA for vitamin C is different than that. Quite different.

It is lower. Much lower. The US RDA for vitamin C for humans is 90 mg for men, 75 mg for women. (If you smoke, they allow an additional 35 mg/day extra. Wow.)

Why are we humans repeatedly urged to consume only the RDA when the RDA is one-tenth or less of that same government's official nutrient requirement for an animal? No wonder so many people are sick and no wonder their medical bills are so high.

If we are going to have health insurance coverage for everyone, wouldn't it be nice for the government to first offer us the same deal it gives to Guinea pigs?

Then why has the government set the "Safe Upper Limit" for vitamin C at 2,000 mg/day?

Perhaps the reason is ignorance. According to nationwide data compiled by the American Association of Poison Control Centers, vitamin C (and the use of any other dietary supplement) does not kill anyone.[5]

Does vitamin C damage DNA?

No. If vitamin C harmed DNA, why do most animals make (not eat, but *make*) between 2,000 and 10,000 milligrams of vitamin C per human equivalent body weight per day? Evolution would never so favor anything that harms vital genetic material. White blood cells and male reproductive fluids contain unusually high quantities of ascorbate. Living, reproducing systems love vitamin C.

Does vitamin C cause low blood sugar, B_{12}-deficiency, birth defects, or infertility?

Vitamin C does not cause birth defects, nor infertility, nor miscarriage. "Harmful effects have been mistakenly attributed to vitamin C, including hypoglycemia, rebound scurvy, infertility, mutagenesis, and destruction of vitamin B_{12}. Health professionals should recognize that vitamin C does not produce these effects."[6]

Does vitamin C . . . Um, uh . . .

In a randomized, double-blind, placebo-controlled fourteen-day trial of 3,000 mg per day of

359

vitamin C the vitamin C group reported greater frequency of sexual intercourse. The vitamin C group (but not the placebo group) also experienced a quantifiable decrease in depression. This is probably due to the fact that vitamin C "modulates catecholaminergic activity, decreases stress reactivity, approach anxiety and prolactin release, improves vascular function, and increases oxytocin release. These processes are relevant to sexual behavior and mood."[7]

Does vitamin C cause kidney stones?

No. The myth of the vitamin C–caused kidney stone is rivaled in popularity only by the Loch Ness Monster. A factoid-crazy medical media often overlooks the fact that William J. McCormick, M.D., demonstrated that vitamin C actually prevents the formation of kidney stones. He did so in 1946, when he published a paper on the subject.[8] His work was confirmed by University of Alabama professor of medicine Emanuel Cheraskin, M.D. Dr. Cheraskin showed that vitamin C inhibits the formation of oxalate stones.[9] Other research reports that: "Even though a certain part of oxalate in the urine derives from metabolized ascorbic acid, the intake of high doses of vitamin C does not increase the risk of calcium oxalate kidney stones. . . (I)n the large-scale Harvard Prospective Health Professional Follow-Up Study, those groups in the highest quintile of vitamin C intake (greater than 1,500 mg/day) had a lower risk of kidney stones than the groups in the lowest quintiles."[10]

Dr. Robert F. Cathcart said, "I started using vitamin C in massive doses in patients in 1969. By the time I read that ascorbate should cause kidney stones, I had clinical evidence that it did not cause kidney stones, so I continued prescribing massive doses to patients. Up to 2006, I estimate that I have put 25,000 patients on massive doses of vitamin C and none have developed kidney stones. Two patients who had dropped their doses to 500 mg a day developed calcium oxalate kidney stones. I raised their doses back up to the more massive doses and added magnesium and B_6 to their program and no more kidney stones. I think they developed the kidney stones because they were not taking enough vitamin C."

Why did Linus Pauling die from cancer if he took all that vitamin C?

Linus Pauling, Ph.D., megadose vitamin C advocate, died in 1994 from prostate cancer. Mayo Clinic cancer researcher Charles G. Moertel, M.D., critic of Pauling and vitamin C, also died in 1994, and also from cancer (lymphoma). Dr. Moertel was 66 years old. Dr. Pauling was 93 years old. One needs to make up one's own mind as to whether this does or does not indicate benefit from vitamin C.

A review of the subject indicates that "vitamin C deficiency is common in patients with advanced cancer. . . . Patients with low plasma concentrations of vitamin C have a shorter survival."[11]

Does vitamin C narrow arteries or cause atherosclerosis?

Abram Hoffer, M.D., has said: "I have used vitamin C in megadoses with my patients since 1952 and have not seen any cases of heart disease develop even after decades of use. Dr. Robert Cathcart with experience on over 25,000 patients since 1969 saw no cases of heart disease developing in patients who did not have any when first seen. He added that the thickening of the vessel walls, if true, indicates that the thinning that occurs with age is reversed. The fact is that vitamin C *decreases* plaque formation according to many clinical studies.

Some critics ignore the knowledge that thickened arterial walls in the absence of plaque formation indicate that the walls are becoming stronger and therefore less apt to rupture. Gokce, Keaney, Frei et al gave patients supplemental vitamin C daily for thirty days and measured blood flow through the arteries. Blood flow **increased nearly fifty percent** after the single dose and this was sustained after the monthly treatment."[12]

What about blood pressure?

A randomized, double-blind, placebo-controlled study showed that hypertensive patients taking supplemental vitamin C had lower blood pressure.[13]

So why the flurry of anti–vitamin C reporting in the mass media? Negative news gets attention. Negative news sells newspapers, and magazines, and pulls in lots of television viewers. Positive *drug* studies do get headlines, of course. Positive vitamin studies do not. Is this a conspiracy? You mean with unscrupulous people all sitting around a shaded table in a darkened back room? Of course not. It is nevertheless an enormous public health problem with enormous consequences.

150 million Americans take supplemental vitamin C every day. This is as much a political issue as a scientific issue. What would happen if everybody took vitamins? Perhaps doctors, hospital administrators and pharmaceutical salespeople would all be lining up for their unemployment checks.

A skeptic might conclude that there is at least some evidence that the politicians are on the wrong side of this. Remember, the US RDA for vitamin C for humans is only 10 percent of the government's USDA vitamin C standards for Guinea pigs.[14] But conspiracy against nutritional medicine? Certainly not. Couldn't be.

References and Additional Reading

1. Cathcart RF. Vitamin C, titration to bowel tolerance, anascorbemia, and acute induced scurvy." *Medical Hypothesis* 7:1359–1376, 1981www.doctoryourself.com/titration.html

See also: http://orthomolecular.org/resources/omns/v05n09.shtml and http://orthomolecular.org/resources/omns/v05n11.shtml

2. Saul AW. Hidden in plain sight: the pioneering work of Frederick Robert Klenner, M.D. J *Orthomolecular Med,* 2007, 22(1):31–38, www.doctoryourself.com/klennerbio.html and http://orthomolecular.org/hof/2005/fklenner.html.

Dr. F.R. Klenner's *Clinical Guide to the Use of Vitamin C* is posted in its entirety at www.seanet.com/~alexs/ascorbate/198x/smith-lh-clinical_guide_1988.htm.

3. Pauling L. *How to Live Longer and Feel Better.* Corvallis, OR: Oregon State University Press, 2006. Reviewed at www.doctoryourself.com/livelonger.html. Linus Pauling's complete vitamin and nutrition bibliography is posted at www.doctoryourself.com/biblio_pauling_ortho.html.

4. The complete text of Irwin Stone's book *The Healing Factor* is posted for free reading at http://vitamincfoundation.org/stone/.

5. http://orthomolecular.org/resources/omns/v06n04.shtml.

6. Levine M et al. *JAMA,* April 21, 1999, 281(15):1419.

7. Brody S. High-dose ascorbic acid increases intercourse frequency and improves mood: a randomized controlled clinical trial. *Psychiatry,* 2002, 52(4):371–4.

8. McCormick WJ. Lithogenesis and hypovitaminosis. *Medical Record,* 1946. 159:410–413.

9. Cheraskin E, Ringsdorf, Jr. M and Sisley E. *The Vitamin C Connection: Getting Well and Staying Well with Vitamin C.* New York: Harper and Row, 1983. Also paperback, 1984: New York, Bantam Books. See: "Vitamin C in the urine tends to bind calcium and decrease its free form. This means less chance of calcium's separating out as calcium oxalate (stones)." [p. 213]. See also: Ringsdorf WM Jr, Cheraskin E. Nutritional aspects of urolithiasis. *South Med J.* 1981, 74(1):41–3, 46.

10. Gerster H. No contribution of ascorbic acid to renal calcium oxalate stones. *Ann Nutr Metab.* 1997, 41(5):269–82. See also: http://orthomolecular.org/resources/omns/v01n07.shtml.

11. Mayland CR, Bennett MI, Allan K. Vitamin C deficiency in cancer patients. *Palliat Med.* 2005, 19(1):17–20. See also: http://orthomolecular.org/resources/omns/v01n09.shtml and http://orthomolecular.org/resources/omns/v04n19.shtml.

12. Free full text paper at http://circ.ahajournals.org/cgi/reprint/99/25/3234. See also: http://orthomolecular.org/resources/omns/v06n20.shtml and http://orthomolecular.org/resources/omns/v01n02.shtml

13. Duffy SJ, Gokce N, Holbrook M, Huang A, Frei B, Keaney JF Jr, Vita JA. Treatment of hypertension with ascorbic acid. *Lancet* 1999, 354(9195):2048–9.

14. http://orthomolecular.org/resources/omns/v06n08.shtml.

"The history of medicine is full of ideas and treatments which are acceptable today but which were rejected out of hand for 40 years and more."

—ABRAM HOFFER, M.D.

Preparation of Sodium Ascorbate for Intravenous and Intramuscular Use

Fully aware that the title of this book is *Doctor Yourself,* this IV preparation guide is not for personal home use. It is for your physician. Intravenous or injectable use of a vitamin absolutely requires your physician's participation. DO NOT ATTEMPT TO SELF-INJECT.

The following is written by Dr. Robert Cathcart and published with his permission. He sent this out in the form of a letter to physicians requesting his guidance on the subject of intravenous vitamin C.

The Stock Bottle of Sodium Ascorbate

Sterilize a 500 cc IV bottle along with a funnel, the rubber stopper, and a spoon. Then fill the bottle to the 300 cc line with sodium ascorbate fine crystals. (I weighed the sodium ascorbate out one time and 250 gm came up to the 300 cc line.) Then add $1/3$ of the 20 ml bottle (6.6 cc) of edetate disodium injection, USP 150 mg/ml. Then add water for injection q.s. 500 cc. Shake up the bottle and if there is 1 mm of crystals left on the bottom, add 1 mm of water to the top. It turns out that sodium ascorbate is soluble to almost exactly a 50 percent concentration at room temperature. I do not worry about the sterility of this because this is very bacteriocidal. Perhaps it should be filtered to get out particulate matter but I have never seen this to be a problem. The pH of this has always turned out to be 7.4. My nurse discovered recently that if you do not shake the mixture to make it go into solution until after you refrigerate it and are ready to use it that the solution is less yellow. I presume that this is good because sodium ascorbate is clear and dehydroascorbate is yellow. The made up solutions are always a little yellow but refrigeration before mixing results in a far less yellow mixture.

Preparation of the IV Bottle

I recommend that the above stock bottle solution be added to lactated Ringer's such that 30 g (grams) (60 cc) to 60 g (120 cc) this be added to a quantity of lactated Ringer's sufficient to make 500 cc of the final solution to be injected IV. I had been using water for injection some time ago because this solution is several times hypertonic already and I did not want to add more tonicity. However, recently I have found that lactated Ringer's feels better to patients so I use that for the final dilution (not the stock solution described above).

Intramuscular Injections

IM injection material for infants is made from the stock solution diluted 50 percent in water giving a 25 percent solution. Generally, the size of the injection can be 2 cc in each buttocks.

362

Ice may be applied if it hurts to much. This may be given every hour or so, frequently enough to bring the fever or other symptoms of excessive free radicals down rapidly.

General Comments

I have not had any trouble with these solutions. I hear all sorts of weird stories from patients who have gotten ascorbate elsewhere. I do not know if it is an acid problem (because ascorbic acid was used rather than sodium ascorbate) or whether some colleges get carried away with what other things they add to the intravenous solutions.

I think that there may be, at times, minor troubles with commercially prepared solutions because of the following. I understand that the U. S. Pharmacopeia specifies that the solutions be made from ascorbic acid and then buffered with sodium hydroxide or sodium bicarbonate to a pH between 3.5 and 7.0. I worry that 60 grams of ascorbate at a pH of 3.5 is too acid. I know that Klenner (the first physician who used high dose intravenous ascorbate by vein) also made his solutions from sodium ascorbate powder.

I watch patients for hypocalcemia (although I have not seen it), hypoglycemia (I encourage patients to eat while taking the IV), and dehydration (I encourage water and slow the IV down.) I also see headaches afterward but not so much since I have been emphasizing the continuing high doses of oral ascorbic acid as soon as the IV is over. Actually I give oral ascorbic acid while the IV is going to get a double effect. Bowel tolerance goes up while the IV is running but one has to be careful to stop giving oral C about an hour before the IV stops or else you may get diarrhea as soon as the IV stops. The oral ascorbic acid is then started again one-half to one hour after the IVC stops.

If the physician does not want to make their sodium ascorbate stock solutions from scratch like I recommend (and I can well understand why you might not), you can order from several suppliers. Ask for "Sodium Ascorbate Fine Crystals."

Above by Robert F. Cathcart, M.D. Reprinted with permission of the author.

Additional Notes

This is Andrew Saul speaking again. I would like to emphasize that ascorbate (vitamin C) for intravenous use is not at all difficult for a physician or hospital to obtain from various suppliers. An Internet search is recommended. I wish to reassert that I have no financial connection whatsoever with any health products company.

Vitamin C in high, **very frequent** oral doses will achieve blood plasma concentrations approaching, but not equaling, intravenous infusion.

By "high," I mean in the range of 30,000 to 100,000 milligrams per day, and 1,000–2,000 milligrams **per dose**.

By "very frequent," I mean taking 1,000–2,000 mg **every ten minutes** you are awake.

How do you know if you took enough? You feel better.

How do you know if you took too much? You will have loose stools. At that point, of course, you back off and take less.

How much less? Enough to still feel better, and not so much as causes loose stools.

If you do not think this will work, it is probably because you have not tried it.

Or, perhaps because you need to read the following especially important and helpful material:

Hickey S and Roberts H. *Ascorbate: The science of vitamin C.* 2004. Lulu Press. Reviewed at www.doctoryourself.com/ascorbate. html.

Duconge J et al. Pharmacokinetics of vitamin C: insights into the oral and intravenous administration of ascorbate. *PR Health Sciences Journal,* 2008. 27:1, March.

Cathcart RF. Vitamin C, titrating to bowel tolerance, anascorbemia, and acute induced scurvy. *Med Hypotheses.* 1981 Nov;7(11):1359–76. Free access to full text paper at www.doctoryourself.com/titration.html

See also: Cathcart RF. The third face of vitamin C. *Journal of Orthomolecular Medicine,* 7:4;197–200, 1993. Free access to full text paper at www.orthomoleculartherapy.net/library/jom/1992/pdf/1992-v07n04-p197.pdf or www.doctoryourself.com/cathcart_ thirdface.html

Other papers by Dr. Cathcart are posted at www.orthomed.com and www.doctoryourself.com/biblio_cathcart.html.

For Further Reading

1. Rath M, Pauling L. Immunological evidence for the accumulation of lipoprotein(a) in the atherosclerotic lesion of the hypoascorbemic guinea pig. *Proc Natl Acad Sci U.S.A.,* 1990 (23):9388–90. PMID: 2147514. Free full text download: www.pnas.org/content/87/23/9388.full.pdf.

2. Rath M, Pauling L. Hypothesis: lipoprotein(a) is a surrogate for ascorbate. *Proc Natl Acad Sci U.S.A.* 1990 87(16):6204–7. [Erratum in: *Proc Natl Acad Sci U S A* 1991 88(24):11588.] PMID: 2143582. Free full text download: www.pnas.org/content/87/16/6204.full.pdf.

3. Rath M, Pauling L. Solution to the puzzle of human cardiovascular disease: Its primary cause is ascorbate deficiency leading to the deposition of lipoprotein(a) and fibrinogen/fibrin in the vascular wall. *J Orthomolecular Med,* 1991, 6:125. Free full text download: http://orthomolecular.org/library/jom/1991/pdf/1991-v06n03&04-p125.pdf.

4. Pauling L, Rath M. An orthomolecular theory of human health and disease. *J Orthomolecular Med,* 1991, 6:135. Free full text download: http://orthomolecular.org/library/jom/1991/pdf/1991-v06n03&04-p135.pdf.

5. Rath M, Pauling L. Apoprotein(a) is an adhesive protein. *J Orthomolecular Med,* 1991, 6:139. Free full text download: http://orthomolecular.org/library/jom/1991/pdf/1991-v06n03&04-p139.pdf.

6. Rath M, Pauling L. Case Report: Lysine/ascorbate related amelioration of angina pectoris. *J Orthomolecular Med,* 1991. 6: 144. Free full text download: http://orthomolecular.org/library/jom/1991/pdf/1991-v06n03&04-p144.pdf.

7. Rath M, Pauling L. A unified theory of human cardiovascular disease leading the way to the abolition of this diseases as a cause for human mortality. *J Orthomolecular Med,* 1992, 7:5. Free full text download: http://orthomolecular.org/library/jom/1992/pdf/1992-v07n01-p005.pdf.

8. Rath M, Pauling L. Plasmin-induced proteolysis and the role of apoprotein(a), lysine and synthetic lysine analogs. *J Orthomolecular Med,* 1992, 7:17. Free full text download: http://orthomolecular.org/library/jom/ 1992/pdf/1992-v07n01-p017.pdf.

For More Information

Fonorow O. Practicing Medicine *Without a License? The Story of the Linus Pauling Therapy for Heart Disease.* 2008. Lulu.com. Reviewed in *J Orthomolecular Med,* 2009. Vol 24, No 1, pp 51–5.

Hickey S and Roberts H. *Ascorbate: The Science of Vitamin C.* 2004. Lulu.com. This book contains 575 references, and is reviewed at www.doctoryourself.com/ascorbate.html.

Hickey S, Saul AW. *Vitamin C: The Real Story.* Laguna Beach, CA: Basic Health Publications, 2008. This book contains 387 references, and is reviewed at www.doctoryourself.com/realstory.html.

Levy TE. *Stop America's #1 Killer: Reversible vitamin deficiency found to be the origin of all coronary heart disease.* 2006. (Dr. Levy is a board-certified cardiologist.) Reviewed in *J Orthomolecular Med,* 2006. Vol 21, No 3, pp 177–178. This book contains 60 pages of references. To download the review: http://orthomolecular.org/ library/jom/2006/pdf/2006-v21n03-p175.pdf.

Pauling L. *How to Live Longer and Feel Better* (Revised edition). Oregon State University Press, 2006. Reviewed in *J Orthomolecular Med,* 2006. Vol 21, No 3, pp 175–177. To download the review: http://orthomolecular.org/ library/jom/2006/pdf/2006-v21n03-p175.pdf.

How to Get Intravenous Vitamin C Given to a Hospitalized Patient

"The three most important considerations in effective vitamin C therapy are dose, dose, and dose. If you don't take enough, you won't get the desired effects."
—THOMAS LEVY, M.D.

For very serious illnesses, parenteral (infused or injected) administration of vitamin C is more effective than even the largest of oral doses. While I personally have seen aggressive oral doses beat illnesses as bad as viral pneumonia, the vitamin C specialists (such as William McCormick, Frederick Klenner, Robert Cathcart, and Hugh Riordan) all give megavitamin C therapy by intravenous infusion or intramuscular injection. Since electing this procedure necessarily makes you dependent on a doctor, I have some very specific ideas and instructions as to how you can arrange for an IV of vitamin C.

1. Know before you go. It is immeasurably easier to get what you want if you contract for it beforehand. Prenuptial agreements, new car deals, roofing and siding estimates, and hospital care need to be negotiated in advance. When the tow truck comes, it is too late to complain about who's driving. Same with an ambulance, or a hasty hospital admission. You have to pre-plan, and here's how:

2. Get a letter. Yes, a "note from the doctor" still carries clout. Have your general practitioner sign a letter stating that he backs your request for a vitamin C IV drip, 10 grams (10,000 mg) per 12 hours, should you (or your designated loved one) require hospitalization. Have copies made and keep them handy. Update the letter annually. You now have your G.P.'s permission. Good start, but not enough.

3. Get some more letters. Try to obtain a similar letter from every specialist that you have used, are using, or may use in the foreseeable future. This sounds cumbersome, but is no more unmanageable than most people's grocery lists. Keep it in perspective: this is just as important as wearing a medical-alert bracelet or keeping a fresh battery in Grandpa's pacemaker.

4. Make some calls. Telephone a representative or two from every hospital within fifty miles of your home. Find out which wants your business the most. When you find a "live one" on the phone, write down their name and title, and follow up with a letter.

5. Write for your rights. In your letter, ask for the hospital's permission to have a vitamin C IV drip, infusion, push, or injection, as well as oral vitamin C, should you or your designated family member(s) come in to that hospital. *You must get this in writing.* Now, do *not* say, "I want that in writing," because people do not like that. But if you write to them by U.S. Mail, they will naturally write back to you. Bingo. Don't correspond by e-mail; you want a real signature on hospital letterhead. (And no, don't ask for that either. It will happen automatically if you write first.)

You might be wondering, What if they write back, "No, we won't." Hold onto that letter. You can make a real stink with it should you need to play hardball in court, and I don't mean a handball court. More likely, however, they simply won't write back. Would you entrust your life to a hospital that refuses to even answer their mail? Make a point to go somewhere else. If you live in a rural community or smaller city, you might be thinking that you do not have a choice of hospitals. But people can be moved. It happens all the time.

Maybe not for the first twenty-four hours in an unexpected circumstance. But people can be moved. That's what modern transportation is for. Famous hospitals get people from all over. How many people do you know that live within walking distance of Sloan-Kettering, Roswell, the Brigham, or the Mayo Clinic?

What is most likely is that the hospital's representative will send you a garbage answer, so noncommittal as to be unusable. Try this: have your doctor "write" the letter. The doctor's letterhead and signature; your composition. You can give a professional a rough draft of what you want said. I had a lawyer ask me to do exactly that when I sought (and succeeded in getting) a vitamin C IV for my hospitalized father. I wrote it and faxed it to the attorney; his staff rewrote it on his stationery and he signed it. It saves time. Be sure your doctor's letter clearly requests a reply.

It is also quite possible that they will ask for more information. This could be a genuine interest, but it is more likely a stall. If you think Nero fiddled while Rome burned, you should see what medical bureaucrats can do. To cut through the treacle, you need to understand the nature of the beast. The first rule of lion taming is, You have to know more than the lions. Therefore:

6. Know the law. Many states have enacted legislation that makes it possible for a physician to provide any natural therapy that a patient requests without fear of losing his or her license. If your state has such a law, it will make it easier to get a doctor to prescribe a vitamin C IV.

7. Know the power structure. Find out who is in charge. I have heard doctors say that they'd be happy to start a vitamin C IV, but the hospital will not let them. Then, when asked, I have heard the hospital say that they allow vitamin C IVs but the doctors won't do them. To avoid an endless Catch-22 situation, you have to know the ropes and where everybody stands. Go to the person that can do you the most good (or harm) and start your negotiations there. If you can persuade the king, the castle is yours.

On the hospital side, which of the administrators has the clout? Talk to their secretaries (they are the people who really run things anyway) and you will find out. It could be that the most influential person for you may be the hospital's patient rights advocate or VP for customer service. It might even be the public relations director. Who knows? You sure don't, so remove the veil of anonymity and find out.

The patient, if conscious, has all the power because it is her body. If a patient insists loud and long enough, she can get almost anything. Since patients tend to be sick, and therefore easily slip into becoming noncombatants, a family member has to get in there and pitch for them. A highly experienced nurse told me that she would never leave a family member in a hospital without a twenty-four-hour-a-day guard in the form of a friend or family member or other advocate. That is sound advice from a lady who's seen it.

Next to the patient, the most powerful family member is the spouse. After that, it would be children. You do not have to have power of attorney, but it helps. If the patient is unable to speak, act, or think, it may be essential. Do not wait until the patient is incapacitated to plan this. Your family needs to come together and present a preplanned, unified front to the medical and administrative people. You may think I am overstating the case, but I have seen patients die simply because no one took the reins and got the C in the veins. I have seen vitamin C IVs halted simply because the patient was moved to intensive care. Think that one over. I have seen vitamin C prescriptions overruled by a nurse or pharmacist. You would not think that possible, would you? Well, it is. There is no nice way to phrase this. Stay on top of the situation or you will have a premature burial on your hands.

8. Know your recourse. If you are getting nowhere, and also rich, get your lawyer on the phone. Better yet, bring your lawyer to the hospital. If you are like the rest of us, you may simply have to bluff if you threaten to call your attorney. The purpose here is to save the life of your loved one, not to make a buck from a malpractice suit. Personally, I think malpractice suits are a sign of the most abject failure on the part of the family, as well as the medical profession. In the same way that accident insurance does not prevent accidents but only pays the costs, so do malpractice settlements fail to resuscitate a dead family member. "Death control" is somewhat like birth control in that you have to act before the event takes place. If we push the analogy, we realize a grim truth: there is no such thing as a "morning after" pill for rigor mortis.

9. Know the facts about vitamin C IVs. For this, there is absolutely no alternative to reading up on the subject. You will want to begin with medical papers written by Frederick Klenner, Robert Cathcart, Ewan Cameron, and Hugh Riordan. This book's bibliography contains many titles you can begin with.

10. Know how to avoid the run-around. Doctors and hospitals are quick to offer rather bogus reasons why they would deny your request for a vitamin C IV. Each of these arguments is a lot of bull, and easily refuted.

Their argument: "We do not have vitamin C for intravenous infusion in our pharmacy."

Your response: "So get some. Or just make it yourselves." From another hospital; by Fed Ex, by medevac helicopter. Or, just make it yourselves. Instructions on how to prepare it, written by a highly experienced physician, begin on page 362.

Their argument: "We've never done this before."

Your response: "Then this is a wonderful opportunity to learn. I've never lost a (insert family member's position here) before."

Their argument: "The patient is too ill."

Your response: "That's why we want the vitamin C IV."

Their argument: "We might get into trouble if we do this."

Your response: "You will be in legal trouble for sure if you don't."

Their argument: "There is no scientific evidence that this is safe, effective, appropriate for this case, blah, blah, blah . . . "

Your response: "Read this." (This short phrase is to be spoken as you produce a large stack of actual studies written by medical doctors who have successfully used vitamin C IVs. See references mentioned above.)

Their argument: "But we do not have time to read all those papers."

Your response: "That's okay. I already have, and it's my body (or my father's, or my mother's). Run the vitamin C IV. Start with 10 grams every 12 hours and do not stop it without my written authorization."

Their argument: "This hospital operates under our authority, these are our rules, and this is the way it is done."

Your response: "This is my mother. If you deny her the treatment the family requests, you will be sued, and we will win. Do you really want to go to the wall on this one?"

Confrontational? Yes. But I have seen too many people die too soon. Frederick Klenner was right when he said, "Some physicians would stand by and see their patient die rather than use ascorbic acid."

Don't let it happen to your family.

Further Reading

Duconge J, et al. Pharmacokinetics of vitamin C: insights into the oral and intravenous administration of ascorbate. *PR Health Sciences Journal,* 2008. 27:1.

Hoffer A, Saul AW, Hickey S. *Hospitals and Health: Your Orthomolecular Guide to a Shorter, Safer Hospital Stay.* Laguna Beach, CA: Basic Health Publications, 2011.

Vitamin C and the Law

by Thomas E. Levy, M.D., J.D.

"In health there is freedom. Health is the first of all liberties."
—HENRI-FREDERIC AMIEL

As a patient, you have the right to any therapy that is established to be effective, not prohibitively expensive, and not prohibitively toxic.

Any physician, or panel of hospital-based physicians, claiming that vitamin C is experimental, unapproved, and/or posing unwarranted risks to the health of the patient, is really only demonstrating a complete and total ignorance or denial of the scientific literature. A serious question as to what the real motivations might be in the withholding of such a therapy then arises.

A doctor has the right to refuse to see you or treat you. A doctor does not have the right to deny you any therapy that is inexpensive and known to be effective and nontoxic; if there is toxicity involved, the patient can discharge his responsibility for such toxicity with proper informed consent. A doctor does not have the right to deny you consultation with another doctor that may have conflicting medical points of view.

Just as ignorance of the law is no sound defense to legal charges brought against you, ignorance of medical fact is ultimately no sound defense for a doctor withholding valid treatment, especially when that information can be easily accessed

While a hospital may or may not have a legal right to dictate to its physicians what they may or may not do, the patient and the family of the patient have the legal right to sue that hospital for any negative outcome that is perceived to directly result from such interference in patient care.

The patient and the family of the patient also have the right to sue any physician that refuses to administer an inexpensive, nontoxic therapy that is established to be of use in the medical literature, such as vitamin C, especially when no other options other than permitting the patient to die are offered. Doctors have a very strong herd mentality, and they do not thrive well when forced to deal with a lawsuit alone, and possibly not even with the backup of their malpractice insurance company, which would seriously question why an approved medicine such as vitamin C was withheld from the patient. Remember that any insurance company always looks for a legal way not to pay expenses or settlements.

In a court of law, legal decisions regarding medical issues are usually decided by comparing a doctor's actions (or inactions) to the accepted standards of medical practice in the community in question. The legal sticking points relate to how different that community might be from others, and whether the accepted standard of practice is too far deviated from overall mainstream medicine norms.

The legal system struggles with reconciling something well-established in the medical literature, but not reflected in the standard medical textbooks. A case involving withheld vitamin C would not currently have any direct legal precedent of which I am aware, but there are multiple reasons to believe that the time is ripe for the law to rule for the patient's right to receive vitamin C in the hospital over the doctor's "right" to withhold it.

369

The time for changing the view of vitamin C by the law and mainstream medicine has arrived. Over the past twenty years, many more doctors have begun to routinely give 50 grams (50,000 mg) or more of vitamin C intravenously on a regular basis to patients with the entire gamut of medical conditions. These doctors have come from the same medical schools and postgraduate training programs as their unlike-minded mainstream counterparts, meaning they have the same traditional credentials and warrant equal consideration.

The law recognizes that there is no one perfect medical approach to a patient. Having an increasingly large body of doctors who recognize the importance of vitamin C will allow the courts to permit an additional "school of thought" as long as enough traditionally trained doctors think that way. The question yet to be legally determined is: How many such doctors is "enough?"

Under United States law, the long-standing *Frye* standard (1923) held that expert opinion based on a scientific technique is admissible only where the technique is generally accepted as reliable in the relevant scientific community. This standard made it almost impossible for any technique embraced by a minority, however competent or appropriately trained, to ever coexist with, much less supersede, a technique embraced by the larger scientific community. Basically, majority always wins, and minority always loses.

The *Daubert* standard (1993) finally replaced the *Frye* standard. *Daubert* held that the court should:

1. Evaluate whether the science can be or has been tested

2. Determine whether the science has been published or peer-reviewed

3. Consider the likelihood of error (quality and quantity of the data)

4. Evaluate the general acceptance of the theory in the scientific community

If the court is so inclined, the evaluation of general acceptance in the scientific (medical) community does not have to invoke the "majority rules" nature of the earlier *Frye* standard. Rather, it can allow the consideration that enough scientific studies embraced by enough qualified doctors could prevail legally. However, any final ruling would be heavily dependent on the particular facts of the case and the precise intervention requested of the court.

The principles of *Daubert* do not assure a victory for vitamin C proponents in a court of law, but they do allow an objective judge to see that the body of evidence supporting vitamin C usage is clearly established in the mainstream medical literature, warranting a thorough legal evaluation as to why it is not yet a permissible therapy. These principles allow for much more flexibility than the earlier *Frye* "majority rules" standard. Also, with any individual case in which a doctor refuses to administer vitamin C and serious damage (including death) occurs, a strong legal case can be now be made that the burden of proof falls with the doctor to show:

1. that the therapy was exceptionally expensive, toxic, and/or unproven

2. that the patient's best interests were somehow best served by withholding vitamin C

Always try to make an alliance with your doctor and avoid an adversarial relationship if at all possible. Theoretically, if your doctor really wants to do what is best for the patient and is not more concerned with being told what to do, much stress and conflict can be avoided by all. However, do not hesitate to let your doctor know directly that you will avail yourself of all your rights or your family member's rights as a patient to optimal health care if so forced.

A very common "out" in all of these scenarios is to suggest that "further studies" should be done. More information is always useful, but vitamin C has already been researched more than any other supplementor even most pharmaceutical drugsin the history of the planet. Don't allow another seventy years of research to transpire before its proper use begins.

Stand up for your rights today. The way medicine is practiced will never change until the public demands it and the law legitimizes it. Remember, it's your body and your health. Doctors are answerable to you, not you to them.

Thomas Edward Levy, M.D., J.D. is certified in Internal Medicine and is also a Fellow of the American College of Cardiology. He was admitted to the Colorado Bar in 1998 and the District of Columbia Bar in 1999.

References

Frye v. United States, 293 F. 1013 (D.C. Cir. 1923)

Daubert v. Merrell Dow Pharmaceuticals, 509 U.S. 579 (1993)

An expanded version of "Vitamin C and the Law" by Dr. Levy is available as a free pdf download at www.tomlevymd.com/downloads/VC.NZ.Sept.2010.pdf or www.doctoryourself.com/VC.NZ.Sept.2010.pdf.

Safety of Nutritional Supplements

"An important scientific innovation rarely makes its way by gradually winning over and converting its opponents. What does happen is that its opponents gradually die out and that the growing generation is familiar with the idea from the beginning."

—MAX PLANCK

If you have been told that high-dose nutrient therapy is useless or harmful, this is the chapter for you. Compared to death, little else is all that important. So let's look first at the greatest safety concern: mortality.

NO DEATHS FROM VITAMINS—NONE AT ALL IN TWENTY-EIGHT YEARS

Over a twenty-eight year period, vitamin supplements have been alleged to have caused the deaths of a total of eleven people in the United States. A new analysis of US poison control center annual report data indicates that there have, in fact, been no deaths whatsoever from vitamins . . . none at all, in the 28 years that such reports have been available.

The American Association of Poison Control Centers (AAPCC) attributes annual deaths to vitamins as:

2010 zero	2003: two	1996: zero	1989: zero
2009: zero	2002: one	1995: zero	1988: zero
2008: zero	2001: zero	1994: zero	1987: one
2007: zero	2000: zero	1993: one	1986: zero
2006: one	1999: zero	1992: zero	1985: zero
2005: zero	1998: zero	1991: two	1984: zero
2004: two	1997: zero	1990: one	1983: zero

Even if these figures are taken as correct, and even if they include intentional and accidental misuse, the number of alleged vitamin fatalities is strikingly low, averaging less than one death per year for over two and a half decades. In 19 of those 28 years, AAPCC reports that there was not one single death due to vitamins.[1]

Still, one might be curious: Did eleven people ***really*** die from vitamins? And if so, how?

Vitamins Not *THE* Cause of Death

In determining cause of death, AAPCC uses a four-point scale called Relative Contribution to Fatality (RCF). A rating of 1 means "Undoubtedly Responsible"; 2 means "Probably Responsible"; 3 means "Contributory"; and 4 means "Probably Not Responsible." In examining poison control data for the year 2006, listing one vitamin death, it was seen that the vitamin's Relative Contribution to Fatality (RCF) was a 4. Since a score of "4" means "Probably Not Responsible," it quite negates the claim that a person died from a vitamin in 2006.

Vitamins Not *A* Cause of Death

In the other seven years reporting one or more of the remaining ten alleged vitamin fatalities, studying the AAPCC reports reveals an absence of any RCF rating for vitamins in any of those years. If there is no Relative Contribution to Fatality at all, then the substance did not contribute to death at all.

Furthermore, in each of those remaining seven years, there is no substantiation provided to demonstrate that any vitamin was a cause of death.

If there is insufficient information about the cause of death to make a clear-cut declaration of cause, then subsequent assertions that vitamins cause deaths are not evidence-based. Although vitamin supplements have often been blamed for causing fatalities, there is no evidence to back up this allegation.

In 2009, two people died from non-nutritional mineral poisoning, one from a sodium salt, and one from an iron salt or iron. On page 1139, the AAPCC report for that year[2] specifically indicates that the iron fatality was not from a nutritional supplement. One other person is alleged to have died from an "Unknown Dietary Supplement or Homeopathic Agent." This claim remains speculative, as no verification information was provided.

By the Numbers

Sixty poison centers provide coast-to-coast data for the U.S. National Poison Data System, "one of the few real-time national surveillance systems in existence, providing a model public health surveillance system for all types of exposures, public health event identification, resilience response and situational awareness tracking."

Over half of the U.S. population takes daily nutritional supplements. Even if each of those people took only one single tablet daily, that makes over 160,000,000 individual doses per day, for a total of nearly 60 billion doses annually. Since many persons take more than just one vitamin or mineral tablet, actual consumption is considerably higher, and the safety of nutritional supplements is all the more remarkable.

If nutritional supplements are allegedly so "dangerous," as the FDA and news media so often claim, then **where are the bodies?**

> **WARNING: Please do not take this box too seriously! It is satire.**
> **It may ring mighty true, but it is still fiction. Mostly.**
>
> ### CONFIDENTIAL MEMORANDUM FROM THE WORLD HEADQUARTERS OF PHARMACEUTICAL POLITICIANS, EDUCATORS AND REPORTERS (WHOPPER)
>
> **Most Secret: Your Eyes Only**
> Distinguished members, our decades of disparaging nutritional therapy have paid off at last. The public, and their healthcare providers, are completely hoodwinked. By pushing "evidence based medicine" on the medical professions, we have elegantly slipped in our choice of evidence to base medicine on. And this is no mere journeyman accomplishment: this is high art. Mr. Machiavelli would be pleased. Certainly the pharmaceutical cartel is. We are well on our way to eliminating the competition, namely that increasingly irritating "orthomolecular medicine" faction.
>
> Here's how we are winning the Vitamin War: It is entirely too obvious, from our reading the

nutritional literature, that vitamins and minerals are a well-proven, safe and effective therapy. Of course, anyone knows that to work they must be employed in appropriate doses, just as any drug must be given in an appropriate dose. That is the problem, but it is also our opportunity. Since high nutrient doses work all too well, we eliminate all those embarrassing positive high-dose results simply by ignoring them. By selecting, pooling and analyzing only unsuccessful low dose studies, our conclusions exactly fit what we want the public to believe.

We also make certain to use either synthetic or fractional vitamin E to "prove" that that nutrient not only has no therapeutic value, but is actually dangerous and can kill! Sure, it is an onion in the ointment that there have been no deaths from vitamin E in 28 years of poison control center reporting. But that's a mere fact, and easily ignored.

We are not going to rest on our proverbial laurels. Now that we have set the precedent for shaping medical practice into pharmaceutical hustling, there's even more we can accomplish.

Here is our master plan. We have solidly established that research data can be selected, pooled, meta-analyzed and then dictate solidly "scientific" conclusions. It is now a mere step to do the same in other disciplines, including education, politics, and the social sciences. For example:

- Using data only from poorly-funded urban schools, we can prove mathematically, by statistical analysis of grade-point-averages, that inner-city kids have no academic future.

- By collecting data as to how many 19th century women graduated from college, we can show that women then were not as qualified to vote as men are today, and overturn the 19th amendment.

- If we assemble data on screen time and analyze actors' roles from Hollywood movies made in the 1920s and 1930s, we can demonstrate that some races are best qualified to be domestic workers, tap dancers or to operate laundries.

- By giving a large sample of the homeless 25 cents each, we can show that higher personal income is ineffective against poverty.

- If we tabulate inventory at Ferrari dealerships exclusively, we can prove Hondas are scarce.

- Repeatedly taking the temperature of thousands of cadavers is justification that funeral homes do not need central heating, at least not at night.

Here is unlimited opportunity for social engineering, and we owe it all to S-EBM: Selective Evidence Based Medicine. Yes indeed: it logically proceeds from our widely-publicized analyses of vitamin supplementation, analyses that were limited to studies that used low doses. Math is a wonderful thing: when we sliced statistics into sound-byte-sized pieces, we even proved that vitamin E kills; vitamin C is worse; don't even THINK of taking those B-vitamin supplements; and even multivitamin pills are dangerous. Give us a just while longer: we will rip the carbons out of vitamin D next.

There is so much to look forward to!

References

1. Download any Annual Report of the American Association of Poison Control Centers from 1983–2009 free of charge at www.aapcc.org/dnn/NPDSPoisonData/NPDSAnnualReports.aspx. The "Vitamin" category is usually near the very end of the report.

2. Bronstein AC, Spyker DA, Cantilena LR Jr, Green JL, Rumack BH, and Giffin SL. 2010. 2009 Annual Report of the American Association of Poison Control Centers' National Poison Data System (NPDS): 27th Annual Report. *Clinical Toxicology* 48: 979–1178. The full text article is available as a free download at www.aapcc.org/dnn/Portals/0/2009%20AR.pdf. The data mentioned above are found in Table 22B, journal pages 1138–1148.

You may download any Annual Report of the American Association of Poison Control Centers from 1983–2010 free of charge at www.aapcc.org/dnn/NPDSPoisonData/NPDSAnnualReports.aspx.

374

Spin-Doctor Yourself

"No amount of evidence can persuade anyone who is not listening."
—ABRAM HOFFER, M.D., PH.D.

Pharmaceutical medicine daily attempts to monopolize the media. The vast amount of cash the drug industry puts out to purchase drug advertisements underwrites much of the broadcasting and publishing industries. Advertiser income garners fealty from newspapers, magazines, and television. Not surprisingly, they have done a fairly good job of ignoring the benefits of nutritional medicine.

It is not working. You cannot fool all of the people all of the time.

Perhaps they think that no one is searching the Internet for a second opinion, and that people only read and believe what they, the major magazines and newspapers, select as fit to print. Maybe the TV networks have forgotten about YouTube, and websites where there is a growing presence of free-access orthomolecular video. One especially noteworthy example is a free-access collection of intravenous vitamin C instructional videos for doctors at http://orthomolecular.org/resources/omns/v07n03.shtml.

On the other hand, there are popular but unreliable Internet sources, like Wikipedia. If you want to read what cliques of amateurs have need to say about subjects that do or do not fit their belief systems, be my guest. I taught for the State University of New York for nine years, and I never met a single faculty member that would pay the slightest heed to a Wikipedia reference. They know better. You know better. That is why I urge you to go directly to academics, researchers, and physicians for information and commentary. Many years ago, my father taught me that when you want to know, "Go to the organ grinder, not the monkey."
Let's do that right now.

Doctors Say: Vitamins Are Safe and Effective

The news media regularly proclaim that taking vitamin supplements is of no value and, somehow, actually dangerous. You have likely already heard an earful from reporters. Now let's hear from doctors.

Michael Janson, M.D.

The standard American diet does not provide even the RDA. Two-thirds of all meals are eaten outside the home, and nearly half of them are in fast-food joints. You can't expect this to provide all the necessary nutrients, and many studies show that it does not. A large number of people admitted to hospitals are found to have deficiencies, and the problems worsen in the hospital. Those given supplements have a lower rate of complications, faster discharge from the hospital, and fewer deaths. Vitamin companies do not send doctors on expense-paid vacations or "seminars," as do the drug companies for prescribing their drugs, and vitamins are safe and cheap. But surely this does not influence pharmaceutical-advertising-paid-for media!

Vitamin E in high doses (800 IU) enhances immunity in healthy elderly subjects. Vitamin C in doses (2,000 mg) far above the RDA (90 mg) significantly reduces allergic rhinitis and asthma and speeds the recovery from airway constriction induced by histamine. Vitamin B$_1$ (thiamin) was used successfully to treat trigeminal neuralgia, as described in an article published in the *Journal of the American Medical Association* way back in 1940.

Many people are losing their faith in the medical profession because many doctors are unwilling to accept what is becoming common knowledge: nutrition and nutrient therapies are safer, cheaper, and more effective than most other medical treatment. It is clear that most media reporters do not know the current nutrition literature, they do not know the old literature, and they do not know the middle-aged literature. If they do not know the literature, they should not be writing articles.

Martin Gallagher, M.D., D.C.

I have been a practicing physician for thirty-seven years. During that time, I have directly treated and supervised over 12,000 patient encounters per year. With each patient, I have prescribed a variety of vitamins, minerals, homeopathic medicines, and herbs. I have to date not encountered a single complication, anaphylactic reaction, or death. The doses have been well above the RDA's for vitamins and minerals. In fact, the IV treatments include doses of ascorbate (vitamin C) that vary from 10,000 to over 100,000 mg per treatment session.

At a time when the leading cause of death in the US is correctly prescribed medication, we need to embrace, not chastise, nutritional supplements.

Robert G. Smith, Ph.D.

Most people in modern societies have vitamin and mineral deficiencies because these nutrients are removed by industrial food processing. Vitamin and mineral supplements are effective in preventing deficiencies that cause major illness such as heart disease, cancer, diabetes, arthritis, osteoporosis, dementia, and many others. Supplements of vitamins and minerals, when taken in proper doses large enough to work (for example: vitamin C for an adult at 3,000 to 6,000 mg/day, and much more when stressed or sick), are safe and effective—and far less expensive than taking prescribed drugs overblown by the medical profession and media.

Michael J. Gonzalez, Ph.D.

Research in Europe has shown that long-term users of antioxidant vitamin supplements have a 48 percent reduced risk of cancer mortality and 42 percent lower all-cause mortality.[1] The media did not bother to mention it. There is in fact overwhelming clinical evidence to justify the use of nutritional supplements for the prevention of disease and the support of optimal health. The Lewin Group estimated a $24 billion savings over five years if a few basic nutritional supplements were used in the elderly.[2] On the other hand, prescription medication kills over 100,000 people a year.[3]

Thomas Levy, M.D.

There are more politics in modern medicine than in modern politics itself. Today's average physician deserves even less trust than today's average politician, as doctors continue their refusal to allow the scientific data on the profound benefits of vitamins and other antioxidant supplements to reach their eyes and brains. And the staunch support of a press, which collectively no longer has a shred of journalistic or scientific integrity, completes the framing of today's colossal medical fraud. Money always rules the day: properly dosed vitamins would eliminate far too much of the profit of prescription-based medicine.

William B. Grant, Ph.D.

Modern lifestyles including wearing clothes and sunscreen and working and living largely indoors have led to widespread vitamin D deficiencies. Numerous ecological and observational studies have found correlations between higher solar UVB doses and vitamin D concentrations and reduced risk of many types of cancer, cardiovascular disease, diabetes mellitus, bacterial and viral infectious diseases, autoimmune diseases, falls and fractures, cognitive impairment, and many more types of disease. To compensate for lack of sun exposure, 1,000 to 5,000 IU per day of vitamin D_3 should be taken to raise serum 25-hydroxyvitamin D concentrations to at least 30–40 ng/ml (75–100 nmol/L). These amounts are safe for all but those with granulomatous diseases, who can develop hypercalcemia. 1,000 to 5,000 IU/day of vitamin D is effective in reducing risk of many types of diseases, as shown in a number of randomized controlled trials, such as cancer, falls and fractures, type A influenza, and pneumonia.

W. Todd Penberthy, Ph.D.

Niacin in particular has been shown to provide exceptional benefit in treating cardiovascular disease in clinical trial after clinical trial[4]. By comparison, the popular diabetes drug Avandia was recently found to cause a 43 percent increase in heart attacks in diabetics.[5] This came out only *after* Avandia had already become the most popular diabetes drug in the world! Never underestimate the power of market-driven forces to sell drugs, and books, such as *The End of Illness* by Dr. Agus, instead of proper information regarding what actually works best.

People are amazed how quickly simply taking supplemental niacin corrects high cholesterol, high triglycerides, low HDL (the good cholesterol), and VLDL. All of these parameters are pushed in the healthier direction because niacin ultimately functions inside the body in over 450 reactions. There is a reason niacin continues as a preferred therapy for doctors in the know, using niacin therapy for over fifty years now. Niacin works better than any drug to correct dyslipidemia.

One thing to always remember is this. You can "prove" that any drug or vitamin does *not* work if you are not using high enough doses to achieve the correct concentration of the molecule. Furthermore, all biochemical pathways rely on more than one molecule to function properly, so generally one drug/vitamin is not enough for optimal health. Our bodies rely on vitamins, not drugs, to routinely stave off illness by means we often take for granted. Sometimes we need much more of these essential molecules. This is common sense, and it is known as orthomolecular medicine.

James A. Jackson, Ph.D.

For over twenty years, I was the laboratory director of a federally approved clinical reference laboratory. We accepted samples from all the United States and foreign countries. We measured all the fat-soluble and water-soluble vitamins in blood and urine. It was common to find vitamin deficiencies in both males and females, whether children or adults. The most common vitamin deficiencies were vitamin C and vitamin D_3. The clinic's physicians treated the patients with the appropriate vitamins and were monitored by our laboratory. Many were helped by the vitamin replacement treatment, including those with complaints such as headache, joint and muscle pain, chronic fatigue syndrome, and ADHD. We published many of these cases in the *Journal of Orthomolecular Medicine*. (http://orthomolecular.org/library/ jom/index.shtml).

377

Ian Brightbope, M.D.

Over 70 percent of Australians consume vitamins on a regular basis. A search of the department of health's database reveals no serious adverse reactions or deaths have occurred in the Australian population over the past ten years from the use of complementary medicines. There is an extreme bias against very low- to extremely low-risk products by government regulators and health professionals working within and outside the establishment institutions.

Robert Jenkins, D.C., M.S.

I have been in practice for fifty-two years and have treated thousands of patients with diet and nutritional supplements for numerous health conditions ranging from hypertension, diabetes, hypercholesterolemia, metabolic syndrome, irritable bowel syndrome, and many others. I have yet to experience adverse patient reactions from taking nutritional supplements. I have lectured second year medical students at two medical schools in the Philadelphia, PA, area. When I asked those students how much nutritional training they had received, they all held up their hands with the sign of zero. The pharmaceutical industry makes sure medical students are trained in how to prescribe their drugs, while no positive mention is made of nutritional supplements. Why would anyone think that our modern medical doctors are to be considered authorities on nutritional supplementation for health conditions when they are not trained to do so? When this lack of nutritional education is combined with the news media's ignorance of supplements and their benefits, we have "the blind leading the blind."

Gert Schuitemaker, Ph.D.

In the Netherlands, a report of the Dutch Health Council states that less than 2 percent of the population is eating according to official dietary guidelines.[6] Moreover, the authorities state that, even if a person is eating according to the dietary guidelines, he is not getting enough vitamin A, D, folic acid, iron, selenium, and zinc.[7] Research in a Dutch hospital showed that 40 percent of patients at the time of admission were malnourished.[8] So, dietary supplements are necessary. Usually, chronic diseases, developing with increasing age, are treated with medicines, inevitably accompanied with the risk of severe side effects and unnecessary deaths. While the basis of many chronic diseases is a metabolic disturbance and nutritional deficiencies, the best treatment approach is good nutrition, including the use of dietary supplements. The "danger" of vitamins and minerals lies in chronic deficiencies, *not* in alleged toxic effects. Following the scientific literature on a daily basis, in thirty years I have not seen any harmful effect from supplements.

Damien Downing, M.D.

The more toxins you are exposed to, the more nutrients you will use up in dealing with them. Every year, we are exposed to more and more toxins, and our DNA has had no time to adapt: heavy metals such as lead, mercury, and fluorine; pesticides including the newer ones like glyphosate ("Roundup"); flame retardants that are even contaminating the Arctic; and hundreds of thousands of other new-to-nature molecules that every human has to deal with. And like it or not, pharmaceutical medications are mostly toxins too.

At the same time, intensive farming, soil depletion, and poor diets (often foisted on us for spurious reasons such as fear of cholesterol) mean that it's normal to be deficient now. We are deficient in vitamins, minerals, and other nutrients as well.

What chance does a human have? A much better one if she doesn't buy the hype from big companies, the dogma from pharma-paid scientists, and the bullying from governments. Take your vitamins.

Steve Hickey, Ph.D.

Over the past three centuries, the frequency of deficiency and infectious diseases has been reduced through improved nutrition and better hygiene. Throughout this time, however, the role of nutrition has been belittled by the authorities. These same authorities now reject the idea that nutritional supplements can prevent our current chronic diseases. Thus, as a result of such authoritarian medicine, we may have replaced the horrors of pellagra, scurvy, and rickets with those of dementia, heart disease, and cancer. If so, it is likely that people in the future will look back with similar dismay on the current and needless destruction of health. How will we answer them, when they ask how could we have allowed this to happen?

Carolyn Dean, M.D., N.D.

I've recommended vitamin and mineral supplements, herbs and homeopathy safely and effectively for 33 years with never a complaint or adverse reaction. In that same time every patient that comes to me has had a negative story to tell about prescription drugs and allopathic doctors. Patients should be informed that there are extremely safe, non-drug alternatives available to them. However, their rights are being denied for no other apparent reason than corporate greed. The rights and freedom of doctors to practice non-drug medicine are also being violated, which effectively keeps us all in the dark ages of medicine.

Dean Elledge, D.D.S., M.S.

The high-carbohydrate, nutrient-poor diet is a primary contributing factor in dental diseases.[9] Vitamin D and vitamin C are safe to use in dentistry to help the patient recover from dental diseases. Vitamins in general help reduce inflammation, and antioxidant vitamins reduce the inflammation in periodontal disease. Vitamin supplements improve antioxidant reserves.

Michael Ellis, M.D.

I see so many patients in conventional general practice who are deficient in vitamins. I had one patient who had ended up in a hospital neurosurgical unit only to be found to have severe B_{12} deficiency. The foods that most people eat are high in sugar, processed, and denatured of essential nutrients. All patients need, at the very least, daily multivitamins.

Ralph Campbell, M.D.

We have had lots of talk of the alleged "toxicity" of vitamins over the decades I have been in pediatric practice. I remain leery of the validity of such accusations. Most are just uninformed regurgitation of poorly designed studies. If alert, a clinician can easily detect vitamin deficiencies, and with experience, quickly spot suboptimal vitamin levels. The medical establishment seems to be increasingly aware of vitamin D, B_{12}, and folic acid deficiency. What is taking the media so long?

Karin Munsterhjelm-Ahumada, M.D.

I have been a physician for thirty-five years. For the last twenty years, I have worked with combining general medicine with nutritional (orthomolecular) medicine, the practice of preventing and treating disease by providing the body with optimal amounts of substances that are natural to the body, principally vitamins and minerals. I have had good opportunity to *compare* the results of my work as a GP from the time *before* I got knowledge of vitamins and minerals as therapeutic substances with the time *after* I had learned to integrate them in my work with patients. I can today certify that I have seen a great number of very positive results after beginning to integrate vitamins in my clinical work. The results have been particularly fine in neurologic and psychiatric conditions, including schizophrenia, and in hormonal and infectious diseases. During these last twenty years I have not seen severe side effects of orthomolecular substances. On the contrary, I have often been able to decrease the dosage of strong pharmaceutical drugs that carry severe side effects. This has led to a completely new and better quality of life for my patients, and for myself as a doctor.

Conclusion

The old saying remains true: the person who says it can't be done should not interrupt the person successfully doing it. Progressive doctors prescribe vitamins because they work. If your doctor doesn't "believe" in vitamins, maybe it is time for him or her to change such an antiquated belief system in favor of the true clinical evidence.

References

1. Li K, Kaaks R, Linseisen J, and Rohrmann S. Vitamin/mineral supplementation and cancer, cardiovascular, and all-cause mortality in a German prospective cohort (EPIC-Heidelberg). *Eur J Nutr.,* 2011, Jul 22.

2. Suh DC, Woodall BS, Shin SK, and Hermes-De Santis ER. Clinical and economic impact of adverse drug reactions in hospitalized patients. *Ann Pharmacother,* 2000, 34(12):1373–9.

3. Lazarou J, Pomeranz BH, and Corey PN. Incidence of adverse drug reactions in hospitalized patients: a meta-analysis of prospective studies. *JAMA,* 1998, 279(15):1200–5.

4. Carlson LA: Nicotinic acid: the broad-spectrum lipid drug. A 50th anniversary review. *J Intern Med,* 2005, 258: 94–114.

5. Nissen SE, and Wolski K: Effect of rosiglitazone on the risk of myocardial infarction and death from cardiovascular causes. *N Engl J Med,* 2007, 356:2457–2471.

6. Significant trends in food consumption in the Netherlands. The Hague: Health Council of the Netherlands, 2002; publication no. 2002/12.

7. Voedingscentrum. Richtlijnen goede voedselkeuze [The Netherlands Nutrition Centre. Guidelines Good Nutritional Choice]. 2011.

8. Naber TH, Schermer T, de Bree A, et al. Prevalence of malnutrition in nonsurgical hospitalized patients and its association with disease complications. *Am J Clin Nutr.,* 1997, 66(5):1232–9.

9. Elledge DA. Effective hemostasis and tissue management. *Dentistry Today,* Oct 2010, p.150.

(Used with permission of the Orthomomecular Medicine News Service)

Interpreting Research and Spotting Political Conclusions

Science is a great servant but a poor master. Not infrequently, it can exemplify what Harvard math professor Tom Lehrer satirized as where "the important thing is to understand what you're doing, rather than to get the right answer." Just because a published study suggests something does not make it true.

I never liked math very much, and I still don't. But I am indebted to dedicated math teachers who taught me in spite of myself. Decades ago, one such teacher gave me wise advice that spans all disciplines: "Look at your answer. Does your answer make sense?"

So when research suggests that vitamins somehow may actually cause cancer, it is time to hit the books. It may even occasionally be necessary to hit them right out of the way, and use common sense instead.

FOLIC ACID DOES NOT CAUSE CANCER

Folate, once known as vitamin B_9, is named after the dark green leafy vegetables it was first extracted from. *Folium* is Latin for "leaf." Leaves and greens are high in folate. Herbivorous animals get plenty of folate because they eat plenty of foliage. Carnivorous animals also get plenty of folate, because they consume herbivorous animals. In the wild, this means the entire animal, including its abdominal organs full of the prey's last meal of partially digested vegetation. Indeed, the viscera are typically the first thing a predator eats.

If folate caused cancer, the whole animal kingdom would have a lot of it. And while wild animals have their own problems, cancer is rarely one of them.

If you look at the research suggesting a human cancer connection (1,2), it does not say that folate in food causes cancer. The research only points to **folic acid**, as specifically found in supplements, as the bogeyman.

But there is virtually no difference whatsoever between the two forms of this nutrient. Folate and folic acid are different only in whether the carboxylic acid groups have dissociated or not. Folic acid's molecular formula is C19, **H19**, N7, O6. Folate's is C19, **H18**, N7, O6. The difference? Folate has one less hydrogen cation (H+). A hydrogen cation is a proton. A single proton. I have never seen evidence that protons cause cancer.

If folate/folic acid somehow caused cancer, it would have to be the rest of the molecule that is the problem. But most research shows that folic acid/folate prevents cancer. It is well-known that persons eating plant-based diets have a significantly lower risk of cancer. In addition to providing nutrients, eating more vegetation means more fiber and less constipation, valuable for preventing colon cancer. Herbivorous animals are definitely not constipated. Ask any dairy farmer, and you can start with me: many years ago, I used to milk 120 cows twice daily. When you walk behind Bossy, look out.

As for lung cancer, the research accusing folic acid also happens to show that 94 percent of the study subjects who developed lung cancer were either current or former smokers. Smoking causes cancer. Animals do not smoke. But they do eat a lot of foliage, either by grazing on greens or gorging on guts.

Both studies claiming that folic acid causes cancer were published in the *Journal of the American Medical Association* (*JAMA*), which also contains a large amount of pharmaceutical advertising. *JAMA* is among the journals that peer-reviewed research has shown to be biased against vitamins due to vested interests.[3]

What is more likely: that a small group of scientists made an error or two, or that all of Nature did? On this one, I am backing the animals. 1.8 million species can't be all wrong.

381

References

1. Folic acid, B12 may increase cancer risk. www.webmd.com/cancer/news/20091117/folic-acid-b12-may-increase-cancer-risk. Original study: www.ncbi.nlm.nih.gov/pubmed/19920236

2. High doses of folic acid may increase colon cancer risk. www.foxnews.com/story/0,2933,278237,00.html. Original study: www.ncbi.nlm.nih.gov/pubmed/17551129

3. Pharmaceutical advertising biases journals against vitamin supplements.

http://orthomolecular.org/resources/omns/v05n02.shtml. Original study: Kemper KJ, Hood KL. (2008). Does pharmaceutical advertising affect journal publication about dietary supplements? BMC *Complement Altern Med*. 8:11. Full text at www.biomedcentral.com/1472–6882/8/11 or www.pubmedcentral.nih.gov/articlerender.fcgi?tool=pubmed&pubmedid=18400092

A Closet Full of Drugs

"The best doctor gives the least medicines."
—BENJAMIN FRANKLIN

Once upon a time there was a young couple with two children in diapers. Across the hall from their ground-floor apartment lived a pharmaceutical salesman. He was a nice young fellow, quiet and easy to talk to. Since he was obviously single, the couple asked him over for some home-cooked meals now and again, and they all became good acquaintances.

The pharmaceutical salesman, also called a "detail man" in the profession, was on the road a lot, and not home to receive the many shipments that his employer sent him. Most of these were cases of drug samples to give away to physicians to promote the latest and greatest medicine of the month. Large trailer trucks would somehow negotiate their way through the narrow apartment complex access roads, twist their way around cars in the parking lot, and back up to the apartment building. Up went the back of the truck and off came boxes and boxes of drug samples, addressed to the man who was rarely home. Did the truckers go away with the cargo undelivered? Not likely, when there was a stay-at-home mother with two toddlers next door. Again and again they would knock on her door, explain that the delivery was for 5B across the hall, and ask her to sign for the shipment. She figured, why not? and accepted a handtruck or two of prescription chemicals. Sometimes they left them in the unlocked apartment hall closet outside her door. Sometimes it was full, so they left the big cartons stacked in her living room, as the kids waddled around.

You may have already guessed: This, many years ago, played out in my apartment building and I knew all the participants personally.

If some military supplies' mail-order warehouse delivered a few crates of guns and ammunition like this, there would be a public outcry fed by *60 Minutes* reports. The legal drug pushers get away with it.

DRUG ADVERTISING EXPENDITURES: THEN AND NOW

"Advertising spending for all prescription drugs was $55 million in 1991. By 1996, it had risen to $595 million. (Shane S. Depression patients face a blitz of drug advertising. *Baltimore Sun,* July 21, 1997.)

In 2010, prescription drug ad spending was **$4.3 billion**. That's $4300 million—**over 78 times as much**. (http://adage.com/images/bin/pdf/WPpharmmarketing_revise.pdf)

Vitamins are cheaper than drugs. Vitamins are safer than drugs. Vitamins prevent and cure many illnesses. The standard is not perfection; the standard is the alternative.

WHAT KIND OF MEDICAL STUDY WOULD HAVE GRANDMA BELIEVE THAT HER DAILY MULTIVITAMIN IS DANGEROUS?

by Robert G. Smith, Ph.D.

A study suggested that multivitamin and nutrient supplements can increase the mortality rate in older women.[1] However, there are several concerns about the study's methods and significance.

- The study was observational, in which participants filled out a survey about their eating habits and their use of supplements. It reports only a small increase in overall mortality (1 percent) from those taking multivitamins. This is a small effect, not much larger than would be expected by chance. Generalizing from such a small effect is not scientific.

- **The study actually reported that taking supplements of B complex, vitamins C, D, E, and calcium and magnesium were associated with a *lower* risk of mortality.** But this was not emphasized in the abstract, leading the non-specialist to think that all supplements were associated with mortality. The report did not determine the amounts of vitamin and nutrient supplements taken, nor whether they were artificial or natural. Further, most of the association with mortality came from the use of iron and copper supplements, which are known to be potentially inflammatory and toxic when taken by older people, because they tend to accumulate in the body.[2,3,4] The risk from taking iron supplements should not be generalized to imply that all vitamin and nutrient supplements are harmful.

- The study lacks scientific plausibility for several reasons. It tabulated results from surveys of 38,000 older women, based on their recall of what they ate over an eighteen-year period. But they were only surveyed three times during that period, relying only on their memory of what foods and supplements they took. This factor alone causes the study to be unreliable.

- Some of these women smoked (~15 percent) or had previously (~35 percent), some drank alcohol (~45 percent), some had high blood pressure (~40 percent), and many of them developed heart disease and/or cancer. Some preexisting medical conditions were taken into account by adjusting the risk factors, but this caused the study to contradict what we already know about efficacy of supplements. For example, the study reports an increase in mortality from taking vitamin D, when adjusted for several health-relevant factors. However, vitamin D has recently been clearly shown to be helpful in preventing heart disease[5] and many types of cancer,[6] which are major causes of death. Furthermore, supplement users were twice as likely to be on hormone replacement therapy, which is a more plausible explanation for increased mortality than taking supplements.

- The effect of doctor recommendations was not taken into account. By their own repeated admissions, **medical doctors and hospital nutritionists are more likely to recommend a daily multivitamin, and only a multivitamin, for their sicker patients**. The study did not take this into account. All it did was tabulate deaths and attempt to correct the numbers for some prior health conditions. The numbers reported do not reflect other factors such as developing disease, side effects of pharmaceutical prescriptions, or other possible causes for the mortality. The study only reports statistical correlations, and gives no plausible cause for a claimed increase in mortality from multivitamin supplements.

- The effect of education was not taken into account. When a doctor gives advice about illnesses, well-educated people will often respond by trying to be proactive. Some will take drugs prescribed by the doctor, and some will try to eat a better diet, including supplements of vitamins and nutrients. This is suggested by the study itself: the supplement users in the survey had more education than those who did not take supplements. It seems likely, therefore, the participants who got sick were more likely to have taken supplements. Because those who got sick are also more likely to die, it stands to reason that they would also be more likely to have taken supplements. This effect is purely statistical; it does not represent an increase in risk that taking supplements of vitamins and essential nutrients will cause disease or death. This type of statistical correlation is very common in observational health studies and those who are health-conscious should not be confounded by it.

- The known safety of vitamin and nutrient supplements when taken at appropriate doses was not taken into account. The participants most likely took a simple multivitamin tablet, which contains low doses. Much higher doses are also safe,[4,7] implying that the low doses in common multivitamin tablets are very safe. Further, because each individual requires different amounts of vitamins and nutrients, some people must take much higher doses for best health.[8]

Summary: In an observational study of older women in good health, it was said that those who died were more likely to have taken multivitamin and nutrient supplements than those who did not. The effect was small, and does not indicate any reason for disease or death. Instead, the study's methods suggest that people who have serious health conditions take vitamin and mineral supplements because they know that supplements can help. Indeed, the study showed a benefit from taking B complex, C, D, and E vitamins, and calcium and magnesium. Therefore, if those wanting better health would take appropriate doses of supplements regularly, they would likely continue to achieve better health and longer life.

References

1. Mursu J, Robien K, Harnack LJ, Park K, Jacobs DR Jr (2011) Dietary supplements and mortality rate in older women. The Iowa Women's Health Study. Arch Intern Med. 171(18):1625–1633.

2. Emery, TF. (1991). *Iron and your health: Facts and fallacies.* Boca Raton, FL: CRC Press.

3. Fairbanks, VF. (1999). Iron in medicine and nutrition." Chapter 10 in *Modern Nutrition in Health and Disease,* editors ME Shils, JA Olson, M. Shike, et al., 9th ed. Baltimore, MD: Williams & Wilkins.

4. Hoffer, A. and Saul, A.W. (2008). *Orthomolecular Medicine for Everyone: Megavitamin Therapeutics for Families and Physicians.* Laguna Beach, CA: Basic Health Publications.

5. Parker J, Hashmi O, Dutton D, Mavrodaris A, Stranges S, Kandala NB, Clarke A, Franco OH.(2010). Levels of vitamin D and cardiometabolic disorders: systematic review and meta-analysis. *Maturitas* 65(3):225–36.

6. Lappe, JM, Travers-Gustafson D, Davies KM, Recker RR, Heaney RP. (2007). Vitamin D and calcium supplementation reduces cancer risk: results of a randomized trial. *Am J Clin Nutr.* 85(6):1586–91.

7. Padayatty, SJ, Sun AY, Chen Q, Espey MG, Drisko J, Levine M. (2010). Vitamin C: intravenous use by complementary and alternative medicine practitioners and adverse effects. *PLoS One* 5(7):e11414.

8. Williams, RJ and Deason, G. (1967). Individuality in vitamin C needs. Proc Natl Acad Sci, USA. 57:1638–1641.

Also of Interest

Orthomolecular Medicine News Service, April 29, 2010. Multivitamins Dangerous? Latest News from the World Headquarters of Pharmaceutical Politicians, Educators, and Reporters: http://orthomolecular.org/resources/omns/v06n15.shtml.

Scientific Snobbery

The human body has not changed much over the past few decades. Indeed, it has not changed all that much for hundreds of thousands of years. Still, some medical apologists actually say that they only consider research of value if it is 1) only from the top medical journals and 2) only published in the last ten years. This is an interesting bit of bias. The top medical journals are specifically those that have been shown to be the most biased against nutritional therapy. And not surprisingly, the major journals are, correspondingly, the very ones with the most pharmaceutical ads.

In their article for *BMC Complementary and Alternative Medicine,* "Does Pharmaceutical Advertising Affect Journal Publication about Dietary Supplements?, the authors wrote: "In major medical journals, more pharmaceutical advertising is associated with publishing fewer articles about dietary supplements" and instead publishing more articles drawing "negative conclusions about dietary supplement safety. . . . Journals with the most pharmads published no clinical trials or cohort studies about supplements. The percentage of major articles concluding that supplements were unsafe was 4% in journals with fewest and 67% among those with the most pharmads." The authors further stated that "the ultimate impact of this bias on professional guidelines, health care, and health policy is a matter of great public concern."

Bo H. Jonsson, M.D., Ph.D., says: "Positive reports about the effects of high-dose vitamins have long been ignored by the medical establishment instead of being further examined scientifically."

The largest underreported scandal rocking the scientific world is medical research fraud due to financial conflicts of interest. It may be outright falsification of the data from drug studies to make them look favorable. It may also be publishers' refusal to publish research contrary to the interests of their largest advertisers.

385

References

Kemper KJ, Hood KL. Does pharmaceutical advertising affect journal publication about dietary supplements? *BMC Complement Altern Med.* 8:11, 2008. www.biomedcentral.com/1472–6882/8/11 or www.pubmedcentral.nih.gov/articlerender.fcgi?tool= pubmed&pubmedid=18400092.

Orthomolecular Medicine News Service, November 5, 2008. Rigged Trials: Drug Studies Favor the Manufacturer. http://orthomolecular.org/resources/omns/v04n20.shtml.

Drug studies skewed toward study sponsors. Industry-funded research often favors patent-holders, study finds. Vedantam S. *Washington Post,* April 11, 2006. www.msnbc.msn.com/id/12275329/from/RS.5/.

Heres S, Davis J , Maino K, et al. Why Olanzapine Beats Risperidone, Risperidone Beats Quetiapine, and Quetiapine Beats Olanzapine: An Exploratory Analysis of Head-to-Head Comparison Studies of Second-Generation Antipsychotics. *Am J Psychiatry* 163:185–194, February 2006. http://ajp.psychiatryonline.org/cgi/content/full/163/2/185.

Angell M. *The Truth about the Drug Companies.* New York: Random House, 2004. See also: Angell M. Is academic medicine for sale? *N Engl J Med.* 342(20):1516–8, 2000.

And these problems have been at their absolute worst in the last ten years.

Therefore, the promoters of so-called evidence based medicine are themselves relying on poor evidence. When they attack vitamin therapy, they are proceeding from false assumptions and flimsy bases. At best, for this is assuming no deliberate monopolistic intent.

Question Authority

Trust no one, including me. One especially wants to avoid putting their faith in so-called "consumer protection" folks who want you to fall in line and march in step. Having told you what is true, "consumer protectors" then tell you what to think. They want intellectual communism. They do not want well-informed consent. They want poorly informed compliance.

Cow cookies. Never give up your autonomy. Never! Protection is for children. They require it. You do not.

One day, when I was at a large furniture store, I heard a salesman speaking to a hesitant customer. She obviously loved the living room set he had shown her, but was reluctant to buy. She hedged by saying, "I have to bring a friend in to look at it." The salesman's response was, with a big smile: "Why? Does she have better taste than you?" Taken aback, the woman fell back on the unassailable alternative defense: "Well, I certainly have to bring my husband in first." The salesman replied, with an even bigger grin, "Why? Is he in charge of everything you do?" I thought for sure she was going to sock him one. She did not. She bought the living-room suite, and enjoyed every minute of it.

If you think I am trying to persuade you, you are correct. But I am not trying to persuade you to do what this book says. No, I am trying to persuade you to investigate what is reported in this book. Aha! Sneaky, yes? For all the case stories, dosage information and research references I have provided to you, by far the most subversive aspects of this book are its title and its key premise: think and do for yourself.

The elderly, distinguished, and perennially controversial journalist Helen Thomas was asked by a college student how, with all the divergent information out there, could one decide what to believe? Ms. Thomas's answer was, "Just read and make up your own mind. I trust you."

This book dares to trust your curiosity and your judgment. So do I.

Linus Pauling put it best, saying: "Do not let either the medical authorities or the politicians mislead you. Find out what the facts are, and make your own decisions about how to live a happy life and how to work for a better world."

Why I Did Not Die in Bio Lab

"It is time to lay to rest the notion that germs jump into people and cause diseases."

—EMANUEL CHERASKIN, M.D., D.M.D.

Let me tell you about the kid who was my lab partner in high school biology class, and who was always, always sick. Mike came to class hacking on what seemed to be an everyday basis. Naturally, his assigned seat was right next to me, at the shiny black-topped table-for-two that was so common in science classrooms. All through lectures, he sniffed, snorted, and sneezed. All through lab, he hacked, coughed, and gagged. This kid was sickly. You've got to give him high marks for showing up at all, but he had annoyingly good attendance, which was just my luck.

One day we were doing agar culture plates. This means you mix up some diarrhea-colored, Jell-O–like stuff, heat it, and pour it into shallow, round, four-inch-diameter glass dishes. After it cools, you add some bacteria or whatever microorganism you wish to grow. We'd stocked the incubator with a nice variety of specimens, and had a few extra, unused culture plates all dressed up and nowhere to go.

The lab manual said to leave one out in the classroom, uncovered, and see if a culture could be obtained from what settled out from the air. We went it one better.

We used Mike.

Almost at the same moment, we all came to the realization that Mike was our local one-stop source of pathogens. And, Mr. Thorensen being out of the room at that particular moment, our chance had come. We had Mike cough all over a couple of agar plates. I mean, he really let it all out. The girls turned away into their handkerchiefs. The boys grimaced and kept watching, wincing when a really shattering blast erupted from Mike's capacious lungs.

As Mike was mopping up the table in front of him, we light-footed it to the rear of the lab, covered our extracurricular cultures, and stuck them in the incubator, on the bottom shelf, way in the back. Visions of a Nobel dancing in our heads, we zipped back to our seats just as Mr. Thorensen walked in. We gave him our best cheesy smiles and folded our hands to await his next pronouncement, or the bell, whichever came first.

Naturally, we completely forgot about those culture plates. They were unlabeled, so nobody claimed them, but nobody threw them out, either.

Considerable time went by.

When Mr. Thorensen was out of the room again one day, we recalled our impromptu research project. My pal Sid and I went back to the old gray incubator, opened it, and reached all the way in. Ah yes, there they were, still. We brought the two dishes out and everyone gathered around to see some real science.

It was just gorgeous. Big, hairy black growths, white puffballs, and layers of milky slime covered the culture surface. Ugh. It looked like you'd exhumed the guts of a rotting carp. Gross. Then and there, we knew two things. First: Mike should, by all logic, be dead. Second: all too obviously, he wasn't.

Being Mike's closest friend, in a geographical sense, I had a personal stake in this. I should, at the very least, have had Mike's symptoms in spades.

But I didn't. Somehow, my body was keeping me healthy, in the face of the worst that Mike's propagated population of pathogens could do.

My life in natural healing began that very moment. Now, decades later, and with a duly reverent sense of history, I offer a view of the germ theory as Abraham Lincoln might have phrased it: *You can infect some of the people all of the time, and all of the people some of the time, but you cannot infect all of the people all of the time.* The elderly Pasteur was right: it is not the seed; it's the soil. You can cough on a steel plate and the culture will fail to thrive. If your body gets what it needs, it will stay healthy, no matter what lurks in the lungs of your neighbor.

AFTERWORD

Your Decision, Your Health, Your Life

"If you have a garden and a library, you have everything you need."
—MARCUS TULLIUS CICERO

The whole idea of doctoring yourself is to promote health self-reliance. I like to call it "health homesteading." This is easy talk when you are well, but admittedly a tougher row to hoe when you are sick. As I've stressed throughout this book, it is vital to have reliable information at hand so that you can confidently make decisions about your family's health. Here are some real ways to get detailed, accurate answers to your health questions. All require a measure of personal commitment:

1. Do a search at your local public library, and ask your librarian for assistance. Your library cannot possibly be smaller than the two-room Hamlin Public Library I use in upstate New York, and even out here we have five computer terminals and some of the most helpful librarians I've seen anywhere (and I've met a lot of librarians in my time). This will cost you no money at all.

2. Do a thorough search on the Internet, using several major search engines. In the age of computers, it is easier than ever to quickly mine the vaults of learning. But it helps to know where to do the digging. Give a hungry person a fish and he will be hungry again tomorrow. Teach a person how to fish, and he will always have food. Do not stop at only one or two websites; check them all. The following cautions apply:

• Beware of websites that have a product for sale. Such sites will not be objective. You may have to look very carefully to find the product affiliation within a website, but it is worth the search.

• Beware of so-called consumer-protection sites warning of the dangers of vitamin use. Such misinformation is sixty years out of date. If a site tells you *not* to read something, you should make a point to go and read it immediately.

• Be cautious of sites run by private physicians or other individuals who make their money through consultation services. Such professionals have an interest in offering you some promising free information, and then charging you for the real service.

- For that matter, be cautious about *any* site run by *anyone*. This includes my own website, DoctorYourself.com. Use my CELERY system: **C**heck **E**very **L**iterature reference and personal **E**xperience, and **R**ead for **Y**ourself.

If this all sounds like work, well, of course it is. Life is work. You have to eat anyway; you might as well eat right. You have to spend time on your health; better the library than the doctor's waiting room. Consider the actual time-saving benefits: improving your health will pay you back, not only with more years of life but better years of life. If this is too much for you, then you are ready to die. If you are not ready to die, learn to love libraries, bibliographies, and reading. If I gave your topic of interest short shrift in this book, you can be sure that the library and the Internet do not.

I am daily inundated with people wanting to skip the time-consuming research steps outlined above and instead ask me, in passing, what to do for their health problem. It is called "curbside advice," and I can't blame them for trying. Still, it takes no time at all to formulate the question: "What should I do for so-and-so?" Now, after years of deliberation, I finally have what may be the closest thing to a concise answer:

You need to change your entire life.

Change your life. If you want to get better, that is what you have to do. The first step is to read a lot, a whole lot. But that is only the beginning.

If you've never tried being a vegetarian, start.

If you've never juiced vegetables, start.

If you've never read the *Journal of Orthomolecular Medicine,* start.

If you've never taken vitamin C to saturation, start.

If you've never taught your doctor something, start.

If you've never taken a course in how to meditate or otherwise reduce stress, start.

If you've never done a half-hour fitness workout each day, start.

If you've never given up alcohol or smoking, start. (No, wise guy. I don't mean that you should start the habits in order to give them up.)

If you've never used an interlibrary loan to get a valuable health book, start.

If these things sound impossible to you, then what are you asking the question for? If you have already limited your response, why inquire at all?

To quickly cut through the treacle, I ask clients this most pointed of questions early in a consultation: "What are you willing to do to get better?" The answer I want, of course, is, "Anything." But as with New Year's resolutions, I know better than to hold people too rigorously to their dreams. Flexibility was never more necessary than with self-health care. I will accept a two-thirds effort, for, as a teacher of some experience, I pass anyone at a grade of 65. More is better, but if you were to entirely change two-thirds of your life, I'd be satisfied and impressed. Especially if you held to it for more than a year.

I think you'd be even more impressed with the results.

As Carl Pfeiffer, M.D., said, there is a nutritional alternative for most drugs. You have to dig a bit for the details, but the work has been done. You will find very few negative effects from vitamins in the Physicians' Desk Reference (PDR), but you will see column after column and page after page of side effects, contraindications, and warnings for drugs.

Not surprisingly, I have two kinds of readers: the willing and the not-so-willing. There are two kinds of people who buy luxury cars: those that can afford them and those that cannot. There are two kinds of sick people: those that do not want to change their lifestyle and those that do, but don't know where to start. Prospecting for gold and seeking better health are similar in three ways:

1. You need the motivation to get rich.

2. You need information on where to dig.

3. You need to do the digging.

It takes curiosity, time, and effort. There is no such thing as a free lunch, a quick fix, or a magic wand to cure illness. I wish there were easy answers to people's health questions. There aren't. There are answers, all right, but they are not easy. Modern medicine has created more codependents even than copays. We've learned to hold out for the magic bullet, the new miracle drug, the breakthrough surgical procedure. We've also "learned" to discount the healing power of nature, and the tremendous therapeutic benefit of lifestyle changes, vegetarian diet, raw food juices, and vitamin supplements.

But times are changing. There is a new paradigm, an entirely new way of seeing health, opening in front of us. You may have heard that the Chinese word for "crisis" is the same as the word for "opportunity." There, in a nutshell, lies the *Doctor Yourself* philosophy. Whatever opportunity you are looking for, you must follow leads and dig. Whether it is for oil, gold, information, or health, it requires action. Your action. If you want to change your health, you have to change your life.

391

For Further Information Online

The Orthomolecular MedicineNews Service archives are posted for free access at http://orthomolecular .org/resources/omns/index .shtml.

Thirty-four years of peer-reviewed research articles on therapeutic nutrition, including intravenous vitamin C and cancer: www.riordanclinic.org/research/journal-articles or www.riordanclinic.org/research.

Instructional videos for doctors on why and how to use intravenous vitamin C: http://orthomolecular .org/ resources/omns/v07n03.shtml. These are also on YouTube at www.youtube.com/playlist?list= PL4CA-531C7A3B0D954&feature=viewall and www.youtube.com/playlist?list=PL953B95B3BB977F54 &feature=viewall.

Download the Riordan Intravenous Vitamin C protocol free of charge at www.doctoryourself.com/RiordanIVC.pdf or www.riordanclinic.org/research/vitaminc/protocol.shtml.

Forty-one years of nutrition therapy papers (nearly 500 of them) from the peer-reviewed *Journal of Orthomolecular Medicine:* http://orthomolecular.org/library/jom/ The archive is easily searchable and access is free.

Peer-reviewed vitamin C research papers from 1935 to 1999: www.seanet.com/~alexs/ascorbate/. Clicking the link in the "subject" index will bring up a title listing by decade (yes, there are that many articles). Then, clicking the title link in the decade listing will bring up the full text paper.

The complete seven-year Orthomolecular Medicine News Service archive of over 100 peer-reviewed articles: http://orthomolecular.org/resources/omns/index.shtml.

Video clip: Is Vitamin C Better than Chemo for Cancer? www.youtube.com/watch?v=ZxveVAMir 4o&feature=related or www.youtube.com/watch?v=KfJLpPs1gTQ&NR=1.

YouTube access to Riordan IV-C Symposium Videos. www.youtube.com/results?search_query=riordan+ivc+symposium&aq=f.

If your hospital or doctors say that they cannot obtain injectable vitamin C: www.orthomed.com/ civprep. htm or www.doctoryourself.com/vitciv.html.

If your hospital or doctor says that the hospital will not allow IV vitamin C: www.doctoryourself .com/ strategies.html.

If your hospital or doctor says that IV C is illegal: www.doctoryourself.com/VC.NZ.Sept.2010.pdf .

Dr. Frederick R. Klenner's *Clinical Guide to the Use of Vitamin C* is posted in its entirety at www.seanet. com/~alexs/ascorbate/198x/smith-lh-clinical_guide_1988.htm.

The complete text of Irwin Stone's book *The Healing Factor* is posted for free reading at http://vitaminc-foundation.org/stone/.

A very large number of free-access, full-text papers on curing illness with vitamin C are posted www. seanet.com/~alexs/ascorbate.

For more information on Vitamin C: www.vitamincfoundation.org/ and www.cforyourself.com .

Read Linus Pauling's complete 1968 paper on vitamin therapy at www.orthomed.org/home/pauling2 .html.

A 1974 Pauling paper on the same subject is posted at www.orthomed.org/home/pauling.html.

Linus Pauling and colleagues show how vitamin C and the amino acid lysine may prevent and cure atherosclerosis. www.internetwks.com/pauling/.

Heart Health: www.health-heart.org/aFullSitePDF.pdf is a free pdf download of a full-color book on preventing and reversing heart disease nutritionally.

Dr. Abram Hoffer explains why there is so much opposition to vitamin therapy at www.internetwks .com/ pauling/hoffer.html.

Feingold Association: "Numerous studies show that certain synthetic food additives can have serious learning, behavior, and/or health effects for sensitive people." Learn what to do at www.feingold .org/ research.php and www.feingold.org/newsletters.php Free email newsletter available at www. feingold. org/ON.html.

There are doctors supportive of vegetarianism, and here they are: The Physicians' Committee for Responsible Medicine www.pcrm.org. Free download of their "New Four Food Groups at www.pcrm.org/health/ veginfo/vsk/4foodgroups.pdf.

An expanded version of "Vitamin C and the Law" by Dr. Levy is available as a free pdf download at www.tomlevymd.com/downloads/VC.NZ.Sept.2010.pdf or www.doctoryourself.com/VC.NZ.Sept.2010. pdf.

Multiple Sclerosis: The vitamin-based treatment plan of Frederick Robert Klenner, M.D. is a free download at www.townsendletter.com/Klenner/KlennerProtocol_forMS.pdf.

Cardiovascular Disease: Vitamin E dosages as written and used by Drs. Evan and Wilfrid Shute are posted at www.doctoryourself.com/shute_protocol.html.

En español

Video de los comentarios del Dr. Victor Marcial: www.youtube.com/watch?v=JbOXgG998fl.

Presentan primera guía ortomolecular para el manejo del cancer: www.wapa.tv/noticias.php?nid= 20100428195518.

Archiv der deutschsprachigen Artikel, auf DoctorYourself.com (Archive of Natural Health Articles, in German): www.doctoryourself.com/DeutschIndizieren.html.

APPENDIX

Personal Spiritual Wellness

"If not you, who? If not here, where? If not now, when?"
—ATTRIBUTED TO THEODORE ROOSEVELT

I'd been looking all over Brockport State College for a faculty member named Professor John Mosher and my search finally took me to the science building's basement. He had to be in here somewhere, because he was not in the other science building and not any other faculty office locations. He was not on any of the three floors of this building, either, if the lobby directory was to be trusted. That left the basement.

No windows; cracked linoleum on the floors; asbestos-wrapped pipes along the low ceilings of diarrhea-yellow hallways; the smell of the animal rooms and traces formaldehyde from assorted biology labs; and me approaching the end of a hallway so neglected that every third lightbulb was out. There were no names or room numbers on the stark gray metal doors. This was about the last place anyone would look for a senior college professor, but I was a slightly homesick teenage college freshman, and the intrigue of the practical puzzle at hand kept my mind focused. Finding the Prof was a relatively pleasant challenge in an otherwise deadly boring week of college classes that were, if you were to trust the admissions office, stimulating and edifying. Well, not all of them were. That's why I wanted to study overseas, and Dr. John I. Mosher was head of the college's international education programs for biology majors like me.

For whatever reason, the college evidently had stuck his office somewhere in the basement. So far, every door down there was either locked or contained either mops, sinks, metal barrels, preserved fish in jars, 16mm movie reels, or a custodian eating a late bagged lunch. It was that custodian that pointed me down this last hall, to the door that I now stood before, knocking.

"Come on in," a voice called from the other side of the door. I opened it and walked in. It was a scholarly mess. The room was absolutely packed with papers and books. There was a desk partially submerged amidst the clutter with a tallish, unprepossessing, late-thirties-age man sitting comfortably leaning back in his chair with his hands behind his head.

He smiled. I spoke. "I want to study abroad, and the International Education secretary told me to go see you."

"Well, that's fine, he said. "Please have a seat."

There was nowhere *to* sit but on a single rickety lab stool leaning against the wall. The stool looked as if it would not support the dust on it, let alone me. I mounted it and cautiously settled my skinny body, expecting each creak to indicate not only cracks but inevitable collapse.

The stool held. I put my feet up on the footrest and watched Dr. Mosher, mammalogist, ecologist and ethologist, walk around the room. He did so, stepping over books open on the floor, and place a number of long, thin sticks to protrude between the pages of stacked journals, shelved books, manuscripts, cracks in the beige cement wall, and anywhere else he could fit them. Eccentricity being a given part of many a professor's job description, I was patient and not particularly surprised until he whipped out a big box of strike-anywhere matches and lit each thin stick. Smoke and scent filled the room; they were sticks of incense. Sandlewood incense. Lots of sandlewood incense.

My grandfather having been a fireman, I was beginning to worry that this meeting was all going to quickly end in flaming disaster. Those incense sticks were burning so near so much paper I expected that the room was going to go up like a torch, with us in it. What a way to go: incinerated by and with a hippie professor.

But nothing burned but the incense and the conversation immediately turned to the task of creating a special study program for me. The professor was polite and all business, and he gave me a great deal of good, practical advice.

Initial planning completed, the conversation took a cosmic, spiritual turn. From that, it never reversed. It's been forty-one years since I met Dr. Mosher in 1971. He has been a major influence on my professional life, as well as being a most valued personal friend. In addition to serving for thirty years as Professor of Biology at SUNY Brockport, Dr. Mosher was also my doctoral mentor. Not one to let retirement slow him up, he continues to serve as a popular and highly skilled counselor. His focus is spiritual development, and this topic is a lot more tied into health self-reliance than it may first seem. I therefore include this executive summary of what you'd learn talking with Dr. Mosher, assuming you could find what room he's in. As for me, I am glad I did not give up the search.

THE HERO'S JOURNEY

by John I. Mosher, Ph.D.

Visualize this: You are the hero. You were born from the realm of spirit into the relative or physical world. That act is a sacrifice, a heroic deed. Now that you are in the physical world with a physical body, your hero's journey has begun. The journey is to awaken to your true nature and act accordingly. Nature intends for you to awaken. All of the conditions and experiences in your life are meant to channel you into a position where you want to go beyond, or transcend, the "suffering" of the mind. Sometimes, it seems to take privation and suffering to open our mind to that which is hidden to those who do not seek awakening. To want to transcend this suffering is one of the first steps to awakening to living in spiritual wellness.

Regardless of one's station in life, no matter how favored one is with material comfort, loving family and friends, no matter how powerful one is, occasionally illness is experienced, one grows old, and everyone will die. In addition, there are the smaller psychological sufferings, frustrations, not being able to do what we think we want to do, anger of experiencing what we do not like, the envy of desiring what we do not have, the fear of losing what we do have. We all long for happiness, yet we are constantly laying the foundations for unrest through habitual conditioning of our minds. When we realize that we seem to be in an endless cycle of rising and falling emotions that offers no sense of fulfillment or lasting happiness, many of us look for a remedy. We look for another way to live. We eventually realize what we thought was a normal condition is, in fact, suffering. We realize that aversion and attachment (desire) both cause suffering. It is our ego-centered attitude (our ignorance) that causes the reaction of liking and disliking, attachment and aversion. These causes of suffering are based in our belief that we are separate from others. Taking everything as it appears is an error. By presuming that "I" am the most important object in "my" world, we blind ourselves to the truth that everything is connected and interdependent. Suffering also arises when one is not living in the present: not being right here, right now. When the ego is in charge, it can wander in its thinking to the past and become angry or upset about some event long gone. Or the thinking mind can worry about what might be or might happen. In either case, there is suffering because one is not living in the present, the NOW, this minute.

We can use our disturbing emotions as a catalyst for transformation. As we thoughtfully, consciously, and actively replace our disturbing mental activity with consciously chosen aware, awake, and enlightened responses, we will become spontaneously and naturally liberated from our old habits. Thus, our hero's journey with all of its trials and tribulations are but incidences along the way to awakening. The journey is one of transforming the mind. The great teachers of all time, the awakened ones, have stated that it is the mind that experiences suffering but also that the mind can be taught a way of viewing the world and of behaving in it that ends personal suffering.

This brief introduction to developing spirituality is intended to remind you of what has long been called the Way.

THE MIND-EGO

Opportunity continuously presents itself for each of us to fall into negative states of mind. Fear of not getting what one wants, or losing what one has, is ever present in those not practicing the cultivation of deeper, happier states of mind. The more the mind (or ego) is in charge, the more one is controlling, has fear, and suffers. Through regular practice, the soul is gradually put in charge and the more and more "soul qualities" shine forth. In this state, the individual has put the mind in its proper place as servant to the soul. The ego as a servant is wonderful. It helps you plan, accomplishes scientific wonders, reminds you to take care of your physical self, and daily prods you to get out of bed and get on with it. Yes, the ego is a wonderful servant . . . but a terrible master. Put in charge, the ego can easily destroy ones happiness, and cause much anguish and suffering. Looking at the world, or at the lives of many that we know, we can all too easily see the results of the mind and ego being in charge.

There is no law that states or enforces the idea that life and events must always be as we wish them.

RELATIONSHIPS

A relationship between two people can be a spiritual path, a yoga. It certainly can be a way to grow in love and happiness. However, it is also a difficult path. Some sages say the "Yoga of Relationships" is the toughest of all because it deals with the most powerful emotions on the planet. Your relationship with others, especially those closest to you, is your spiritual workspace.

Relationships are really good places for ego-sightings. Relationships can be destroyed by the mind-ego being in charge. On the other hand, a relationship can change for the better when the soul, the spirit, the heart is in charge. The ego wants control. Control of others often comes from inner fears, which is a mind-ego quality. Trying to control others is a waste of time. Efforts to control another result in stressing yourself and often by garnering anger and resentment from the other. Nothing positive is accomplished.

HOW TO COMMUNICATE BETTER

The communication process begins with our perceptions. The senses, our contact points with the world, are like five doors which open to gather information about the world. Each of us seem to trust one sense of perception somewhat more than the others. When we access information through our most "trusted" sense, we absorb, process and remember that information more efficiently.[1] Therefore, if you want to communicate more effectively with another person, here are some hints:

- Use words that will facilitate understanding of your message. Words can be used to access a person's most trusted sense.

- If an individual thinks in pictures, visual words, like *see, watch, appear, look, inspect,* etc. will access the visual person. This person will retain the written word better than the spoken word. If you see how clear that is from what you just read, perhaps you are a visual person.

- An auditory person can best be accessed by sound words, like *hear, listen say, state, talk, speak,* etc., and will retain spoken words better than written words. If what I am saying here sounds good to you, you may be an auditory person.

- A person who is kinesthetic will respond best to feeling and texture words, such as *feel, grasp, out, feel, touch,* etc., and learns by doing. If you are kinesthetic, you have the grasp of this idea and it might feel like it would be worth trying out.

By really paying attention to your words, and having patience and sensitivity, you may find that communicating with access words can help you express yourself better, and understand others better as well.

References

Bandler, R. & Grinder, J. (1979) *Frogs Into Princes.* Moab, Ut., Real People Press. See also:

Bandler, Grinder, J. & Sativ, V. (1976) *Changing With Families.* Palo Alto, Science & Behavior Books.

Satir, V. (1972) Peoplemaking. Palo Alto, Science & Behavior Books.

In a relationship with another, it is important to turn your attention inward and work on yourself. When anger and frustration or anything less than love arises in ones feeling toward the other, that is a signal. It is a signal to look within. It takes courage to face one's self and be totally honest about what perception or attitude must be change to be in line with the practice of unconditional love.

Play-acting will not do. Denial will not do. One can you can work on yourself. That is one of the best thongs you can do for another. And if both partners in a relationship are doing their inner spiritual homework, cultivating the positive and being in the present, the relationship has a tremendous advantage for each and for both.

SUFFERING AND ATTACHMENT

Suffering arises from attachment to desire. One example is the desire that things have to be the way one thinks they ought to be.

Suffering arises when one is not living in the present: not being right here, right now. When the mind-ego is in charge it can wander in its thinking to the past and become angry or upset about some event long gone. Or the thinking mind can worry about what might be or might happen. In either case there is suffering because one is not living in the present, the now, this minute.

Qualities of the heart, the spirit or soul are compassion, selflessness, tolerance, equanimity, fearlessness, nonattachment, and love without condition. All of these qualities are facilitated and brought forth by the practice of regular meditation, regular prayer, remembering the Divine, and self-discipline—that is, practice being in the present, practice having compassion, being selfless, tolerant, and having equanimity. Practice fearlessness, nonattachment, and love without condition. Cultivating these positive states of mind may be considered one of the most effective ways for obtaining the state of happiness.

Here are some important things to remember during your journey:

- Enjoy life as it occurs. To flow with life is rejuvenating.

- Make plans, set goals, do the best you can, and then take it as it comes.

- Flexible trees and people survive the storms of life.

- Liking and disliking are stressful and tiring.

- What is the benefit of a judging mind? Are you happier for judging yourself? Are you happier by judging your fellow beings?

The impulses of life are put in the realm of enjoying without attachment. The awakened person participates fully in life, having conquered fear, attachment, and having selflessness, unconditional love, equanimity, and being of greatest use to his/herself and others The hero's journey is the journey of self-awakening.

QUIETING THE MIND

The gateway to cultivating spirituality is a tranquil, peaceful, serene mind. The uncultivated human mind has been likened to a wild monkey. Like a wild monkey, the mind jumps here and there from one thought to another causing turbulence and confusion. The serene mind, on the other hand, experiences tranquility and has focus and control of its thoughts. Therefore, the first step in developing one's spirituality is to quiet the "coarse mind," which is ego oriented, and cultivate the subtle, intuitive mind, which is spirit oriented. There are many books and techniques available to help you quiet your mind. Please consider well the Recommended Reading list below.

You have to work on yourself.
No one can do the work for you, and you cannot do it for them.
As Alan Watts said,
'Kindly let me help you or you will drown'
said the monkey, putting the fish safely up a tree."

The well-known French author and monk Teilhard de Chardin said, *"Change yourself and you change the world."* By taking one step at a time, we indeed do change ourselves and, in fact, change the world as we see it. By continued regular practice of quieting techniques, you bring forth more of your essential nature to express itself and thereby transforming your mind. The more awake the mind is to the reality of your true nature, the less "suffering" there is in your life.

The following help me to keep a perspective on things during my journey, and perhaps they will help you on your journey as well:

- You are not your body. You *have* a body.

- Our job is to be loving and understanding, not to judge, blame, criticize or condemn.

- Death is a good advisor. Compared to death, what is so important?

- When we are attached to things being a certain way, we suffer and often cause suffering to others.

- Everyone wants to be loved, and everyone wants to be happy.

- There is no universal law that says "things" must go the way we wish them to go; they go as they go. If we are wise, we do the best we can and take it as it comes and not be attached to the action or the outcome of the action.

- When we act from the heart and give love without expectation or anything in return, we grow in love, maturity, and spirituality.

These reminders work only if you use them. Using them means practice and practice again. It takes time, and excuses abound. The mind-ego wants "me first, as I see it, when I want it" and that is a formula for problems, pain, and alienation. Do not fall for that old trap. Instead, increase your inner self awareness, right here, right now. It is a very good way to build a happier life.

Recommended Reading with Comments

Chopra, Deepak. *Perfect Health.* New York: Harmony Books, 1990.

A practical guide to using the healing power of the mind, based on the principles of Ayurveda (a 5,000-year-old system of mind/body medicine. This is an excellent book to help you understand about keeping yourself healthy.

Chopra, Deepak. *Seven Spiritual Laws of Success.* Novato, CA: New World Library/Amber-Allen Publishing, 1994. Also: New York: Harmony Books, 2001.

An excellent guide on ways of thinking and being that reduce stress, touch your spirit, and help with the awakening process.

Easwaran, Eknath. *Take Your Time.* Tomales, CA: Nilgiri PressTomales, 1994.

The book outlines practical tools for slowing down our thinking. A very useful book for coming to the quiet.

Gangaji. *You Are That.* Boulder, CO: Satsang Press, 1995.

An excellent book that answers questions about your real identity, who you really are. Provides answers to questions about many of life's problems and how they stem from one's ignorance of not knowing who they are.

Ram Dass. *Grist For the Mill.* Bantam Books, 1979.

This classic offers a greater understanding of what life is all about and how to live in peace and harmony. Ram Dass is an American (former Harvard Professor Dr. Richard Alpert) who lived the "Hero's Journey" to awakening.

Tolle, Eckert. *The Power of Now.* Novato, CA: New World Library, 2004.

Transformative insight delivered in a manner that those of us from the western materialistic culture can easily relate. You can begin to heal yourself from the inside out. The secret is to go within. I also recommend Mr. Tolle's other book, Practicing the Power of Now.

Bibliography

Adams R and Murray F. *Megavitamin Therapy.* New York: Larchmont, 1973.

Airola P. *Health Secrets from Europe.* New York: Arco, 1972.

Airola P. *How to Get Well.* Phoenix, AZ: Health Plus, 1980.

Bailey H. *The Vitamin Pioneers.* Emmaus, PA: Rodale Books, 1968.

Bailey H. *Vitamin E for a Healthy Heart and a Longer Life.* New York: Carroll and Graf, 1993.

Balch J and Balch P. *Prescription for Nutritional Healing.* Garden City Park, NY: Avery, 1990.

Barnett LB. New concepts in bone healing. *Journal of Applied Nutrition* 7 (1954): 318–23.

Belfield WO. Vitamin C in treatment of canine and feline distemper complex. *Veterinary Medicine/Small Animal Clinician* (April 1967): 345–48.

Bernier RH, et al. Diphtheria-tetanus toxoids-pertussis vaccination and sudden infant deaths in Tennessee. *Jour Pediatrics* 101 (1982): 419–21.

Bicknell F and Prescott F. *The Vitamins in Medicine,* 3rd ed. Milwaukee, WI: Lee Foundation, 1953.

Billings E and Westmore A. *The Billings Method.* New York: Ballantine, 1983.

Bircher R. A Turning Point in Nutritional Science. Undated reprint (c. 1950) by Lee Foundation for Nutritional Research, Milwaukee, WI.

Bland J. *The Key to the Power of Vitamin C and Its Metabolites.* New Canaan, CT: Keats Publishing, 1989.

Block G, et al. (1991) Epidemiological evidence regarding vitamin C and cancer. *American Journal of Clinical Nutrition* 54 (December 1991): 1310S–314S.

Brighthope I. *The Vitamin Cure for Diabetes.* Laguna Beach, CA: Basic Health Publications, 2011.

Burgstahler A. Water fluoridation: promise and reality. *National Fluoridation News* (Summer 1985).

Burns D, ed. *The Greatest Health Discovery: Natural Hygiene and Its Evolution, Past Present and Future.* Chicago: Natural Hygiene Press, 1972.

Campbell R, Saul AW. *The Vitamin Cure for Children's Health Problems.* Laguna Beach, CA: Basic Health Publications, 2012

Cameron E. Vitamin C and cancer: an overview. *International Journal of Vitamin and Nutrition Research* Suppl. 23 (1982): 115–127.

Cameron E. "Protocol for the Use of Intravenous Vitamin C in the Treatment of Cancer." Palo Alto, CA: Linus Pauling Institute of Science and Medicine, undated (c.1986–88).

Cameron E. Protocol for the use of vitamin C in the treatment of cancer. *Medical Hypotheses* 36 (1991): 190–94.

Cameron E and Baird G. Ascorbic acid and dependence on opiates in patients with advanced and disseminated cancer. *Journal of International Research Communications* 1 (1973): 38.

Cameron E and Campbell A. The orthomolecular treatment of cancer II. Clinical trial of high-dose ascorbic supplements in advanced human cancer. *Chemical-Biological Interactions* 9 (1974): 285–315.

Cameron E and Campbell A. Innovation vs. quality control: an "unpublishable" clinical trial of supplemental ascorbate in incurable cancer. *Medical Hypotheses* 36 (1991): 185–189.

Cameron E and Pauling L. Ascorbic acid and the glycosaminoglycans: An orthomolecular approach to cancer and other diseases. *Oncology* (Basel) 27 (1973): 181–192.

Cameron E and Pauling L. The orthomolecular treatment of cancer. 1. The role of ascorbate in host resistance. *Chemical-Biological Interactions* 9 (1974): 273–83.

Cameron E and Pauling L. Supplemental ascorbate in the supportive treatment of cancer: prolongation of survival times in terminal human cancer. *Proceedings of the National Academy of Sciences USA* 73 (1976): 3685–689.

Cameron E and Pauling L. Supplemental ascorbate in the supportive treatment of cancer: Reevaluation of prolongation of survival times in terminal human cancer. *Proceedings of the National Academy of Sciences USA* 75 (1978): 4538–542

Cameron E and Pauling L. *Cancer and Vitamin C,* revised edition. Philadelphia: Camino Books, 1993.

Campbell A, Jack T, and Cameron E. Reticulum cell sarcoma: two complete "spontanous" regressions, in response to high-dose ascorbic acid therapy. A report on subsequent progress. *Oncology* 48 (1991): 495–97.

Canter L. *Assertive Discipline for Parents,* revised edition. New York: Harper and Row, 1985.

Carnegie D. *How to Win Friends and Influence People*. New York: Pocket Books, 1981.

Carper J. *Food: Your Miracle Medicine*. New York: Harper-Collins, 1993.

Carter CW. Maintenance nutrition in the pigeon and its relation to heart block. *Biochemistry* 28 (1934): 933–39.

Case HS. *The Vitamin Cure for Women's Health Problems*. Laguna Beach, CA: Basic Health Publications, June 2012.

Cathcart RF. Clinical trial of vitamin C. [Letter to the editor.] *Medical Tribune* (25 June 1975).

Cathcart RF. The method of determining proper doses of vitamin C for the treatment of disease by titrating to bowel tolerance. *Journal of Orthomolecular Psychiatry* 10 (1981): 125–132.

Cathcart RF. Titration to bowel tolerance, anascorbemia, and acute induced scurvy. *Medical Hypotheses* 7 (1981): 1359–376. www.doctoryourself.com/titration.html.

Cathcart RF. Vitamin C in the treatment of acquired immune deficiency syndrome (AIDS). *Medical Hypotheses* 14 (1984): 423–33.

Cathcart RF. Vitamin C, the nontoxic, nonrate-limited antioxidant free radical scavenger. *Medical Hypotheses* 18 (1985): 61–77.

Cathcart RF. The vitamin C treatment of allergy and the normally unprimed state of antibodies. *Medical Hypotheses* 21 (1986): 307–21.

Cathcart RF. A unique function for ascorbate. *Medical Hypotheses* 35 (May 1991): 32–37.

Cathcart RF. The third face of vitamin C. *Journal of Orthomolecular Medicine* 7 (1993): 197–200.

Chakrabarti RN and Dasgupta PS. Effects of ascorbic acid on survival and cell-mediated immunity in tumor bearing mice. *IRCS Med Sci* 12 (1984): 1147–148.

Challem JJ. *Vitamin C Updated*. New Canaan, CT: Keats Publishing, 1983.

Chan AC. Vitamin E and atherosclerosis.[Review.] *J Nutr* 128 (October 1998):1593–596.

Chapman-Smith D. Cost effectiveness: the Manga report. *The Chiropractic Report* (1993): 1–2.

Cheney G. Rapid healing of peptic ulcers in patients receiving fresh cabbage juice. *California Medicine* 70 (1949): 10–14.

Cheney G. Anti-peptic ulcer dietary factor. *J Am Diet Assoc* 26 (1950): 668–72.

Cheney, G. Vitamin U therapy of peptic ulcer. *California Medicine* 77 (1952): 248–52.

Cheraskin E and Ringsdorf WM. *New Hope for Incurable Diseases*. New York: Exposition Press, 1971.

Cheraskin E, et al. *The Vitamin C Connection*. New York: Harper and Row, 1983.

Chopra D. *Perfect Health*. New York: Harmony Books, 1991.

Clarke JH. *The Prescriber*. Essex, England: C. W. Daniel, 1972.

Cleave TL. *The Saccharine Disease*. New Canaan, CT: Keats, 1974.

Cleigh Z. Laetrile. *Well Being Magazine* 26 (November 1977): 29–33.

Coulter H. *Homeopathic Influences in Nineteenth-Century Allopathic Therapeutics*. Falls Church VA: American Institute of Homeopathy, 1973.

Coulter H. *Homoeopathic Science and Modern Medicine*. Richmond, CA: North Atlantic Books, 1981.

Coulter H and Fisher B. *A Shot in the Dark*. Garden City Park, NY: Avery,1991.

Cowley G. Healer of hearts. *Newsweek* (16 March 1998): 50–56.

Cumming F. Vaccinations: A health hazard? *Sydney Sunday Herald* (4 April 1993): 41–42, 79.

Dahl H and Degre M. The effect of ascorbic acid on production of human interferon and the antiviral activity in vitro. *Acta Pathologica et Microbiologica Scandinavica* 84 (1976): 280–84.

Dannenburg AM, et al. Ascorbic acid in the treatment of chronic lead poisoning. *JAMA* 114 (1940): 1439–440.

Davis A. *Let's Get Well*. New York: Signet, 1965.

Davis A. *Let's Eat Right to Keep Fit*. New York: Signet, 1970.

Dawson EB, et al. Effects of ascorbic acid on male fertility. In "Third Conference on Vitamin C," *Annals of the New York Academy of Sciences* 498 (1987).

Dawson W and West GB. The influence of ascorbic acid on histamine metabolism in guinea pigs. *British Journal of Pharmacology* 24 (1965): 725–34.

Downing D. *The Vitamin Cure for Allergies*. Laguna Beach, CA: Basic Health Publications, 2010.

Dufty W. *Sugar Blues*. New York: Warner Books, 1975.

Dworkin S and Dworkin F. *The Good Goodies*. New York: Fawcett Crest, 1974.

Dworkin S and Dworkin F. *The Apartment Gardener*. New York: Signet, 1974.

Eby G, Davis D, and Halcomb W. Reduction in duration of common colds by zinc gluconate lozenges in a double blind study. *Antimicrobal Agents and Chemotherapy* 25 (January 1984). Eby G, Davis D, Halcomb W. Reduction in duration of common cold symptoms by zinc gluconate lozenges in a double-blind study. *Antimicrobial Agents in Chemotherapy* (25):20–24, 1984.

Edward JF. Iodine: its use in the treatment and prevention of poliomyelitis and allied diseases. *Manitoba Medical Review* 34 (1954): 337–39.

Enstrom JE, Kanim LE, and Klein MA. Vitamin C intake and mortality among a sample of the United States population. *Epidemiology* 3 (1992):194–202.

Farrell W. *Why Men Are the Way They Are.* New York: McGraw-Hill, 1986.

Farrell W. *The Myth of Male Power.* New York: Simon and Schuster, 1993.

Feingold BF. *Why Your Child is Hyperactive.* New York: Random House, 1985.

Ford MW, et al. *The Deaf Smith Country Cookbook.* New York: Collier, 1973.

Fredericks C and Bailey H. *Food Facts and Fallacies.* New York: Arco, 1965.

Free V and Sanders P. The use of ascorbic acid and mineral supplements in the detoxification of narcotic addicts. *Journal of Orthomolecular Psychiatry* 7 (1978): 264–70.

Fritsch A and The Center for Science in the Public Interest. *99 Ways to a Simple Lifestyle.* New York: Anchor-Doubleday, 1977.

Furgurson EB. *Chancellorsville, 1863.* New York: Alfred A. Knopf, 1992.

Gerson M. *A Cancer Therapy: Results of Fifty Cases,* 3rd ed. Del Mar, CA: Totality Books, 1977.

Gerson C and Walker M. *The Gerson Therapy.* New York: Kensington Publishing Corp., 2001.

Ghosh J and Das S. Evaluation of vitamin A and C status in normal and malignant conditions and their possible role in cancer prevention. *Japanese Journal of Cancer Research* 76 (December 1995): 1174–178.

Goldbeck N and Goldbeck D. *The Supermarket Handbook.* New York: Signet, 1976.

Gonzalez M, Miranda-Massari J, Saul AW. *I Have Cancer: What Should I Do? Your Orthomolecular Guide for Cancer Management.* Laguna Beach, CA: Basic Health Publications, 2009.

Goodman S. *Vitamin C: The Master Nutrient.* New Canaan, CT: Keats Publishing, 1991.

Graves SB. Carrots and cancer: the surprising connection. *Family Circle* (1 July 1982).

Greenwood J. Optimum vitamin C intake as a factor in the preservation of disk integrity. *Med. Ann. D.C.* 33 (June 1964).

Gregory D. *Dick Gregory's Natural Diet for Folks Who Eat.* New York: Harper and Row, 1973.

Griffin MR, et al. Risk of sudden infant death syndrome after immunization with the diphtheria-tetanus-pertussis vaccine. *New Engl Jour Med* 319 (1988): 618–23.

Gross L. The effects of vitamin deficient diets on rats, with special reference to the motor functions of the intestinal tract in vivo and in vitro. *Journal of Pathology and Bacteriology* 27 (1924): 27–50.

Growdon A. "Neurotransmitter Precursors in the Diet". In *Nutrition and the Brain,* edited by Wurtman and Wurtman, 117–81. New York: Raven Press, 1979.

Guenther RM. Alcoholism and nutrition. *International Journal of Biosocial Research* 4 (1983): 3–4.

Gupta RS, et al. The prevalence, severity, and distribution of childhood food allergy in the United States. *Pediatrics* 128(1): e9–e17, 2011. See also: Tanner L. Study says 1 in 13 U.S. children have food allergy. Associated Press, 6/19/2011.

Harrell RF, et al. Can nutritional supplements help mentally retarded children? An exploratory study. *Proceedings of the National Academy of Sciences USA* 78 (1981): 574–78.

Harris A, Robinson A, and Pauling L. Blood plasma l-ascorbic acid concentration for oral l-ascorbic acid dosage up to 12 grams per day. *International Research Communications System* (December 1973):19.

Hart BF and Levensdorf M. Is there an alternative to surgery for angina pectoris? *Let's Live* (October 1977).

Hawkins DR, Bortin AW, Runyon RP. Orthomolecular psychiatry: niacin and megavitamin therapy. *Psychosomatics* 11(1970): 517–21.

Hawkins DR and Pauling L. *Orthomolecular Psychiatry.* San Francisco: Freeman, 1973.

Hemil H. Vitamin C and the common cold. *British Journal of Nutrition* 67 (1992): 3–16.

Hickey S. *The Vitamin Cure for Migraines.* Laguna Beach, CA: Basic Health Publications, 2010.

Hickey S, Saul AW. *Vitamin C: The Real Story.* Laguna Beach, CA: Basic Health Publications, 2008.

Hillemann HH. The illusion of American health and longevity. *Clinical Physiology* 2 (1960): 120–77.

Hoffer A, Osmond H, Callbeck JM, and Kahan I. Treatment of schizophrenia with nicotinic acid and nicotinamide. *Journal of Clinical Experimental Psychopathology* 18 (1957): 131–58.

Hoffer A. (1958) "Relation of Epinephrine Metabolites to Schizophrenia." In *Chemical Concepts of Psychiatry,* edited by M Rinkel and HGB Denber. New York: Mowell-Obolensky Inc., 1958.

Hoffer A. *Niacin Therapy in Psychiatry.* Springfield, IL: Charles S. Thomas, 1962.

Hoffer A. Use of ascorbic acid with niacin in schizophrenia. *Canadian Medical Journal* (6 November 1971).

Hoffer A. Treatment of schizophrenia. *Orthomolecular Psychiatry* 3 (1974): 280–90.

Hoffer A. *Vitamin C and Cancer: Discovery, Recovery, Controversy.* Kingston, ON: Quarry Press, 1999.

Hoffer A, Foster HD. *Feel Better, Live Longer with Vitamin B-3: Nutrient Deficiency and Dependency.* CCNM Press, 2007.

Hoffer A and Osmond H. Treatment of schizophrenia with nicotinic acid: a ten-year follow-up. *Acta Psychiatr Scand* 40 (1964): 171–89.

Hoffer A and Osmond H. *New Hope for Alcoholics*. New Hyde Park, NY: University Books, 1968.

Hoffer A, Saul AW. The Vitamin Cure for Alcoholism. Laguna Beach, CA: Basic Health Publications, 2009. Reviews at http://www.doctoryourself.com/alcoholcure.html

Hoffer A, Saul AW. Orthomolecular Medicine for Everyone: Megavitamin Therapeutics for Families and Physicians. Laguna Beach, CA: Basic Health Publications, 2008.

Hoffer A and Pauling L. Hardin Jones biostatistical analysis of mortality data for cohorts of cancer patients with a large fraction surviving at the termination of the study and a comparison of survival times of cancer patients receiving large regular oral doses of vitamin C and other nutrients with similar patients not receiving those doses. *Journal of Orthomolecular Medicine* 5 (1990): 143–54.

Hoffer A and Pauling L. Hardin Jones biostatistical analysis of mortality data for a second set of cohorts of cancer patients with a large fraction surviving at the termination of the study and a comparison of survival times of cancer patients receiving large regular oral doses of vitamin C and other nutrients with similar patients not receiving those doses. *Journal of Orthomolecular Medicine* 8:157–167, 1993.

Hoffer A, Saul AW, Foster HD. *Niacin: The Real Story*. Laguna Beach, CA: Basic Health Publications.

Hoffer A, Saul AW, Hickey S. *Hospitals and Health: Your Orthomolecular Guide to a Shorter, Safer Hospital Stay*. Laguna Beach, CA: Basic Health Publications, 2011.

Hoffmann-La Roche. "Marginal Vitamin Deficiency: The Gray Area of Nutrition." [Reprint.] La Canada, CA: Bronson Pharmaceuticals, (undated brochure).

Horwitt MK. Vitamin E: a reexamination. *American Journal of Clinical Nutrition* 29 (5 May 1976).

Horwitz N. Vitamins, minerals boost IQ in retarded. *Medical Tribune* 22 (1981): 1, 19.

Huggins H. *It's All in Your Head. Diseases Caused by Silver-Mercury Fillings*. Colorado Springs, CO: Life Sciences Press, 1990.

Hume ED. *Bechamp or Pasteur? A Lost Chapter in the History of Biology*. London: C.W. Daniel, 1923.

Humer RP. Brain food: Neurotransmitters make you think. *Let's Live* (December 1981).

Hunter BT. *The Natural Foods Cookbook*. New York: Pyramid, 1961.

Hutton E. The fight over vitamin E. *Maclean's Magazine* (15 June 1953).

Illich I. *Deschooling Society*. New York: Harper and Row, 1970.

Illich I. *Medical Nemesis*. New York: Bantam, 1976.

Inglis B. *The Case for Unorthodox Medicine*. New York: Putnam, 1965.

Issac K and Gold S, ed. *Eating Clean 2: Overcoming Food Hazards*. Washington, D.C.: Center for Study of Responsive Law, 1987.

Jarvis DC. *Folk Medicine*. New York: Holt, 1958.

Johnston EA. Vitamins and their relation to diseases of the alimentary tract. *Journal of the American College of Proctology* [Undated reprint].

Jungeblut CW. Inactivation of poliomyelitis virus by crystallin vitamin C (ascorbic acid). *Journal of Experimental Medicine* 62 (1935): 517–21.

Jungeblut CW. Further observations on vitamin C therapy in experimental poliomyelitis. *Journal of Experimental Medicine* 65 (1939):127–46.

Jungeblut CW. A further contribution to the vitamin C therapy in experimental poliomyelitis. *Journal of Experimental Medicine* 70 (1939): 327.

Kalokerinos A. *Every Second Child*. New Canaan, CT: Keats Publishing, 1981.

Kaufman W. *Common Forms of Niacinamide Deficiency Disease: Aniacin Amidosis*. New Haven, CT: Yale University Press, 1943.

Kaufman W. *The Common Form of Joint Dysfunction: Its Incidence and Treatment*. Brattleboro, VT: E. L. Hildreth and Co., 1949. The book's full text is posted at doctoryour self. com.

Kirschner HE. Comfrey. *Let's Live* (October–December 1958).

Klenner FR. Treating multiple sclerosis nutritionally. *Cancer Control Journal* 2[3]:16–20 [Undated].

Klenner FR. Virus pneumonia and its treatment with vitamin C. *Southern Medicine and Surgery* 110(2):36–38, 46, February, 1948.

Klenner FR. The treatment of poliomyelitis and other virus diseases with vitamin C. *Southern Medicine and Surgery* 113 (1949):101–107.

Klenner FR. Massive doses of vitamin C and the virus diseases. *Southern Medicine and Surgery* (1951). *Southern Medicine & Surgery* 103(4):101–107, April, 1951/

Klenner FR. The use of vitamin C as an antibiotic. *Journal of Applied Nutrition* 6 (1953): 274–78.

Klenner FR. The history of lockjaw. *Tri-State Medical Journal* (June 1954).

Klenner FR. Recent discoveries in the treatment of lockjaw. *Tri-State Medical Journal* (July 1954).

Klenner FR. The role of ascorbic acid in therapeutics. *Tri-State Medical Journal* (November 1955).

Klenner FR. Observations on the dose of administration of ascorbic acid when employed beyond the range of a vitamin in human pathology. Journal of Applied Nutrition. Vol 23, Number 3 & 4, (Winter 1971): 61–68.

Klenner FR. Response of peripheral and central nerve pathology to megadoses of the vitamin B complex and other metabolites. *Journal of Applied Nutrition* 25 (1973):16.

Klenner FR. "Significance of High Daily Intake of Ascorbic Acid in Preventive Medicine." In *A Physician's Handbook on Orthomolecular Medicine,* edited by RJ Williams and DK Kalita. New Canaan, CT: Keats, 1979.

Kordish J. *The Juiceman's Power of Juicing.* New York: William Morrow, 1992.

Kulvinskas V. *Survival into the 21st Century.* Wethersfield, CT: Omangod Press, 1975.

Landrigan PJ and Witte JJ. Neurologic disorders following live measles-virus vaccination. *JAMA* 223 (1973):1459–1462.

Lasagna L. One-a-day, plus C. *The Sciences* (November 1981), 35.

Lasky MS. *The Complete Junk Food Book.* New York: McGraw-Hill, 1977.

Law D. *A Guide to Alternative Medicine.* Garden City, NY: Dolphin, 1976.

Lee R. *Clinical Nutrition: Food vs. Drugs.* Milwaukee, WI: Lee Foundation for Nutritional Research, [undated].

Lee R. Vitamins in dental care. *Health Culture* (May 1955).

Levin M and Hartzell W. Ascorbic acid: the concept of optimum requirements. In "Third Conference on Vitamin C," *Annals of the New York Academy of Sciences* 498: (1987).

Levy T. *Vitamin C, Infectious Diseases, and Toxins: Curing the Incurable.* Philadelphia, PA: Xlibris, 2002.

Lewin S. *Vitamin C: Its Molecular Biology and Medical Potential.* London: Academic Press, 1976.

Lin D. Extensive clinical uses of vitamin E. *Nutritional Perspectives* (July 1992): 16–28.

Abrupt termination of high daily intake of vitamin C: the rebound effect. *Linus Pauling Institute of Science and Medicine Newsletter* 2 (1985): 6.

Loeffler W. Department of Education and Human Development Lecture. State University College at Brockport, New York (3 November 1986).

Lupulescu A. The role of vitamins A, beta-carotene, E and C in cancer cell biology. *International Journal of Vitamin and Nutrition Research* 64 (1994): 3–14.

Lust JB. *The Herb Book.* New York: Bantam, 1974.

MacAlister CJ and Titherley AW. *Narrative of an Investigation Concerning an Ancient Medicinal Remedy and its Modern Utilities Together with an Account of the Chemical Constitution of Allantoin.* London: John Bale, Sons, and Danielsson, 1936.

Machlin LJ. Beyond deficiency: new views on the function and health effects of vitamins. [Introduction.] *Annals of the New York Academy of Sciences* 669 (1992): 1–6.

Massell BE, Warren JE, Patterson PR, et al. Antirheumatic activity of ascorbic acid in large doses. *New England Journal of Medicine* (1950).

McCormick, WJ. Lithogenesis and hypovitaminosis. *Medical Record* 159:7, 1946.

McCormick WJ. The changing incidence and mortality of infectious disease in relation to changed trends in nutrition. *Medical Record* (September 1947).

McCormick WJ. Ascorbic acid as a chemotherapeutic agent. *Archives of Pediatrics of New York* 69 (April 1952): 151–55.

McCormick WJ. Coronary thrombosis: the number one killer. *Insurance Index* (May 1953): 88–91.

McCormick WJ. Cancer: The preconditioning factor in pathogenesis. *Archives of Pediatrics of New York* 71 (1954): 313.

McCormick WJ. Intervertebral disc lesions: a new etiological concept. *Archives of Pediatrics of New York* 71 (1954): 29–33.

McCormick WJ. Coronary thrombosis: a new concept of mechanism and etiology. *Clinical Medicine* 4(7), 1957. [Pages unavailable; taken from a reprint.]

McCormick WJ. Have we forgotten the lesson of scurvy? *Journal of Applied Nutrition* 15 (1962): 4–12.

Physician's Desk Reference. Montvale, New Jersey: Medical Economics Data Production Company, 1994.

Meares A. *Relief without Drugs.* London: Souvenir Press, 1994.

Mendelsohn RS. *Confessions of a Medical Heretic.* Chicago: Contemporary Books, 1979.

Mendelsohn RS. *How to Raise a Healthy Child in Spite of Your Doctor.* New York: Ballantine Books, 1985.

Miller NZ. Vaccines and natural health. *Mothering* (Spring 1994): 44–54.

Miller NZ. *Immunization: Theory vs. Reality—Expose on Vaccinations.* Santa Fe, NM: New Atlantean Press, 1996.

Monte T. An interview with Dr. Anthony Sattilaro. *East-West Journal* (March 1981): 24–29.

Morishige F and Murata A. Prolongation of survival times in terminal human cancer by administration of supplemental ascorbate. *Journal of the International Academy of Preventive Medicine* 5 (1979): 47–52.

Moss R. *The Cancer Syndrome.* New York: Grove Press, 1980.

Moss R. *The Cancer Industry.* New York: Paragon Press, 1989.

Dr. Harold W. Manner: the man who cures cancer. *Mother Earth News* (November-December 1978): 17–24.

Andrew Saul: You can be your own doctor. *Mother Earth News* 85 (January-February 1984): 17–23.

Mothering Magazine. *Vaccinations: The Rest of the Story.* Chicago: Mothering Books, 1993.

Mousain-Bosc M, Roche M, Rapin J, and Bali JP. Magnesium Vit B_6 intake reduces central nervous system hyperexcitability in children. J Am Coll Nutr. 23(5):545S– 548S, 2004.

Mowat F. *Never Cry Wolf.* New York: Dell, 1970.

Mullins E. *Murder by Injection; The Medical Conspiracy against America.* Staunton, VA: National Council for Medical Research, 1988.

Murata A. Virucidal activity of vitamin C: Vitamin C for the prevention and treatment of viral diseases. *Proceedings of the First Intersectional Congress of Microbiological Societies, Science Council of Japan* 3 (1975): 432–42.

Murata A, Morishige F, and Yamaguchi H. Prolongation of survival times of terminal cancer patients by administration of large doses of ascorbate. *International Journal of Vitamin and Nutrition Research Suppl.* 23 (1982): 103–113.

Murray F. *Program Your Heart for Health.* New York: Larchmont, 1978.

Murray M. *The Complete Book of Juicing.* Rocklin, CA: Prima Publishing, 1992.

Myers JA. The role of some nutritional elements in the health of the teeth and their supporting structures. *Annals of Dentistry* 22 (1958): 35–47.

Natenberg M. *The Legacy of Dr. Wiley.* Chicago: Regent House, 1957.

Natural vitamin E for heart diseases. *Popular Science Digest* (March 1953): 4–6.

Newmark HL. Stability of vitamin B_{12} in the presence of ascorbic acid. *American Journal of Clinical Nutrition* 29 (1976): 645–49.

Null G, et al. Vitamin C and the treatment of cancer: abstracts and commentary from the scientific literature. *The Townsend Letter for Doctors and Patients* (April-May 1997).

Osmond H and Hoffer A. Massive niacin treatment in schizophrenia: review of a nine-year study. *Lancet* 1 (1962): 316–19.

Parham B. *What's Wrong with Eating Meat?* Denver, CO: Ananda Marga, 1979.

Park CH. Biological nature of the effect of ascorbic acids on the growth of human leukemic cells. *Cancer Research* 45 (1985):3969–973.

Parsons W., Jr. *Cholesterol Control Without Diet.* Lilac Press, 2000.

Passwater R. *Supernutrition.* New York: Dial, 1985.

Pauling L. Orthomolecular psychiatry. *Science* 160 (1968): 265–71.

Pauling L. *Vitamin C, the Common Cold, and the Flu.* San Francisco: W. H. Freeman, 1976.

Pauling L. Plowboy interview: Dr. Linus Pauling. *Mother Earth News* (January-February 1978): 17–22.

Pauling L. On good nutrition for the good life. *Executive Health* 17(4): 6, (Jan 1981).

Pauling L. On vitamin C and infectious diseases. *Executive Health* 19(4): 1–5, (Jan 1983).

Pauling L. (1986; revised ed. 2006). *How to Live Longer and Feel Better.* Corvallis, OR: Oregon State University Press.

Pauling L and Rath M. An orthomolecular theory of human health and disease. *Journal of Orthomolecular Medicine* 6 (1991): 135–138.

Pauling L, et al. Effect of dietary ascorbic acid on the incidence of spontaneous mammary tumors in RIII mice. Proceedings of the National Academy of Sciences. 82 (August 1985): 5185–189.

Pfeiffer CC. "Mental Illness and Schizophrenia." In *The Nutrition Connection.* New York: Thorsons, 1987.

Price W. *Nutrition and Physical Degeneration.* La Mesa, CA: Price-Pottenger Nutrition Foundation, 1970.

Prien EL and Gershoff SF. Magnesium oxide-pyridoxine therapy for recurrent calcium oxalate calculi. *J Urol* 112 (1974): 509–12.

Prousky J. *The Vitamin Cure for Chronic Fatigue.* Laguna Beach, CA: Basic Health Publications, 2010.

Quigley DT. *The National Malnutrition.* Milwaukee, WI: Lee Foundation for Nutritional Research, 1948.

Raasch C and Cochran W. Millions injected into health care debate. *Democrat and Chronicle* [Rochester, New York]. 17 April 1994.

Ratcliff JD. For heart disease: vitamin E. *Coronet* (October 1948).

Rath M. *Eradicating Heart Disease.* San Francisco, CA: Health Now, 1993.

Rattan V, et al. Effect of combined supplementation of magnesium oxide and pyridoxine in calcium-oxalate stone formers. *Urol Res* 22 (1994): 161–165.

Ray O and Ksir C. *Drugs, Society, and Human Behavior,* 5th ed. Mosby, St. Louis: Times Mirror, 1990, 198.

Rehert I. Doctor finds cure in macrobiotic diet. *Los Angeles Times.* 13 December 1981.

Riker J. The Salk vaccine. *New Directions* (Summer 1991): 21–25.

Rimm EB, et al. Vitamin E consumption and the risk of coronary heart disease in men. *New England Journal of Medicine* 328 (1993): 1450–456.

Rinse J. Atherosclerosis: prevention and cure [parts 1 and 2]. *Prevention* (November/December 1975).

Rinse J. Cholesterol and phospholipids in relation to atherosclerosis. *American Laboratory Magazine* (April 1978).

Riordan HD. *Medical Mavericks.* Wichita, KS: Bio-Communications Press, c.1988.

Riordan HD, Jackson JA, and Neathery S. Vitamin, blood lead, and urine pyrrole levels in Down's syndrome. *American Clinical Laboratory* (January 1990): 8–9.

Riordan HD, Jackson JA, Schultz M. Case study: high-dose intravenous vitamin C in the treatment of a patient with adenocarcinoma of the kidney. *J Ortho Med* 5 (1990): 5–7.

Riordan NH, et al. Intravenous ascorbate as a tumor cytotoxic chemotherapeutic agent. *Medical Hypotheses* 44 (1995): 207–13.

Riordan N, Jackson JA, Riordan HD. Intravenous vitamin C in a terminal cancer patient. J Ortho Med 11(1996): 80–82.

Rivers JM. Safety of high-level vitamin C injection. In "Third Conference on Vitamin C," *Annals of the New York Academy of Sciences* 498 (1987): 95–102.

Roberts H, Hickey S. *The Vitamin Cure for Heart Disease.* Laguna Beach, CA: Basic Health Publications, 2011.

Robertson L, et al. *Laurel's Kitchen.* New York: Bantam, 1976.

Rodale JI. *The Healthy Hunzas.* Emmaus, PA: Rodale Press, 1948.

Rogers LL, Pelton RB, and Williams RJ. Voluntary alcohol consumption by rats following administration of glutamine. *J Biol Chem* 214 (1955): 503–06.

Rogoff JM, et al. Vitamin C and insulin action. *Pennsylvania Medical Journal* 47 (1944): 579–82.

Sabin AB. Vitamin C in relation to experimental poliomyelitis. *Journal of Experimental Medicine* 69 (1939): 507–515.

Sandler BP. Treatment of tuberculosis with a low carbohydrate, high protein diet. *Diseases of the Chest* 17 (1950): 398.

Saul AW. Plowboy interview: You can be your own doctor. *Mother Earth News* 85 (January-February 1984): 17–23.

Saul AW. *Paperback Clinic.* Seneca Falls, NY: New York Chiropractic College Press, 1994.

Saul AW. *Fire Your Doctor! How to be independently healthy.* Laguna Beach, CA: Basic Health Publications, 2005.

Saul AW. *Liberati dal Dottore [Fire Your Doctor].* Diegarodi Cesena (FC): Macro Edizioni. 2009. Italian.

Scher J, et al. Massive vitamin C as an adjunct in methadone maintenance and detoxification of narcotic addicts. *Journal of Orthomolecular Psychiatry* 5 (1976): 191–198.

Schlegel Pipkin GE, Nishimura R, Shultz GN. The role of ascorbic acid in the prevention of bladder tumor formation. *Trans Amer Assn Genitourin Surg* 61 (1969).

Schlegel JU, Pipkin GE, Nishimura R, Shultz GN. The role of ascorbic acid in the prevention of bladder tumor formation. *J. Urol.* 103 (1970): 155.

Shafer CF. Ascorbic acid and atherosclerosis. *American Journal of Clinical Nutrition* 23 (1970): 27.

Shute E, et al. *The Heart and Vitamin E.* London, Canada: The Shute Foundation for Medical Research, 1963.

Shute E. Proposed study of vitamin E therapy. *Can Med Assoc J* 106 (May 1972): 1057.

Shute E. Vitamin E fatigue? [Letter.] *Calif Med* 119 (1973): 73.

Shute E. *The Vitamin E Story: The Medical Memoirs of Evan Shute.* Burlington, Ontario: Welch Publishing, 1985.

Shute WE and Taub HJ. *Vitamin E for Ailing and Healthy Hearts.* New York: Pyramid House, 1969.

Shute WE. *Health Preserver.* Emmaus, PA: Rodale Press, 1977.

Shute WE. *The Vitamin E Book.* New Canaan, CT: Keats Publishing, 1978.

Shute WE. *Your Child and Vitamin E.* New Canaan, CT: Keats Publishing, 1979.

Smith L, ed. *Clinical Guide to the Use of Vitamin C: The Clinical Experiences of Frederick R. Klenner, M.D.* Tacoma, WA: Life Sciences Press, 1988.

Smith JL and Hodges RE. Serum levels of vitamin C in relation to dietary and supplemental intake of vitamin C in smokers and nonsmokers. In "Third Conference on Vitamin C," *Annals of the New York Academy of Sciences* 498 (1987).

Smith SF and Smith CM. *Personal Health Choices.* Boston: Jones and Bartlett, 1990.

Smith RG. *The Vitamin Cure for Eye Disease.* Laguna Beach, CA: Basic Health Publications, June 2012.

Solomon J. (1982) Placebo revisited: An update on a very useful agent. *Consultant* (December 1982): 220–29.

Spittle CR. Atherosclerosis and vitamin C. *Lancet* 2 (1971): 1280–281.

Spittle CR. The action of vitamin C on blood vessels. *American Heart Journal* 88 (1974): 387–88.

Spock B. *Baby and Child Care.* New York: Pocket Books, 1976.

Stampfer MJ, et al. Vitamin E consumption and the risk of coronary disease in women. *New England Journal of Medicine* 328 (1993):1444–449.

Stahelin HB, et al. Vitamin C levels lower in cancer group. *J Nat Canc Inst* 73 (1984): 1463–468.

Stoll W. *Saving Yourself from the Disease-Care Crisis.* Panama City, FL: [Self-published], 1996.

Stone I. *The Healing Factor.* New York: Putnam, 1972.

Straus H. *Dr. Max Gerson: Healing the Hopeless.* With Barbara Marinacci. Kingston, Ontario: Quarry Press, 2002.

Sugiura K. On the relation of diets to the development, prevention, and treatment of cancer, with special reference to cancer of the stomach and liver. *Journal of Nutrition* 44 (1951): 345.

Taub HJ. *Keeping Healthy in a Polluted World.* New York: Penguin, 1975.

Torch WC. Diphtheria-pertussis-tetanus (DPT) immunization: A potential cause of the sudden infant death syndrome (SIDS). [Abstract.] *Neurology* 32 (1982): A169.

Torch WC. Characteristics of diphtheria-pertussis-tetanus (DPT) postvaccinal deaths and DPT-caused sudden infant death syndrome (SIDS): A review. [Abstract.] *Neurology* Suppl. 1 (1986): 148.

Tsao CS, Dunham WB, and Ping YL. In vivo antineoplastic activity of ascorbic acid for human mammary tumor. *In Vivo* 2 (1988): 147–150.

Turner J. *The Chemical Feast.* New York: Grossman, 1970.

Verlangieri AJ. *The Role of Vitamin C in Diabetic and Nondiabetic Atherosclerosis.* Bulletin, Vol. 21. University of Mississippi: Bureau of Pharm. Services, 1985.

Wachowicz K. Cancer victim endorses raw foods, sprout therapy. *The Colonian* [Albany, NY] (16 November 1981).

Waldbott GL, Burgstahler AW, and McKinney HL. *Fluoridation: The Great Dilemma.* Lawrence, KS: Coronado Press, 1978.

Walker AM, et al. Diphtheria-tetanus-pertussis immunization and sudden infant death syndrome. *Am Jour Pub Health* 77 (1987): 945–51.

Walker M. *Dirty Medicine: Science, Big Business, and the Assault on Natural Health Care.* London: Slingshot Publications, 1993.

Walker NW. *Diet and Salad Suggestions.* Phoenix, AZ: Norwalk Press, 1971.

Wapnick AA. The effect of ascorbic acid deficiency on desferrioxamine-induced urinary iron excretion. *British Journal of Haematology* 17 (1969): 563–68.

Warmbrand M. *Encyclopedia of Health and Nutrition.* New York: Pyramid, 1962.

Werbach M. *Nutritional Influences on Illness.* New Canaan, CT: Keats Publishing, 1988.

Werbach M. *Textbook of Nutritional Medicine.* Tarzana, CA: Third Line Press, 1999.

Whitaker J. Act now to protect your health. *Health and Healing Newsletter* Suppl. (September 1993): 1–4.

White K. PACs on precise missions. *Democrat and Chronicle* [Rochester, NY] (6 March 1994).

Wigmore A. *Why Suffer?* New York: Hemisphere Press, 1964.

Wigmore A. *Recipes for Longer Life.* Garden City Park, NY: Avery, 1982.

Wigmore A. *Be Your Own Doctor.* Garden City Park, NY: Avery, 1983.

Wilcox A, Weinberg C, and Baird D. Caffeinated beverages and decreased fertility. *The Lancet* 8626–7 (December 1988): 1473–476.

Wiley HW. *The History of a Crime Against the Food Law.* Washington, D.C.: [Self-published] 1929. Reprinted Milwaukee, WI: Lee Foundation for Nutritional Research, 1955. The book's full text is posted at doctoryourself .com.

Williams RJ. *Nutrition and Alcoholism.* Norman, OK: University of Oklahoma Press, 1951.

Williams RJ. *Biochemical Individuality: The Basis for the Genetotrophic Concept.* New York: Wiley, 1956. Reprinted Austin, TX: University of Texas Press, 1973.

Williams RJ. *Alcoholism: The Nutritional Approach.* Austin, TX: University of Texas Press, 1959.

Williams RJ. *Nutrition in a Nutshell.* New York: Dolphin Books, 1962.

Williams RJ. *You Are Extraordinary.* New York: Random House, 1967.

Williams RJ. *Nutrition Against Disease.* New York: Pitman, 1971.

Williams RJ. Biochemical individuality: A story of neglect. *Journal of the International Academy of Preventive Medicine* 1 (1974): 99–106.

Williams RJ. The neglect of nutritional science in cancer research. *Congressional Record* (16 October 1974): S.19204.

Williams RJ. *Physicians' Handbook of Nutritional Science.* Springfield, IL: Charles C. Thomas, 1975.

Williams RJ. *The Prevention of Alcoholism through Nutrition.* New York: Bantam, 1981.

Williams RJ and Kalita DK, eds. *A Physician's Handbook on Orthomolecular Medicine.* New Canaan, CT: Keats, 1977.

Williams SR. *Nutrition and Diet Therapy,* 7th edition. St. Louis: Mosby, 1993.

Willis GC. The reversibility of atherosclerosis. *Canadian Medical Association Journal of Nutrition* 77 (1957): 106–109.

Winacour J, ed. *The Story of the Titanic as Told by Its Survivors.* New York: Dover, 1960.

Yiamouyiannis J. *Fluoride: The Aging Factor.* Delaware, OH: Health Action Press 1986.

Yonemoto RH, et al. Enhanced lymphocyte blastogenesis by oral ascorbic acid. *Proceedings of the American Association for Cancer Research* 17 (1976): 288.

Yuan JM, et al. Diet and breast cancer in Shanghai and Tianjin, China. *British Journal of Cancer* 71 (1995): 1353–358.

Zannoni VG, et al. Ascorbic acid, alcohol, and environmental chemicals. In "Third Conference on Vitamin C," *Annals of the New York Academy of Sciences* 498: (1987).

Zuskin E, Lewis AJ, Bouhuys A. Inhibition of histamine-induced airway constriction by ascorbic acid. *Journal of Allergy and Clinical Immunology* 51 (1973): 218–26.

Index

About the
Author

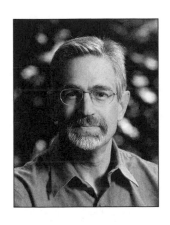

Andrew Saul, Ph.D., a biologist and teacher by training, has been a consulting specialist in natural healing for more than thirty-five years, helping medical doctors' problem patients get better. Dr. Saul has written a dozen books and has published over 170 reviews and editorials in peer-reviewed journals. He is on the editorial board of the *Journal of Orthomolecular Medicine* and is Editor-in-Chief of the *Orthomolecular Medicine News Service.* He was on the faculty of the State University of New York for nine years, has studied in Africa and Australia and has twice won New York Empire State Fellowships for teaching. Firsthand reports from South America confirm that a number of rainforest Indian tribes are now megadosing with vitamins due to his guidance. The result is that these natives' miscarriage and infant mortality rates have plummeted. Dr. Saul has been awarded the Citizens for Health Outstanding Health Freedom Activist Award. *Psychology Today* magazine named him one of seven natural health pioneers, and he is featured in the documentary movie *FoodMatters.* His internationally famous website is DoctorYourself.com, the largest non-commercial natural healing resource on the Internet.